Unhappy mothers

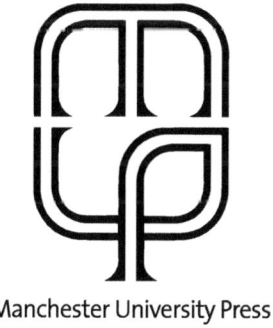
Manchester University Press

SOCIAL HISTORIES OF MEDICINE
Series Editors
David Cantor, Anne Hanley and Elaine Leong

Editorial Board
Diego Armus, Swarthmore College, PA, USA
Rana Hogarth, University of Illinois, Urbana-Champaign, USA
Angela Ki Che Leung, University of Hong Kong, China
Ian Miller, Ulster University, Northern Ireland

Social Histories of Medicine is concerned with all aspects of health, illness and medicine, from prehistory to the present, in every part of the world. The series covers the circumstances that promote health or illness, the ways in which people experience and explain such conditions, and what, practically, they do about them. Practitioners of all approaches to health and healing come within its scope, as do their ideas, beliefs, and practices, and the social, economic and cultural contexts in which they operate. Methodologically, the series welcomes relevant studies in social, economic, cultural, and intellectual history, as well as approaches derived from other disciplines in the arts, sciences, social sciences and humanities. The series is a collaboration between Manchester University Press and the Society for the Social History of Medicine.

To buy or to find out more about the books currently available in this series, please go to: https://manchesteruniversitypress.co.uk/series/social-histories-of-medicine/

Unhappy mothers

Women, motherhood, and social change in postwar Britain

Sarah Crook

MANCHESTER UNIVERSITY PRESS

Copyright © Sarah Crook 2025

The right of Sarah Crook to be identified as the author of this work has been asserted in accordance with the Copyright, Designs and Patents Act 1988.

An electronic version of this book has been made freely available under a Creative Commons (CC BY-NC-ND) licence, thanks to the support of the Wellcome Trust (grant number 099362/Z/12/Z), which permits non-commercial use, distribution and reproduction provided the author(s) and Manchester University Press are fully cited and no modifications or adaptations are made. Details of the licence can be viewed at https://creativecommons.org/licenses/by-nc-nd/4.0/

Published by Manchester University Press
Oxford Road, Manchester, M13 9PL

www.manchesteruniversitypress.co.uk

British Library Cataloguing-in-Publication Data
A catalogue record for this book is available from the British Library

ISBN   978 1 5261 4012 8   hardback

First published 2025

The publisher has no responsibility for the persistence or accuracy of URLs for any external or third-party internet websites referred to in this book, and does not guarantee that any content on such websites is, or will remain, accurate or appropriate.

Typeset by Deanta Global Publishing Services, Chennai, India

To Calum, who changed everything.

Contents

Acknowledgements		*page* viii
Introduction		1
1	Mothers, general practitioners, and the NHS	33
2	Health visitors and the worlds of new mothers	65
3	Expertise and experience: mothers' self-help	94
4	The women's liberation movement and mothers' discontent	137
5	Feminist sociology, research, and visibility	177
Conclusion		215
Bibliography		223
Index		261

Acknowledgements

This book was made possible and enriched by the support, generosity, and wisdom of others. Some of the most important support was behind the scenes, and thus it is to the expert staff at Swansea University Students' Union Day Nursery that I would like to extend my first thanks. Thank you, Tracey Knuszka and team, for your care for Evelyn, Alastair, and Elspeth. Our childminder, Leanne Clulee, has made school pick ups managable and school holidays less frantic. Thank, you, Leanne. My mother, Frances, frequently and unhesitatingly zoomed along hundreds of miles of motorway from London at short notice to offer childcare support. My out-of-law family, Susan and Graeme White, have regularly made the long journey down from Scotland to help, met by our deep appreciation and the kids' adoration. Janice Alexander and Lauren White have cheer-led our family from afar. This book, in many ways, is a reminder of the importance of a village, and we are very lucky to have ours.

This research would not have been possible without Wellcome Trust funding (grant number 099362/Z/12/Z). Thank you to those at Queen Mary and beyond who saw this idea first develop and, slowly, come to fruition: Rhodri Hayward, who supported its early incarnation with patience and a critical eye; Thomas Dixon, who led the Centre for the History of Emotions with great insight; Barbara Taylor, who has inspired me and many others; and the administrative team, who steered the ship with their steadiness and organisation. Stephen Brooke and Sally Alexander gave early feedback that immeasurably improved the book.

Acknowledgements

Research was done at various libraries and institutions, all of which are kept afloat by the tireless work of their wonderful staff. Teams at the Wellcome Archives, the Bishopsgate Institute, the LSE Women's Library, and the Royal College of General Practitioners' archive responded to my requests with calm expertise and deep knowledge: thank you. Staff at the British Library, the Bodleian, the IHR, and Swansea University Library tolerated my many requests with utmost professionalism and kindness. Thanks to the team at APNI who let me explore their archives.

Behind the production of a book is an entire team of experts who steer the process, and Meredith Carroll, my editor at MUP, has been a model of efficiency and patience. The reviewers and series editors provided perceptive and astute suggestions, and I am so grateful.

Friends and colleagues proofread and commented on the text at various points and provided encouragement when I flagged. At Swansea, I owe a debt to Simon John, Martin Johnes, Stephen Harrison (for office DIY assistance as well as emotional and intellectual support), Christoph Laucht, Jo Berry, Adam Mosley, and Nigel Pollard, all of whom have championed the research or given me a healthy nudge when needed. Ryan Murphy, as Pro-Vice Chancellor of the Faculty of Humanities and Social Sciences, ensured that I was given research leave upon return from maternity leave, significantly easing my ability to return to this book. My delightful students, too many to name (but you know who you are!), have consistently helped me to clarify my ideas and to express my thoughts more clearly: thank you.

Thanks are also due to June Purvis for her permission to publish in Chapter 4 some ideas that appeared in an earlier article, 'The Women's Liberation Movement, Activism and Therapy at the Grassroots, 1968–1985', *Women's History Review* 27, 7, 1152–68. June was also an immensely lovely editor for a 'viewpoint' piece on academic mothering I published in the journal during the lockdowns of Covid-19, and I think often of how grateful I am to her for her encouragement at a moment when the two roles – academic and mother – felt incompatible.

I feel hugely lucky to be a part of a supportive scholarly community. Across this book's long gestation Hilary Marland, Pat Thane, Rhodri Hayward, Lynn Abrams, Sue Bruley, Peter Mandler,

Helen Traill, and Fabiola Creed have all read draft chapters, asked questions, and shared insightful criticisms and comments. I eagerly await the publication of Hilary Marland's forthcoming work on postnatal depression, and am very grateful to her for her generosity and intellectual support, as well as her sharp eye on parts of this work. Lynn Abrams's writing and research has been fundamental to my thinking on this project, and she has been a personal inspiration, too. Rhodri Hayward's kindness and belief – and expansive knowledge – made this possible. Helen Traill provided wisdom both maternal and scholarly. Fabiola Creed read a draft of Chapter 4 and responded to it with kindness – thank you, Fabiola. Peter Mandler and Sue Bruley both prompted me to be more interrogative around class, improving my understanding in ways that I hope are reflected here. I am in awe of Pat Thane's generosity in reading Chapter 2 when I provided such an unreasonably sharp turnaround and by the characteristic insight of her response. Working with Caitríona Beaumont, Eve Colpus, and Ruth Davidson towards the publication of a chapter in their edited collection, *Everyday Welfare in Modern British History*, helped to develop my ideas in ways that have enriched this book, and I am grateful to them for their energy, collaborative instincts, and perceptive insights around the interaction between expertise and experience.

The work was presented at a truly embarrassing number of events, seminar series, and conferences, and the audiences at each helped to improve, craft, and nuance my ideas. Thank you to those who listened to me talk about this research, and improved it with generous comments: at the Feminist Thinking Research Seminar in Oxford; at the Social History Society Conference in both Lancaster and Essex; at the Rethinking Contemporary British Political History conference at Queen Mary, University of London; at the IHR Lifecycles Seminar; at the Perceptions of Pregnancy conference at the University of Hertfordshire, and at the University of Manchester CHSTM series, among other places.

I am also grateful for the little acts of kindness that have eased anxiety at key moments. There are very many of these, but one that I think of often is a supportive email I received from Ellie Lee soon after the publication of one of my articles, an act of solidarity that I remain grateful for, and that I try to pay forward. Charmian Mansell and Sarah Kenny both provided empathy and solidarity while they developed their own (wonderful) books. Through her steadfast friendship and empathy Gemma Almond has made my experience of combining writing and motherhood so much lighter, easier, funnier, and calmer – thank you, Gemma, for being an inspiration in so many ways. Charlie Jeffries, you bring joy to every aspect of my life, and the lovely experience of writing with you and thinking with you on our edited collection has shaped me profoundly: thank you.

The title of this book changed relatively late in the process, and several generous scholars have cited it under the working title – I ask for their forgiveness for this.

Calum, you are the love of my life and the most magnificent partner, reviewer, and cheerleader I could possibly imagine. My marvellous children provided the drive to finish this book, and were the major impediment to its completion. Evelyn, Alastair, and Elspeth, you fill every day with wonder, laughter, chaos, and love. Elspeth, you are sleeping on my office floor while I write this. Thank you for being adorable and for napping at convenient times. The three of you – my sweet agents of chaos – have taught me so very much.

Introduction

Nine weeks after playwright and author Vivienne Welburn's second child – a daughter, like her first – arrived, Vivienne sank into a deep depression. Summer was turning to autumn, and she watched leaves fall in a 'heavy, lumpish haze'. 'Each falling leaf was a dead hope, the end of a possibility of better things', she recalled. Her mind raced and time passed irrhythmically. It was 1974 and every task was exhausting. Her depression came on slowly, 'more like one of those leaves, slowly and inevitably drifting down, down'. The second baby came at a time of transition. Writing, a 'solace and joy', had occupied less of her time since the birth of her first daughter. Challenges mounted: her inner life was neglected; her social network faltered; her husband started a new job; her elder daughter got mumps. Vivienne struggled. She made an appointment with her sympathetic and astute general practitioner, who told her postnatal depression was very common, prescribed antidepressants, saw her very regularly, and encouraged a referral to the Marriage Guidance Council in an acknowledgement that the arrival of a new baby was a family event, not a 'woman's problem'. The antidepressants did not help, and Vivienne flushed them down the toilet. Instead, she took her younger child with her to stay with friends. The camaraderie, relaxation, and lightening of responsibilities paid off and the trip marked a turning point. Slowly, the depression started to diminish. She started writing again, and 'learned, slowly and painfully, to recognize that I have needs which must be satisfied if I am to grow and develop'.[1]

Welburn found solace in writing. In 1978, she completed a book on postnatal depression. For this, she conducted formal interviews with twenty-five mothers, talked to many more, and solicited further contributions via an appeal in *Mother and Baby* magazine. She consulted medical experts and sought advice from the National Childbirth Trust (NCT), the Association for Improvements in the Maternity Services (AIMS), and Depressives Associated. The resulting book, first published in 1980, was a study that wore its feminism lightly but insistently.

In many ways Welburn was lucky. She had an understanding general practitioner and was able to access support when she needed it; she was educated, middle-class, and had some financial security. In some ways she was extraordinary: some, but not all, unhappy mothers are inspired to write books as a result of their distress. In other ways, though, she was ordinary. She experienced a painful but common form of distress and worked to recover from, understand, and transform it.

Welburn was not the first nor last mother to find writing to be a balm – perhaps her most famous forerunner was American writer Charlotte Perkins Gilman, whose short story, *The Yellow Wallpaper*, first published in 1892, explored a young mother's psychological struggles when prescribed a 'rest cure' that involved isolation and that prohibited both creative and intellectual work.[2] Neither were the women Welburn interviewed outliers in taking up an opportunity to share their experiences; rather, they were participating in a culture that had, from the 1960s, increasingly acknowledged the expertise that could be derived from experience, and in which women's sharing of information about themselves with researchers allowed them to demonstrate an active form of self-making.[3] The suggestion that she and her husband seek marital help reflected the postwar emphasis on stable intimate relationships as key components of, and evidence for, healthy democratic citizenship.[4] The three organisations she consulted, all of which will surface again in this book, were founded by mothers who recognised the need to organise around the problems they had experienced.

The unravelling of the tight knots around early mothering's difficulties – the loneliness, the boredom, the uncertainty – has been a project to which many mothers across time and place have contributed. This book homes in on this endeavour's more recent past, spanning examples from Scotland, England, and Wales to tell the story of some of the ways that the experience of unhappy mothering was made visible between the mid-1940s and the end of the 1980s. This postwar period saw an increasing acceptance of experiential expertise and the creation of communities around it; saw mothers' work outside the home become normalised; and saw women develop new feminist frameworks to explain and interpret their discontent. But it was also an era of contradictions and tensions. The growing availability of contraception – particularly, from the 1960s, the Pill – meant women could increasingly choose when and if they became mothers, but the overriding social expectation remained that they would eventually do so. The nuclear family was considered to be a private, foundational, and sacred social unit, but it was also perceived to be a brittle arrangement, vulnerable to external threats and trends. Lone motherhood, divorce, births outside marriage, and queer parenthood became increasingly common but were viewed by governments and the press with suspicion and unease. In 1948, at the start of this period, the welfare state inaugurated its most remarkable institution – the NHS – and, in the 1980s, the welfare state faced its most substantive threats to date. Through this period, motherhood remained sanctified and mothers were poorly socially supported.

Unhappy Mothers: Women, Motherhood, and Social Change in Postwar Britain highlights the presence of conversations about discontented motherhood, the creation of mother-led communities of experiential expertise, and the multidisciplinary interest that unhappy motherhood stirred across this span of some forty years. It makes three interrelated arguments around the themes of visibility, expertise, and meanings. First, this book argues that the frustrations and struggles of early motherhood were made visible by mothers, health professionals, researchers, and feminist activists in postwar Britain (notably, of course, these categories overlapped). Second, it suggests that distressed mothers played a crucial role in the increasing visibility of unhappy motherhood, and in doing so, they emphasised the value of their experiential expertise. Third, it points to how the feminist movement of the late 1960s to the 1980s imbued discontented motherhood with political and social meanings. The movement helped to create possibilities for motherhood's transformation through a political assessment of its vicissitudes: of love and joy, but also of pain, isolation, and despair. Many of these possibilities are yet to be realised, I argue in the conclusion. Nonetheless, the labour of visibility matters; this work created the possibility for new conversations about the experience of motherhood and opened new ways of imagining the social world in which women mother.

My focus here is on early mothering, taken here to mean mothering children who are babies or young toddlers (as people gleefully remind me when I am with my very young children, I should *just wait*, for parenting adolescents will bring its own difficulties). The book begins as the psychological importance of mothering to babies' development was emphasised in the wake of the Second World War, and it closes in the 1980s when discussion of unhappy mothering had entered the parenting mainstream.[5] It looks closely at some of the communities – general practitioners, health visitors, self-help and community groups, and feminists outside and then inside the academy – that helped this mainstreaming process. These communities, taken in turn, form the structure of the book. This structure is imperfectly chronological, moving focus through these constituencies as the decades progress. Through these decades, these constituencies developed their own cultures, creating new lines of sight on unhappy motherhood.

In 1978, activist and author Sheila Kitzinger observed that 'mothers are made by the culture in which they have to operate'.[6] Like other women who feature in this book, Kitzinger contained multitudes – she was, among other things, a feminist, an anthropologist, an author, a researcher, a mother of five, and a campaigner around the conditions of pregnancy, childbirth, and mothering. Kitzinger was right. Mothers are made within culture, and their unhappiness is shaped by cultural forces, structural impediments and personal contexts. By looking at what was done with their unhappiness, and who was interested in it across the postwar decades, we can see points of change in cultures of expertise, self-help, the politicisation of emotion, and feminist thought. It is these points of change that *Unhappy Mothers* considers.

Terminology and scope

Unhappy mothering is a spectrum: most mothers of young babies will experience moments, if not days or weeks, when unyielding sleep deprivation, the struggle of feeding, and the monotony of babycare take their toll. Pregnancy and then childbirth – no matter its form, whether vaginal or caesarean – are immensely physical acts, and the rest required for recovery is hard to reconcile with the needs of a newborn. The arrival of a new baby is a time of profound change, shifting family dynamics, exerting new financial pressures, and bringing new rhythms to the passing of time. Things that were once simple, like leaving the house, become administratively complex. The inhospitality of cities and towns to buggies and babies is thrown into sudden relief. Feeding – whether breast or formula – can be a time-consuming struggle. Motherhood changes women's bodies and hormones, and the responsibility for such a delicate, dependent new life can be daunting. The spectrum of emotional responses is wide. Some women's feelings of discontent pass quickly, and they are able to settle into new lives with relative ease.[7] But for other mothers, distress is more profound, enduring, and severe, and moves beyond the common and short-lived 'baby blues'. Those mothers may be diagnosed with postnatal depression.[8] Some mothers in this book received this diagnosis, which as Ellie Lee has identified, first emerged as a psychiatric concept in the 1960s and soon attained widespread cultural circulation; others did not.[9] Some mothers in this book experienced acute distress, while others experienced discontent that inhabited the milder end of the scale. The diagnosis of postnatal depression was taken up by the groups in this book at different moments and used in a variety of ways. Some groups found it validating and helpful; others argued that it medicalised a problem that had social roots and thus obscured its sociopolitical solutions. Postnatal depression is therefore a thread of this book but not its focus; the diagnosis was one of several mechanisms that made maternal unhappiness legible.[10] This expansive approach, untethered from clinical terminology and diagnostic criteria, enables the book to encompass a spectrum of emotions, traversing the often-blurred lines between sadness, loneliness, and anger. Unhappiness and distress tend to be used here interchangeably; depressed is used predominantly in cases where the source applied it. This wide approach is useful not least because women have applied their own vernaculars to their intimate lives (historian Barbara Taylor's mother experienced something she called 'the miseries' after the birth of her second child; Taylor says 'it seems likely that she had a full-blown breakdown').[11] Some mothers repudiated medical languages. 'I didn't suffer from post-natal depression', explained Victoria Hardie, a writer and mother of two, 'more from rage'.[12] Taking in this breadth – despite the particular textures of each evocation of experience, a topic for another historian – brings to the fore more mothers' voices and allows me to venture to broad sites of discussion.

This undogmatic approach to terminology is important given the range of communities that this book homes in on. The expertise, arguments, and experiences articulated by general practitioners, health visitors, self-help groups, women's liberation movement activists, and feminist sociologists helped to forge contemporary understandings of unhappy motherhood. These are not the only interested communities – novelists, poets, psychiatrists, midwives, and psychoanalysts are important omissions – but they are five that played crucial and interlocking roles as vectors for unhappy mothering's visibility and interpretation. They were chosen to demonstrate the breadth of interested constituencies, the range of motivations and investments, and the variety of meanings that mothers' unhappiness acquired. The communities are, of course, not silos, and they worked alongside constituencies who are not my focus here. Notably and predictably, constituencies overlap: some feminist activists were midwives or psychotherapists; some sociologists were novelists or poets, and all interested groups contained mothers. Unsurprisingly, then, this book draws upon a range of materials. These materials include medical journals; sociological studies; health visiting journals and textbooks; women's liberation magazines, books, and pamphlets; the archival records of self-help groups; newspapers; and the archives of social science surveys.

Some of these materials are worth noting here. National newspapers, for example, furthered the visibility of mothers' struggles, but it is the local press that I have particularly attended to. While national newspapers published articles that exposed mothers' distress, these tended – particularly in tabloids – to centre on the rare and tragic instances where its most severe manifestations resulted in the death of a mother or infant. This might be seen to fall within the scope of public interest, or perhaps a less generous interpretation would be that these unusual cases attracted somewhat prurient attention. National newspapers were also provoked to discuss unhappy mothering when a well-known mother drew attention to the issue – usually by talking about her own experience – or when it was the theme of a cultural project, such as a television programme or radio play.[13] Local newspapers, however, highlighted the ordinariness of mothers' distress by publishing pieces about mothers' groups nestled alongside the wider ephemera of community life. While this was likely part of their remit to promote local events and developments, it obliquely conveyed the quotidian nature of unhappy motherhood.

The breadth of material used in this book underlines the dispersed, diffuse nature of the labour of visibility. The work of visibility was not exclusively driven forward by metropoles. The professional communities discussed here – general practitioners, health visitors, academics – were geographically dispersed across Britain. Scottish, English, and Welsh mothers from both rural and urban areas leveraged the tools available to them to articulate their experiences, establish activist networks, and form groups of shared experience.

These groups were part of an increasing acknowledgement of experiential expertise from the 1960s onwards.[14] The concept of experiential knowledge was developed in the 1970s by American sociologist Thomasina Borkman, who defined it as 'truth based on personal experience with a phenomenon'.[15] The concept has been useful to historians, who have used the idea to explore the ways that people have navigated and challenged a range of socio-institutional structures.[16] More recently, Caitríona Beaumont, Eve Colpus, and Ruth Davidson have explored the way experience created 'pathways to activism'; this thread is picked up in *Unhappy Mothers*, showing the ways that mothers organised around their feelings and used them to agitate for change.[17] Nonetheless, across the decades explored here, a heightened awareness of experiential expertise existed alongside, and contested, other types of knowledge. The types of expertise around mothers' unhappiness were heterogeneous in late twentieth-century Britain; by turns intersecting, complementary, and conflicting.

Mothers argued for the knowledge rendered from their interactions with state infrastructures. As Hardie wrote, 'Mothers know quicker than anyone else what is needed, what is unsatisfactory, and what works in the local community, and better than any journalist or politician'.[18] Put another way, mothers' cumulative interactions with the welfare state gave them a distinctive perspective on the design and performance of various bureaucracies. This is as true today as it was in the postwar period. Liz Berry's recent poem 'The Republic of Motherhood' describes standing 'with my sisters in the queues of Motherhood – / the weighing clinic, the supermarket – waiting / for its bureaucracies to open their doors'. Women bear witness while in the 'queues of Motherhood'.[19] They scrutinise the dilapidated walls of the crowded clinic; they map the cracked pavements that jolt sleeping infants awake; they note, with exasperation, when buses suddenly disappear from schedules. Mothers' experience of social conditions is political knowledge. But there is evidence that by the late 1990s, there was some fatigue with mothers making arguments from their own experiences. The *London Review of Books* criticised one author's 'bleak' exploration of middle-class motherhood for leaning too heavily on her own life, and on 'chats with her friends in the kitchen, half-listened-to talk shows on the radio, and casual quotation from a mass of female columnists and magazines'.[20] But each generation of mothers discovers anew how hard mothering is made. As literary critic Jacqueline Rose observed in the same magazine, women who have written searingly about the knottiness of mothers' emotions are 'issuing a political corrective' to the enduring idea of maternal virtue.[21] The home is not the only cradle for the politicisation of mothering, but the kitchen, the radio, and the magazine – all found within its walls – are where unhappy mothers have frequently discovered that they are not alone. At the same time, we are reminded of the many ways that women are made to doubt their expertise. We even use it as a cultural shorthand for a superstitious belief not founded on sound evidence: an old wives' tale. Bad information passed on and down through generations by women.

In many ways, this book charts work around visibility that has not had full effect. Unhappy mothers have no union. There is no 'Department of Motherhood', as invoked by 'The Republic of Motherhood', to whom women can direct their complaints.[22] Despite attempts to mobilise around mothers' unhappiness, mothers' hours are long, the labour is isolated, and the physical toll is exacting. The constituencies discussed in this book worked for ostensibly little practical consequence. Is the testimony of mothers' 'quotidian, unrelieved, anonymous misery', as legal scholar Ruth Cain has considered, too sticky, contagious, and frustrating to tackle? Cain warns that vicarious suffering

> affects not only 'mainstream' perceptions of maternal unhappiness, leading to the common construction of unhappy mothers as deviant, harmful and unproductive citizens; it also afflicts feminism, when the transmission of depressive affect combines with the inescapable mundanity of maternal misery, presenting potential activists with subjects whose 'oppression' seems too dull and elusive to become a subject for advocacy, and who do not fit into readily readable victim-categories.[23]

This book considers attempts to make mothers' unhappiness meaningful despite the quotidian quality of the misery.

Mothers and expertise

In the decades before the Second World War the ground was laid for the subsequent expansion of interest in mothers' emotional lives. The interwar period saw the dissemination and cultural permeation of new psychological ideas, legal changes around infanticide that reflected an increased awareness of the potential for psychological disorders after childbirth, and the emergence of concern about an apparent 'suburban neurosis' in bored and isolated housewives.[24] In the 1920s the advice of New Zealand doctor F. Truby King and American behavioural psychologist John B. Watson became prominent, encouraging mothers to adopt disciplinarian and regimented approaches, enforcing what they argued were positive habits but with a minimum of tenderness.[25] In the 1930s child guidance clinics multiplied and child mental health was seen as vulnerable and precarious, with the onus of the achievement of 'normalcy' and its enemy, maladjustment, placed on mothers.[26] Sex educators and marriage reformers argued that successful marriages underpinned national health, and new interventions were developed to promote marital stability; to this end, the Marriage Guidance Council was established in 1938.[27] During the 1940s anxiety about the family became rife, with cultural commentators wringing their hands about the perceived threat to the nation posed by a low birth rate, illegitimacy, neglect, and delinquency. During the Second World War, the evacuation of working-class, inner-city children focused attention on what were seen to be pre-existing symptoms of their maladjustment, providing further impetus for work on child mental health. As John Stewart has shown, child guidance was embedded in the development of the early welfare state, and consensus solidified around the idea that domestic and childhood emotional stability underpinned national strength.[28] Even once anxiety about the birth rate diminished, the family, marriage, and childrearing occupied a central place in the national psyche.

It was against this background that, after the war, the emphasis on the practices of childrearing shifted away from the desirability of disciplinarian habits and moved towards an onus on mothers to be affectionate, present, and intuitively responsive to their babies. This emotional attentiveness would be situated in a newly meaningful home environment, in which children were conceptualised as future citizens.[29] Quite how these future citizens should be brought up was a topic of lively public interest. American paediatrician Benjamin Spock broke away from the rigidity his predecessors espoused; his comparatively permissive book *Baby and Child Care* (first published as *The Common Sense Book of Baby and Child Care*) became a global phenomenon, selling fifty million copies in over forty languages in the decades that followed its 1946 publication.[30] In Britain, psychologists and psychoanalysts gained access to prominent public platforms and became household names. Psychoanalyst John Bowlby's bestselling *Child Care and the Growth of Love*, published in 1953, argued for a 'warm, intimate, and continuous relationship' between mother and baby.[31] Psychoanalyst Donald Winnicott's BBC radio broadcasts, in which he discussed the 'ordinary devoted mother', reached millions of listeners.[32] Winnicott encouraged new mothers to move away from the prioritisation of 'administrative tidiness, the dictates of hygiene, a laudable urge towards the promotion of bodily health'; instead, he argued for the prioritisation of the mother-baby relationship.[33] Winnicott's emphasis on being 'good enough' was greeted with relief by some mothers, but others worried that the instinctive sensitivity he espoused obscured the ambivalence that so often coexisted with maternal love.[34]

These changes in attitudes to children and childrearing amounted to what historians in the 1980s perceived as demonstrating a bewildering volatility.³⁵ Of course, the extent to which mothers put advice into practice is debatable.³⁶ While some studies found that parents were keen to be seen as abreast of modern ideas about childrearing, even researchers expressed some scepticism about the utility of childrearing guidance.³⁷ John and Elizabeth Newson, psychologists who led a large-scale study of childrearing in Nottingham in the 1960s, saw their first-hand experience of parenthood as 'an almost indispensable professional qualification' and condemned infant care as an area in which 'many different specialists use the full weight of their professional authority to back up their private prejudices'.³⁸ Mothers, when writing about the delicious pleasures and anxious lows of childrearing, pointed to the limits of manuals, as 'books don't tell of the darkness of passions and how to live with them or how to cope with anger and remorse'.³⁹ Feminist sociological studies found that mothers were critical readers, acutely aware of the disparity between professional exposition and personal experience. One 1970s middle-class mother, for example, reflected to the sociologist Ann Oakley that,

> I used to read all the literature available about having a baby, and really there is a tremendous halo of enjoyment about it. No one ever tells you about the hard work. You know you've got to do bottles and nappies and all the rest of it, but no one ever tells you how shattering it is to do it all the time, seven days a week. There are no books anywhere that are realistic. In fact I was thinking the other day, I'd really like to write a paper on it – on having a baby and how it's not all a super enviable state.⁴⁰

This middle-class mother, more than her working-class equivalents, would have had the resources needed to write this dissenting paper, and it is likely that, as the decade progressed, she would see herself reflected in the expansion of literature that made visible the disjuncture between – to borrow American writer Adrienne Rich's famous framing – the experience and the institution of motherhood.⁴¹

Postwar landscapes

This book shows that the work of discussing the travails of mothering was undertaken by the mothers who responded to sociological and media surveys; who told health visitors, general practitioners, and psychiatrists about their feelings; who wrote about their experiences in magazines, newspapers, leaflets, or books; who established support, feminist, and self-help groups; and who entered the academy and developed new understandings and ideas. Some of these women's names have been lost or anonymised. Other names, like that of Adrienne Rich, are well-known. Ann Oakley, whose feminist sociological work has been foundational to the development of more expansive, nuanced, and critical understandings of women's experiences of motherhood and mothering, is another well-known figure. Not only was her work crucial to developing new sociological lenses – as discussed later in this book – but her life course reflects some of the key changes that occurred in postwar Britain. Using Oakley, then, we can survey the social landscape from which interest in unhappy mothering surfaced.

Born in 1944, Oakley was an only child. Her father, Richard Titmuss, was professor in social administration at the LSE, a prominent social policy academic, and an architect of the welfare state, while her mother, Kathleen 'Kay' Titmuss, was a social worker who gave up her career upon marriage. Their marriage was traditional, conforming to the dominant ideal of the mid-century. Kay supported her prolific and eminent husband, sublimating her own health; Oakley found this family environment challenging.[42] But postwar Britain offered increasing opportunities for psychological introspection, and attitudes to mental health were changing. Psychological discourses circulated through society in new ways, driven forward in part by newly prominent psychiatrists and psychoanalysts. Aged eighteen, Oakley was sent to see Donald Winnicott, who referred her to another psychoanalyst whom she would regularly see before, and occasionally after, she took up a place to study Politics, Philosophy, and Economics at Somerville College, Oxford, in October 1962.[43] In going to university in the 1960s, Oakley joined a cohort of young people who progressed into higher education in greater numbers than ever before, enabled by the creation of new universities and the expansion of existing institutions. But a university education for women did not promise an uninterrupted career. Thus in the 1960s Oakley soon found herself becoming, like many other women of her generation, what social researchers had investigated in the previous decade: a graduate wife.[44]

Oakley married and had children in her early twenties. The arrival of her first child in 1967 was personally momentous. Whereas earlier in the century homebirths had been common, the delivery of Oakley's child in a hospital setting was part of a wider trend towards hospitalisation within maternity care that accelerated in the mid-1960s. While, as Joanna Moorhead has observed, the 1960s were a time of optimism about maternity care within the medical profession, the sense that technological innovation and medicalisation was improving the experience of childbirth was not wholly shared by mothers.[45] Indeed, as this book goes on to explore, the medicalisation of childbirth was not accepted without complaint, and the natural birth movement that gained momentum and support after the 1950s offered robust critiques of the perception that childbirth was a medical event. Like many other mothers who gave birth in hospitals during the late-1960s, then, Oakley was 'lonely and lost' during labour, and found the experience of giving birth under intense medical management disorienting and disempowering.[46] Her second child was born at home sixteen months later, in May 1968, signalling the start of a melancholy period of motherhood in which she was diagnosed with postnatal depression, and which she experienced as an 'unhappy haze of nappy-washing and pill-taking'.[47] But the term postnatal depression was, she says, 'a ridiculous term', asking 'Who wouldn't feel some distress when dealing with a genitally mutilated body and suddenly exposed to responsibility for the care of a new and totally dependent human being, a condition which imposes the further symptom of sleep-deprivation lasting for months, if not years?'[48] Her general practitioner prescribed weekly meetings in the surgery and antidepressant medications which enabled her to be a 'mechanical housewife'. Together with her family, Oakley was referred to a psychiatric hospital, and they were, offered inpatient treatment. They declined.[49]

Ultimately, it was not medical interventions that alleviated Oakley's profound unhappiness. Looking back on the prescription given to her by her general practitioner, Oakley suggested that he should instead have drawn out 'the difference between the experience and the institution of motherhood'.[50] Instead, Oakley addressed her unhappiness through work and a developing feminist consciousness. In 1969 she registered for a PhD at Bedford

College, where, a few years earlier, sociologist Hannah Gavron had conducted pioneering research into the lives of working-class and middle-class housewives, and on doing so Oakley 'stopped calling myself depressed and I stopped eating pills'.[51] The field of the social sciences that Oakley entered was experiencing rapid expansion in the 1960s but was, at this point, markedly male-dominated. This masculine orientation was challenged by feminist sociologists across the ensuing decades, and it was while conducting research that Oakley was introduced to the nascent feminist movement. The movement was stirring in the late 1960s and cohered in the early 1970s. Feminism would provide Oakley with community, courage, and inspiration, and its members shared her interest in the consequences of housewifery and motherhood for women.

It was not until the mid-1970s, though, that Oakley's academic work shifted its primary focus to motherhood. Of course, the precursor to this, her doctoral study of housework, tackled some of the issues raised by mothering: all of the forty women in her survey were mothers, and her interviews reflected the conflicting demands of childrearing and housework.[52] However, it was her 'Transition to Motherhood' study, conducted from 1974 to 1979, that focused its whole attention on motherhood. Here she interviewed fifty-five women in London, all first-time mothers, about their experiences of antenatal medical care, childbirth, and early mothering, listening closely to their experiential expertise as a counterpoint to idealised narratives of early motherhood. Each woman was interviewed four times at intervals that spanned their pregnancy and the early months of baby rearing. Oakley also attended six births. The project initially led to two texts, one of which, *Becoming a Mother* (1979, later republished as *From Here to Maternity*), was aimed at a 'lay' audience, and the second of which, *Women Confined: Towards a Sociology of Childbirth* (1980), addressed an academic readership. More recently, Oakley and social scientist Meg Wiggins conducted a follow-up to this study, re-interviewing thirty-six of the original participants.[53] These interviews, both the originals and the follow-up, are drawn upon across this book. By the time Oakley and Wiggins returned to the project in 2012, sociology was no longer a masculine domain. Albeit unevenly, female researchers were well represented in social science and sociology departments across the country. In some ways, this reflected wider shifts in the labour force, which married women entered into in ever greater numbers across the postwar years.

Paid work and unpaid labour

The increasing uptake of paid work by married women and mothers was one of the most profound social shifts of the twentieth century in Britain and one that attracted some of the most emotionally fraught discussion. Mothers' paid work was a tense topic even at the start of the century, and mothers were discouraged from seeking paid employment if at all possible for the sake of their children.[54] While women undertook war work during the First World War, in the interwar period that followed, the housewife-mother continued to dominate ideas about aspirational womanhood.[55] Following the war mothers were seen to play a vital role in safeguarding family health, and through this, to play an important role in the racial health – with all its eugenicist implications – of the nation. The importance of motherhood was buttressed by maternal and child welfare movements, and this emphasis on female domesticity faced little opposition. However, the first half of the twentieth century saw important changes occurring in households. Although some parts of the middle-classes began reducing their family size in the 1860s, this was increasingly widespread by the 1930s, by which point smaller families were increasingly common and normal within all social classes.[56] The presence of live-in domestic servants in middle-class homes, widespread at the beginning of the century but declining to the point of perceived crisis in the interwar years, diminished profoundly during the Second World War and did not recover.[57] The experience of conflict once again necessitated the mobilisation of women into workplaces, but ideas about women's 'natural' interests endured and housewifery and motherhood for women were perceived to be the ideal to which peacetime society should rapidly seek to return.[58] Thus middle-class women who returned to domesticity – or who entered it for the first time – in the wake of the Second World War were obliged *en masse* to take up arduous, physically demanding, and protracted domestic tasks.[59] Gradually, the availability of new household appliances grew for middle-class families, but housework, and the many different tasks that fell under its capacious title, remained time consuming, repetitive, labourious, and, as Ann Oakley's doctoral study found during the 1960s, was frequently disliked by the women to whom it fell.[60] Meanwhile, women's maternal labour was held up to be of major social importance, and the raising of their own young children to be their primary occupation. The stakes were high. In the years that followed the war, mothers' paid work, which necessitated their absence from the home, was pointed to as a contributing factor to juvenile delinquency and national disorder.[61]

However, in the 1950s, an alternative social pattern surfaced. As families became smaller and lifespans longer, mothering emerged as an intense full-time commitment with temporal edges.[62] After a period of full-time domesticity while children were young, mothers increasingly returned to the workforce when their children were of school age. This, as social scientists Alva Myrdal and Viola Klein observed in 1956, allowed women to be with their young children but prevented the wastage of their professional skills.[63] Married women's labour participation trebled from 10 to 32 per cent between 1931 and 1961, enabled in part by the availability of part-time work.[64] In this period access to consumer goods grew and standards of life rose. But women's work was not exclusively driven by material needs or economic aspirations; it was, as historians have argued, a signifier of modern womanhood, undertaken by women for themselves as well as for their families.[65] The unequal distribution of domestic labour was more tenacious: employed wives continued to bear the brunt of the domestic workload.[66] Nonetheless, by 1970, the shift towards married women's work was readily apparent, drawing interest from social researchers, and the stigma around mothers' employment began to diminish.[67] But increasing social acceptance did not precipitate practical ease. The many difficulties faced by working parents, and particularly working mothers, inspired feminist activism in the 1970s.[68]

But on a wide social scale feminist reforms did not come to pass, and in the 1980s society still did little to provide practical support to working mothers. At the start of the decade 60 per cent of married or cohabiting women were in the labour force, although the majority of this work was part-time.[69] In the media, worries duly shifted to the psychological toll on high-achieving working mothers and their children. *The Times* warned in 1987 that 'high-flyers are being brought low by postnatal depression'. These 'high-flying "superwomen", who believe that they can schedule a baby like a business appointment and breastfeed successfully between board meetings' were 'particularly easy prey to postnatal depression', the article cautioned.[70] Little surprise then, that in the 1980s some working mothers felt guilty, and that by the 1990s some feminists were identifying the cultural *leitmotif* of the harried working mother as a significant component of the conservative backlash against women's gains.[71] However, the expectation for mothers was still that they would have a period out of the workforce while their children were young, and it is largely in this time of intensive mothering that we see mothers expressing the unhappiness explored in this book.[72]

Mothers in the workforce were dependent on the availability of formal and informal childcare. Securing childcare, however, was far from straightforward in a postwar Britain. The widespread mobilisation of married women during the Second World War stimulated the establishment of day nurseries.[73] Despite the challenges these wartime nurseries faced, their success was used to underline the benefits of nurseries for working mothers and their children.[74] Nonetheless, after the war their availability contracted drastically.[75] Demand well outstripped supply; in 1946, in Lewisham, a London borough, for example, 250 children were on waiting lists – a number equal to those already in nursery places. Researchers concluded that childcare provision was a significant factor in keeping mothers out of paid work.[76] In the 1960s there were just 22,000 day care places available, despite married women's increasing uptake of part-time work during this decade.[77] Given this, many working mothers needed to look outside this provision, and turned to childminders as a solution to their predicament. Despite offering the reassurance of a setting that mirrored the family home and that entailed the care of a woman who was frequently a mother herself, childminding occupied an uneasy position in postwar Britain. As Angela Davis has shown, childminders were assumed to be in need of regulation in a way that cast doubt on state commitment to the idea of mothers' experiential expertise.[78]

Working mothers who did manage to secure childcare frequently found that it was precarious. On the cusp of the 1990s, *The Times* pointed out that British women workers had the highest rates of absenteeism in the Western world. One explanation put forward for this was that when children fell sick it was mothers who were forced to take time off work.[79] Thus, as a mother wrote in 1989, mothers in her generation found themselves

> juggling full-time or part-time jobs plus family, clearly finding the situation emotionally and physically shattering. In some cases their pay only just covered their child-minding expenses. They vibrated unspoken anxieties and insecurities, as if life would collapse at the sign of a temperature or a disappearing nanny.[80]

These anxieties were not ill-founded. For most women formal childcare was expensive and hard to secure. The cost of this insecurity was unevenly distributed. Single mothers and those living away from kin networks had fewer sources of help to fall back on. Parents of disabled children found that access to childminders or adequate state childcare was frequently out of reach.[81] Black mothers encountered racism within childcare settings. Access to the infrastructures of the 'village', so often lauded as a necessary prerequisite to raising a child, was neither even nor easy.

Class, race, and politics

As Angela Davis observes, in the 1960s, the 'dissatisfied, educated mother was a stereotypical figure'.[82] This figure permeated popular culture: the Valium-dependent housewife was famously depicted by the Rolling Stones in their 1966 single *Mother's Little Helper*. In the late 1970s, Sheila Kitzinger observed that the 'unhappy mother, trapped within the four walls of home, anxious, depressed, or desperate, is a stock figure of the contemporary TV film and the novel'.[83] As with any stock figure though, recognition rested on common characteristics, including class and race. Until the late 1970s, the idea prevailed that educated, middle-class mothers were more vulnerable to depression than working-class mothers. Psychiatrists and psychologists attributed this to middle-class women's higher expectations and their greater sense of control over their lives, which they suggested made them more prone to disappointment and guilt. Even feminist advocates of empowered motherhood acknowledged that middle-class women's education and careers could leave them susceptible to emotional conflict. Sheila Kitzinger, for example, worried that educated middle-class women were torn between the desire for freedom – pursuing paid work and the associated benefits of a consumer lifestyle – and societal expectations to settle down. Educated women, she thought, were made to feel that having a baby was a 'private indulgence', and thus they approached childbirth and motherhood 'in a businesslike spirit, determined to do it well, but concerned to get back to the real challenges of living': childrearing, far from being a central purpose, was a disruption of educated women's 'real' lives.[84] The emphasis on 'self-expression, self-development, and self-fulfilment' had downgraded motherhood to being 'just a mother'.[85] But society was to blame, she said: motherhood was seen as drudgery because it was socially devalued. The world was organised around education and work, not family life; mothers identified that their young children were unwelcome and poorly accommodated in public spaces.[86] Moreover, smaller families meant that middle-class women, despite their take-up of antenatal classes – the provision of which is explored later in this book – were perceived to be increasingly ill-informed about childbirth and unprepared for the reality of mothering.[87]

As the century progressed, it was middle-class women, with their greater access to the resources and platforms needed to articulate their discontent, who most vocally critiqued their experiences within the institution of motherhood. But the stereotype obscured the reality. The archetype of the middle-class depressed mother was challenged in the 1970s when sociologist George Brown and clinical psychologist Tirril Harris's important study in Camberwell found significantly higher rates of depression in working-class mothers than in their middle-class counterparts.[88]

Social researchers had long drawn connections between poverty and mothers' poor health and unhappiness. In 1901 Seebohm Rowntree's study of York observed that poverty drove working-class women to become 'hopeless drudges', and that mothers of young children were rarely afforded time to themselves.[89] In 1915 Margaret Llewelyn Davies caused an outcry when she published letters that detailed the hardships and suffering experienced by impoverished mothers in *Maternity: Letters from Working Women*.[90] Similar experiences and themes were exposed in the 1930s by Margery Spring Rice, who found that working-class mothers struggled with poor housing conditions, poor physical health, a lack of support, and insufficient access to nutritious food. Some of these mothers reported on the effects of this on their mental health. Consider this letter to Spring Rice:

> I believe myself that one of the biggest difficulties our mothers have is our husbands do not realise we ever need any leisure time. My life for many years consisted of being penned in a kitchen 9 feet square, every fourteen months a baby... until what with the struggle to live and no leisure I used to feel I was just a machine, until I had my first breakdown, and as dark as it was and as hard as it was it gave me the freedom and privilege of having an hour's fresh air.[91]

A breakdown provided short-lived respite from this mother's domestic labour. But other working-class mothers struggled on; one Essex-based wife of an unemployed man reported that the 'constant struggle with poverty' had made her 'very nervy and irritable'.[92] Reflecting on life in an Edinburgh tenement, Mary Holligan, born in 1910, recalled that 'I often wonder how I managed through the first years of married life. I often think my husband never realised how I felt, the trauma of post-natal depression. I didn't want to go out. I just seemed to let myself go. Yet I tried to behave normally'.[93] Large-scale studies underlined the extent to which class informed women's experiences of healthcare and maternity. 'In all aspects of maternity care well-to-do mothers get better attention than those who are poor', observed one 1946 study of fourteen thousand mothers.[94] Poor mothers had fewer healthcare options and, as their families grew, faced cumulative health and financial problems.

The establishment of the NHS in 1948 may have alleviated some of these health issues, but poverty still shaped mothers' lives. In 1966 a Nottingham newspaper reported that one depressed mother was found guilty of stealing money from her domestic gas meter. Aged twenty-five, she was pregnant and had three children under four years old. Her husband was unemployed, and the family were in debt. 'It was just before Christmas, and I had nothing for the children', she told the police.[95] Mothers on council estates faced challenges exacerbated by urban design. In 1971 Labour Member of Parliament Frank Allaun observed the lack of child-friendly spaces on council estates, asking in Parliament,

> Does the Prime Minister realise that many blocks of flats have no nursery school and no playground nearby? Does he further appreciate that where there is a playground it is usually impossible for a mother to keep her eye on her child 15 storeys down? Is he further aware that as a result thousands of children are kept in flats throughout the day, with serious mental effects on themselves and their mothers, which could be avoided through the conversion of one of these flats?[96]

Across the twentieth century, then, less affluent mothers faced conditions that exacted an emotional cost. Nonetheless, in the face of the structural oppressions at work in British society, working-class mothers created opportunities to communicate, interpret, and address their distress. Working-class mothers stimulated conversations about the social and economic contexts within which they parented. They wrote about their experiences and established networks to campaign for change. Some of these organisations explicitly drew attention to the struggles of childrearing on a low income and used their experiences as evidence of the need for change. But other working-class mothers established groups to meet more immediate needs, like childcare and sociability. By acknowledging personal needs, these groups enabled working-class mothers to participate in the turn towards the interior that prevailed in postwar Britain, but as Jessica White has shown, such groups were sometimes – but not always – marred by racial exclusion.[97]

Black women's experiences of mothering in postwar Britain were contoured by racism. Immigration from British colonies was stimulated in the 1940s to address postwar labour shortages. But while immigrant women were in demand as workers – particularly within the NHS – Black motherhood was disparaged and discouraged.[98] In the 1970s this was made readily apparent by the disproportionate and unconsenting use of Depo-Provera, a controversial injectable contraceptive, on women of colour.[99] Within the NHS, Black workers were underrepresented in higher grades, were concentrated in less popular nursing specialisms, and were overrepresented on night shifts.[100] Black mothers who fulfilled the demand for healthcare workers found that their rigid hours and low pay posed logistical problems for childcare.[101] Racism was directed at women of colour in the health service as both patients and as workers.[102] Moreover, race structured the visibility of maternal experiences: for example, some of the most important sociological work that made white mothers' distress visible excluded women of colour from being interviewees.[103] Where it was given voice, it is clear that distress in mothers of colour and migrant and minoritised mothers was compounded by racism. In 2018 American scholar Jennifer C. Nash observed that

> In a moment in which the booming maternal memoir genre roots itself in mapping white maternal ambivalence, in treating motherhood as a space that takes—perhaps even steals—from women, black maternal testimonies obsessively track motherhood as a site of spiritual and psychic renewal and steadfastly refuse to document the violence of motherhood apart from the threat of state violence. I find myself wondering: is there space for maternal unhappiness in the black feminist theoretical maternal archive, space for accounts of motherhood that find mothering profoundly unradical, perhaps even tedious, exhausting, or upsetting?

She was, she wrote, 'particularly interested in how feminist accounts – even black feminist accounts – of maternal ambivalence... remain uncited here, thus obscuring the long roots of black feminist engagement with maternal ambivalence'.[104] This question is particularly important here as some of the mechanisms of visibility explored by this book intensified the coding of unhappy motherhood as a white, heterosexual, middle-class experience. Such encoding obscures the 'long roots' in experiences of distress and ambivalence within motherhood of women of colour.

What was new motherhood like for women of colour in Britain? Journalist and writer Yasmin Alibhai (later Alibhai-Brown), born in Uganda's Asian community in 1949 and who moved to Britain in 1972, wrote that after the birth of her son in 1978, she 'cried for two weeks'. She reflected that 'the never-had-it-so-good feelings were constantly being overshadowed by a deep sense of sorrow'.[105] The context, she explains, was a hostile colonial nation, atomising national values, and a white women's movement indifferent or inattentive to the experiences of women of colour. 'This background is essential to understand the feelings of loss and fear I experienced when my son was born', she wrote,

> Especially in terms of what Britain had begun to mean to me then. That had been another psychological earthquake. In the hospital they called it post-natal depression. I think it was a watershed time when my past identity, personal and political, had crashed into new bits and pieces that had begun to grow since I arrived here.

The hospital labelled such a complex convergence of feelings post-natal depression; Alibhai saw it instead as a disassembling and reassembling of identities in an environment that was hostile to her and her child.[106]

But it was not just in labour wards that mothers of colour were vulnerable. Black communities encountered racism elsewhere, not least in work, housing, health, childcare, and education. Given these widespread structural and social obstacles, how did Black women raise the profile of issues that affected themselves and their families and organise around resistance? One path was via the formation of organised groups. The Black Parents Movement, for example, established in 1975, tackled racism in education and the police harassment of young Black people.[107] Another route to visibility was through scholarly and autofictional writing, as Black social researchers, activists, scholars, and novelists explored structural and interpersonal discrimination against Black women and mothers of colour.[108] The development of alternative, feminist, and radical publishing infrastructures aided the dissemination of dissent. In 1982, Protasia Torkington wrote an article about Black women and the NHS in a women's liberation magazine that was subsequently republished by a feminist publishing house. In this Torkington observed that 'for black people there is an added dimension of racism in the wider social, political and economic structure which makes black people... so much more the victims of all major illnesses from infant mortality to post-natal depression than the white working class'.[109] Black mothers also organised playgroups, creches, and mother and toddler groups, enabling them to undertake paid work, have greater independence, and create social networks.[110] As the century progressed, sites for the discussion and analysis of mothers' unhappiness were developed by social movements, and women created networks to meet the needs that medicine, the family, and the state neglected.

Conclusion

This book proposes one answer to a question that Oakley gestured to when she wrote that 'In those days – the late 1960s – it was not yet acceptable for women to admit openly to their dissatisfactions'.[111] Such a claim sits uneasily alongside the assertion that by the late 1960s the figure of the unhappy, tranquilised housewife was a familiar stereotype, a 'stock figure' of popular culture. Surely cultural circulation facilitated a degree of destigmatisation? Alas, not necessarily: stereotypes can prevent emotional disclosure by adding a further layer of embarrassment. They pull towards shame. Thus stock figures and silences can manifest around the same topic. Moreover, stereotypes do not permeate the culture evenly. But, if we take Oakley's claim at face value, we can ask if in the 1960s it was not 'yet' acceptable, when and how did it become acceptable for women and mothers to air their dissatisfactions? How, in Britain, did the five communities discussed in this book give 'the problem with no name' – the discontent of suburban housewives, as identified by American feminist Betty Friedan in 1963 – greater visibility?[112]

This process is still, of course, not complete. But this book offers some ideas about how unhappy motherhood gained attention, visibility, and legibility. It focuses on the communities of people who, for different reasons and within different disciplines and networks, were invested in understanding unhappy motherhood. This process took place against changing attitudes towards experience, expertise, and self-disclosure. In this way, it agrees with Lynn Abrams, who has identified a 'new discursive landscape of emotions that emerged from the late 1950s in Britain' that 'brought forth a tsunami of speaking about feelings amongst ordinary women, both in public and in private'.¹¹³ A driving argument of this book, then, is that mothers took up and created opportunities to explore, share, and critique their own experiences of distress in postwar Britain. The development of grassroots mutual aid and consciousness-raising groups tells a story about maternal unhappiness that takes place outside medical infrastructures. It tells us that mothers played a crucial role in shaping their own social support.

In the late 1980s Victoria Hardie termed the mutual support mothers gave one another a kind of 'constructive anarchy', a form of 'mutual positive help', taking place as it did outside the waged economy.¹¹⁴ Both before and during the retrenchment of state support, mothers formed informal but meaningful communities. My interest in the labour of legibility suggests that recent work around the struggles of mothering should be seen as a continuation of discussions that have evolved across the last seventy years. Generations of mothers contributed to it by giving voice to their experiences. The book looks to sites of visibility across a range of disciplines and social spaces, highlighting how people asserted different types of expertise depending on what was available to them, and thinking in particular about how mothers and women came to use mothers' unhappiness – across a broad sweep of the emotional spectrum – as a lens on the problems of the social world.

Notes

1 Vivienne Welburn, *Postnatal Depression* (Glasgow, 1983 [1980]), 148–159.
2 Charlotte Perkins Gilman, *The Yellow Wallpaper* (London, 2008 [1892]).
3 Helen McCarthy, 'Feminism, Selfhood and Social Research: Professional Women's Organizations in 1960s Britain', in *Precarious Professionals: Gender, Identities and Social Change in Modern Britain*, eds Heidi Egginton and Zoë Thomas (London, 2021), 287–304.
4 Teri Chettiar, *The Intimate State: How Emotional Life Became Political in Welfare-State Britain* (New York, 2023), 112–140.
5 Judy Dunn, 'Unhappy Mothers', *London Review of Books*, 2, 14, 17 July 1980. Retrieved from https://www.lrb.co.uk/the-paper/v02/n14/judy-dunn/unhappy-mothers [Accessed September 2024].
6 Sheila Kitzinger, *Women as Mothers* (Glasgow, 1978), 270.

7 For work that looks at how some postwar women navigated domesticity with ease, see Ali Haggett, *Desperate Housewives, Neuroses and the Domestic Environment, 1945–1970* (Abingdon, 2016 [2012]).
8 National Health Service. 'Postnatal Depression'. Retrieved from https://www.nhs.uk/conditions/post-natal-depression/ [Accessed 1 April 2018].
9 Ellie Lee, *Abortion, Motherhood, and Mental Health: Medicalising Reproduction in the United States and Great Britain* (New York, 2003), 190.
10 See Lee, *Abortion, Motherhood, and Mental Health*. For scholarship on Victorian approaches to motherhood and mental health, see Hilary Marland, *Dangerous Motherhood: Insanity and Childbirth in Victorian Britain* (New York, 2004). Marland has a forthcoming study of the more modern history of postnatal depression that emerges from her large-scale Wellcome Trust-funded study, 'The Last Taboo of Motherhood?'
11 Barbara Taylor, *The Last Asylum: A Memoir of Madness in Our Times* (London, 2015), 34.
12 Victoria Hardie, 'The World Became a More Dangerous Place', in *Balancing Acts: On Being a Mother*, ed. Katherine Gieve (London, 1989), 52–72, 62.
13 For a discussion of one such programme, see Fabiola Creed, 'Nemone Lethbridge's Play Baby Blues on BBC Television: Maternal Mental Illness Narratives, Stigma and Support in 1970s Britain', *Women's History Review*, 34, 2024, 1–25.
14 Jennifer Crane, *Child Protection in England, 1960–2000: Expertise, Experience, and Emotion* (Basingstoke, 2018), 8.
15 Thomasina Borkman, 'Experiential Knowledge: A New Concept for the Analysis of Self-Help Groups', *Social Service Review*, 50, 3, 1976, 445–456, 445.
16 See, for example, Crane, *Child Protection in England*, 2018); Ruth Davidson, 'Working-Class Women Activists: Citizenship at the Local Level', in *Alternatives to State-Socialism in Britain: Other Worlds of Labour in the Twentieth Century*, eds Peter Ackers and Alastair Reid (Basingstoke, 2016), 93–121; Caitríona Beaumont, *Housewives and Citizens: Domesticity and the Women's Movement in England, 1928–64* (Manchester, 2013); Eve Colpus, *Female Philanthropy in the Interwar World: Between Self and Other* (London, 2018).
17 Caitríona Beaumont, Eve Colpus, and Ruth Davidson (eds), 'Introduction', in *Everyday Welfare in Modern British History: Experience, Expertise, and Activism*, ed. Caitríona Beaumont, Eve Colpus and Ruth Davidson (Cham, 2024), 1–24, 14.

18 Hardie, 'The World', 70–71.
19 Liz Berry, 'The Republic of Motherhood', *The Republic of Motherhood* (London, 2018), 1–2, 1.
20 Anna Vaux, 'Motherblame', *London Review of Books*, 20, 10, 21 May 1998. Retrieved from https://www.lrb.co.uk/the-paper/v20/n10/anna-vaux/motherblame [Accessed 25 September 2024].
21 Jacqueline Rose, 'Mothers', *London Review of Books*, 36, 12, 19 June 2014. Retrieved from https://www.lrb.co.uk/the-paper/v36/n12/jacqueline-rose/mothers [Accessed 25 September 2024].
22 Berry, *The Republic of Motherhood*, 1.
23 Ruth Cain, 'A View You Won't Get Anywhere Else'? Depressed Mothers, Public Regulation and 'Private' Narrative', *Feminist Legal Studies* 17, 2009, 123–143, 125–126.
24 For psychological ideas and the interwar period, see Mathew Thomson, 'Psychology and the "Consciousness of Modernity" in Early Twentieth-Century Britain', in *Meanings of Modernity: Britain from the Late-Victorian Era to World War II*, eds Martin Daunton and Bernhard Rieger (London, 2001), 97–115. For infanticide, see Tony Ward, 'The Sad Subject of Infanticide: Law, Medicine and Child Murder, 1860–1938', *Social & Legal Studies*, 8, 2, 1999, 163–180. For the reasons for the legislation, see Daniel Grey, 'Women's Policy Networks and the Infanticide Act 1922', *Twentieth Century British History*, 21, 4, 2010, 441–463; see also HMSO Infanticide Act 1938. For suburban neurosis, see Stephen Taylor, 'The Suburban Neurosis', *The Lancet*, 231, 5978, 1938, 759–762, 761. For more on this, see Rhodri Hayward, 'Desperate Housewives and Model Amoebae: The Invention of Suburban Neurosis in Inter-War Britain', in *Health and the Modern Home*, ed. Mark Jackson (London, 2007), 42–62.
25 Harry Hendrick, *Children, Childhood and English Society, 1880–1990* (Cambridge, 1997), 28–29.
26 John Stewart, *Child Guidance in Britain, 1918–1955: The Dangerous Age of Childhood* (London, 2013), 59–106.
27 Teri Chettiar, '"More than a Contract": The Emergence of a State-Supported Marriage Welfare Service and the Politics of Emotional Life in Post-1945 Britain', *Journal of British Studies*, 55, 3, 2016, 566–591.
28 Stewart, *Child Guidance*, 108–109, 142.
29 Laura King, 'Future Citizens: Cultural and Political Conceptions of Children in Britain, 1930s–1950s', *Twentieth Century British History*, 27, 3, 2016, 389–411, 389; Claire Langhamer, *The English in Love: The Intimate Story of an Emotional Revolution* (Oxford, 2013),

181; see also Claire Langhamer, 'The Meanings of Home in Postwar Britain', *Journal of Contemporary History*, 40, 2, 2005, 341–362.
30 'The Man Who Loved Children', *TIME Magazine*, 10 March 1998. Retrieved from https://time.com/archive/6732499/the-man-who-loved-children-dr-benjamin-spock-1903-1998/ [Accessed 19 September 2024].
31 John Bowlby, *Child Care and the Growth of Love*. 2nd ed. (Harmondsworth, 1973 [1953]), 13; see also John Bowlby, *Maternal Care and Mental Health* (Geneva, 1951).
32 Michal Shapira, *The War Inside: Psychoanalysis, Total War, and the Making of the Democratic Self in Postwar Britain* (Cambridge, 2013), 112–117.
33 D.W. Winnicott, *The Child and the Family*, ed. Janet Hardenberg (London, 1957), 143–144.
34 Julia Vellacott, 'Motherhood in the Imagination', in *Balancing Acts: On Being a Mother* Ed. Katherine Gieve (London, 1989), 177–203, 191.
35 Peter Laslett, 'Mothering', *London Review of Books*, 3, 14, 6 August 1981. Retrieved from https://www.lrb.co.uk/the-paper/v03/n14/peter-laslett/mothering [Accessed 20 September 2024].
36 David Cowan, '"Modern" Parenting and the Uses of Childcare Advice in Post-War England', *Social History*, 43, 3, 2018, 332–355.
37 L.A. Shaw, 'Impressions of Family Life in a London Suburb (Studies of a General Practice IV)', *The Sociological Review*, 2, 2, 1954, 179–194.
38 John and Elizabeth Newson, *Patterns of Infant Care in an Urban Community* (Harmondsworth, 1976 [1963]), 1, 13.
39 Katherine Gieve (Ed.), 'And Not to Count the Cost', in *Balancing Acts: On Being a Mother* (London, 1989), 41–51, 46.
40 Ann Oakley, *Housewife* (London, 1990 [1974]), 120.
41 Adrienne Rich, *Of Woman Born: Motherhood as Experience and Institution* (New York, 1986 [1976]).
42 Ann Oakley, *Man & Wife: Richard and Kay Titmuss: My Parents' Early Years* (London, 1996).
43 Ann Oakley, *Taking It Like a Woman* (London, 1984), 29.
44 See, for example, Judith Hubback, *Wives Who Went to College* (London, 1957).
45 Joanna Moorhead, *New Generations: 40 Years of Birth in Britain* (Cambridge, 1996), 29, 36.
46 Oakley, *Taking It Like a Woman*, 64. For more, see Angela Davis, 'Choice, Policy and Practice in Maternity Care since 1948', *History & Policy*, 30 May 2013. Retrieved from https://www.historyandpolicy

.org/policy-papers/papers/choice-policy-and-practice-in-maternity-care-since-1948 [Accessed 6 August 2024].
47 Ann Oakley, *Becoming a Mother* (Oxford, 1979), 2–3.
48 Oakley, *Father and Daughter*, 177.
49 Oakley, *Taking It Like a Woman*, 68–69.
50 *Ibid.*, 68.
51 *Ibid.*, 74.
52 Ann Oakley, *Housewife* (London, 1990 [1974]), 102.
53 Ann Oakley, 'Interviewing Women Again: Power, Time and the Gift', *Sociology*, 50, 1, 2016, 195–213.
54 Carol Dyhouse, 'Good Wives and Little Mothers: Social Anxieties and the Schoolgirl's Curriculum, 1890–1920', *Oxford Review of Education*, 3, 1, 1977, 21–35, 27.
55 Helen McCarthy, *Double Lives: A History of Working Motherhood* (London, 2020), 158–159.
56 Shani D'Cruze, 'Women and the Family', in *Women's History: Britain, 1850–1945*, ed. June Purvis (London: 1998), 51–3, 56.
57 Judy Giles, 'Help for Housewives: Domestic Service and the Reconstruction of Domesticity in Britain, 1940–50', *Women's History Review*, 10, 2, 2001, 299–324.
58 Penny Summerfield, 'Women and War in the Twentieth Century', in *Women's History: Britain, 1850–1945, an Introduction*, ed. June Purvis (London, 2000), 307–332, 312–313.
59 Giles, 'Help for Housewives'.
60 Ann Oakley, *The Sociology of Housework* (Oxford, 1974), 49.
61 Dolly Smith Wilson, 'A New Look at the Affluent Worker: The Good Working Mother in Post-War Britain', *Twentieth Century British History*, 17, 2, 2006, 206–229, 207.
62 Ann Taylor Allen, *Feminism and Motherhood in Western Europe, 1890–1970: The Maternal Dilemma* (Basingstoke, 2005), 213.
63 Alva Myrdal and Viola Klein, *Women's Two Roles: Home and Work* (London, 1956).
64 Deirdre McCloskey, 'Paid Work', in *Women in Twentieth Century Britain*, ed. Ina Zweiniger-Bargielowska (Essex, 2001), 165–179, 168; Jane Lewis, *Women in Britain since 1945* (Oxford, 1993), 74.
65 Laura Paterson, '"I Didn't Feel Like My Own Person": Paid Work in Women's Narratives of Self and Working Motherhood, 1950–1980', *Contemporary British History*, 33, 3, 2019, 405–426; Florence Sutcliffe-Braithwaite and Natalie Thomlinson, 'Vernacular Discourses of Gender Equality in the Post-War British Working Class', *Past & Present*, 254, 1, 2022, 277–313, 292; McCarthy, *Double Lives*, 30.

66 Oakley, *Housewife*; R. Rapoport and R.N. Rapoport, *Dual-Career Families* (Harmondsworth, 1971); Michael Young and Peter Willmott, *The Symmetrical Family* (London, [1973] 1980), 109–115.
67 Smith Wilson, 'New Look', 216; McCarthy, *Double Lives*.
68 Sarah E. Stoller, *Inventing the Working Parent: Work, Gender, and Feminism in Neoliberal Britain* (Cambridge, MA, 2023), 61–94.
69 McCloskey, 'Paid Work', 169.
70 'Birth of the Blues?', *The Times*, 3 December 1987.
71 Margaret Smith, 'The Best of Both Worlds?', in *Balancing Acts: On Being a Mother*, ed. Katherine Gieve (London, 1989), 160–176, 171. For the argument that there was a conservative backlash against feminism, see for example, Susan Faludi, *Backlash: The Undeclared War Against American Women* (New York, 1991).
72 McCarthy, *Double Lives*, 248–249.
73 Joint Committee of the Royal College of Obstetricians and Gynaecologists and the Population Investigation Committee, *Maternity in Great Britain: A Survey of Social and Economic Aspects of Pregnancy and Childbirth* (London and New York, 1948), 173.
74 Lady Reading, 'While Mothers Work', *Picture Post*, 8, 3, 20 July 1940, 23–25.
75 War-time Nurseries, HC Deb 09 March 1945 vol 408 cc2425-50; 'While Mother Works', *Daily Mirror*, 2 July 1946, 2.
76 Joint Committee of the Royal College of Obstetricians and Gynaecologists and the Population Investigation Committee, *Maternity in Great Britain*, 174–175.
77 Katherine Holden, 'Family, Caring and Unpaid Work', in *Women in Twentieth-Century Britain*, ed. Ina Zweiniger-Bargielowska (Essex, 2001), 134–148, 139.
78 Angela Davis, 'Childminders and the Limits of Mothering as Experiential Expertise, England c.1948–2000', in *Everyday Welfare in Modern British History: Experience, Expertise and Activism*, eds Caitríona Beaumont, Eve Colpus, and Ruth Davidson (Cham, 2024), 95–116.
79 'Caring for the Absent Women', *The Times*, 10 February 1989.
80 Hardie, 'The World', 55.
81 Rahila Gupta, 'Giving Birth Again', in *Balancing Acts: On Being a Mother*, ed. Katherine Gieve (London, 1989), 94–106, 101.
82 Davis, *Modern Motherhood*, 147.
83 Sheila Kitzinger, *Women as Mothers* (Glasgow, 1978), 28.
84 *Ibid.*, 29.
85 *Ibid.*, 46–47.
86 *Ibid.*, 270–271.

87 B. Rathbone, *Focus on New Mothers: A Study of Antenatal Classes* (London, 1973); Royal College of Midwives, *Preparation for Parenthood* (Taunton, 1966).
88 George W. Brown and Tirril Harris, *The Social Origins of Depression: A Study of Psychiatric Disorder in Women* (London, 1989 [1978]), 150. For more on this study, see Rhodri Hayward, 'Sadness in Camberwell: Imagining Stress and Constructing History in Post-War Britain', in *Stress, Trauma and Adaptation in the Twentieth Century*, eds David Cantor and Edmund Ramsden (Rochester, NY, 2014), 320–341.
89 Seebohm Rowntree, *Poverty: A Study in Town Life* (London, 1902 [1901]), 77–78.
90 Margaret Llewelyn Davies, *Maternity: Letters From Working Women* (London, 1978 [1915]).
91 Margery Spring Rice, *Working-Class Wives* (London, 1981 [1939]), 94.
92 *Ibid.*, 69.
93 Helen Clark and Elizabeth Carnegie, *She Was Aye Workin': Memories of Tenement Women in Edinburgh and Glasgow* (Oxford, 2006 [2003]), 89.
94 Joint Committee of the Royal College of Obstetricians and Gynaecologists and the Population Investigation Committee, *Maternity in Great Britain*, 207.
95 '"A Good Mother" Fined for Theft', *Nottingham Evening Post and News*, 29 June 1966.
96 Play Groups, HC Deb 25 May 1971 vol 818 cc229-30.
97 Jessica White, 'Child-Centred Matriarch or Mother Among Other Things? Race and the Construction of Working-Class Motherhood in Late Twentieth-Century Britain', *Twentieth Century British History*, 33, 4, 2022, 498–521.
98 Wendy Webster, *Imagining Home: Gender, Race and National Identity, 1945–1964* (Abingdon, 2023 [1998]), 173-174.
99 Caitlin Lambert, '"The Objectionable Injectable": Recovering the Lost History of the WLM Through the Campaign against Depo-Provera', *Women's History Review*, 29, 3, 2019, 520–539.
100 Editorial, 'Tackling Racism in the NHS', *Health Visitor*, 62, December 1989, 357.
101 Njoki, quoted in Tuula Gordon, *Feminist Mothers* (Hampshire, 1990), 81.
102 See, for example, assessments of the Asian Mother and Baby Campaign, which identified racism directed at both link workers and mothers. 'Antenatal Care: Who Needs It?', *Health Visitor*,

61, 1, January 1988, 29; Yvette Rocheron, 'The Asian Mother and Baby Campaign: The Construction of Ethnic Minorities' Health Needs', *Critical Social Policy*, 8, 22, 1988, 4–23.
103 Gavron, 'The Position', 31.
104 Jennifer C. Nash, 'The Political Life of Black Motherhood', *Feminist Studies*, 44, 3, 2018, 699–712, 711.
105 Yasmin Alibhai, 'Burning in the Cold', in *Balancing Acts: On Being a Mother*, ed. Katherine Gieve (London, 1989), 24–40, 27.
106 *Ibid.*, 30–38.
107 Rob Waters, *Thinking Black: Britain, 1964–1985* (Oakland, CA, 2018), 44.
108 Buchi Emecheta, *Second-Class Citizen* (London, 2021 [1974]); Pauline Davies, *Trapped: Unmarried West Indian Mothers in Handsworth*. Papers on Community & Youth Work, No. 2. Department of Community and Youth Work, Westhill College (Birmingham, 1983); Beverley Bryan, Stella Dadzie, and Suzanne Scafe, *Heart of the Race: Black Women's Lives in Britain* (London, 1985).
109 Protasia Torkington, 'Black Women and the NHS', in *Sweeping Statements: Writings From the Women's Liberation Movement 1981–83*, eds Hannah Kanter, Sarah Lefanu, Shaila Shah, and Carole Spedding (London, 1984), 92–96, 93.
110 White, 'Child-Centred Matriarch'.
111 Ann Oakley, *Becoming a Mother* (Oxford, 1979), 2.
112 Betty Friedan, *The Feminine Mystique* (New York, 1963), 15.
113 Lynn Abrams, *Feminist Lives: Women, Feelings, & the Self in Post-War Britain* (Oxford, 2023), 152.
114 Hardie, 'The World', 71.

1

Mothers, general practitioners, and the NHS

In 1952 two general practitioners based in the working-class community of Ibstock, Leicestershire, stressed the centrality of treating milder forms of mental illness to their practice. Doctors B.M. (Beatrice or 'Betty') Watts and her husband C.A.H. (Arthur) Watts worried that psychological cases were too often seen as 'the bugbear' of general practice, dismissed with a sedative, and hastily dispatched from the doctors' office. Such an approach, they warned, was inadequate. It was in dealing with psychiatric cases that general practitioners could come into their own, they argued. Unlike hospital-based clinicians, the general practitioner lived among their patients, so had a 'more accurate norm' against which to compare them; the general practitioner was familiar with patients' family histories and backgrounds; and the general practitioner had access to the majority of the 'diagnostic weapons' available to the consultant. There were other motivating factors, though, which related to the broader status of a medical specialism in flux. There was 'a danger that we may become finger posts directing our patients to the most appropriate specialist', they warned, 'We are being driven out of the hospitals, and in general our work in one way or another is being curtailed and limited. Here in psychiatry is a new sphere of work for our attention. It is essentially work for general practitioners'. Moreover, general practitioners lived among their practice populations: they knew their patients' backgrounds and extended histories, and thus witnessed their everyday lives, their families, and general dispositions.[1] This facilitated what Rhodri Hayward has termed a 'new kind of psychological intimacy'.[2] The Wattses were not alone in viewing mental health as a promising area for general practitioners' intervention. Attentiveness to psychological issues was taking on a more central role in general practice in the early postwar years – this, when put alongside the rapid development of antidepressants and the interest in the psychological atmosphere of the family, would have important implications for the visibility of mothers' distress.

These intersecting interests were driven forward by vocal general practitioners. Beatrice Watts (née Axton), for example, was an advocate of general practitioners' psychiatric work, and was interested in advancing studies of child development. Born in 1911, she qualified as a doctor in 1935, married C.A.H. Watts in April 1937, and together the couple raised four children.[3] Shortly after she and her husband published *Psychiatry in General Practice* in 1952, her essay on the effect of the emotional atmosphere of the home on children was awarded second place for the Butterworth Prize in a competition organised by the College of General Practitioners. Here she again emphasised the 'special contribution' that could be made by general practitioners to studies of the home, for 'Patients willingly accept routine observation of their infants as part of the service of the family doctor'.[4] But the piece was more expansively about how interest in the home as a mutually interlocking and interdependent emotional unit, rather than as a collection of fragmented individuals, might help to shine new light on effective childrearing. The climate of the home was not just the mother-child dyad, she stressed, but was informed by the other relationships within it, and particularly by the relationship between the mother and father. She encouraged the cultivation of 'real warmth' and close fatherly involvement in childrearing, observing that 'the presence of a good father, as well as mother, appears to be essential for the best development of the children in every sphere'. Beatrice admired John Bowlby's influence, crediting him with popularising the 'revolutionary news' that human relationships lay at the core of family life and childrearing practices. It was within this context and because of him that society had been 'jolted into paying more attention to the atmosphere than to the mechanics of the home, and into viewing the child as a growing thing that is likely to develop satisfactorily if given the right conditions', she argued. Bowlby, she thought, marked a break from expert childrearing advice that had been overly didactic and gloomy in tone. 'So many potentially excellent mothers are worried and robbed of the enjoyment of their children's early years by the welter of articles, talks and instructions on what to do, and what not to do, and on the shocking effects of mistakes', she lamented. Instead, affectionate famiy relationships and an emphasis on enjoying one another should be encouraged, she urged, a shift that could prevent 'untold misery' among these mothers.[5] In the postwar period, then, general practitioners were turning to 'milder' emotional complaints and to the realm of the family as two areas in which they had distinct professional advantages. These overlapping fields – the family and mental health – helped to shape medical awareness of unhappy motherhood and the emotional climate of the family.

But Beatrice Watts signifies something broader. Like other women in the immediate postwar years, she navigated a culture that saw paid work as a potentially noxious distraction from motherhood and domesticity. Despite this, Beatrice, like other mothers, found ways to contribute to her profession. In 1951 women comprised just over 15 per cent of active doctors, rising to 18 per cent in 1971 – increasing from 7,520 to 12,596 across the two decades.[6] General practice was sometimes seen as a comparatively appropriate medical field for married female doctors, offering flexibility and fewer formal training demands. In 1968 women were 11 per cent of all general practitioners, rising slowly to 14 per cent – 3,301 out of 22,015 – in 1976.[7] Women who studied medicine during the Second World War married earlier and at higher rates than those who came before them, leading to a slight rise in medically qualified mothers.[8] In many ways, married female doctors' careers reflected wider trends in married women's employment in the postwar period, with part-time work and periods out of the workforce widespread among these professionals.[9] In the late 1960s and 1970s studies found that a high proportion of medical women found themselves in general practice.[10] Some of these women were combining this paid work with childrearing, or were returning to employment after a period of domesticity, and are thus a reminder that women – despite significant impediments – contributed to the medical landscape during this period. Their presence may also have encouraged an interest in women and the family in the field. But interrupted career patterns mean that medical women appear and then disappear from view. Beatrice Watts co-authored *Psychiatry in General Practice* with her husband, and was named alongside him upon its publication in

1952, but his name alone featured on *Depressive Disorders in the Community* (1966), its intellectual sequel, which, he said, 'could never have been done without the unstinted help and co-operation of my wife, Dr B.M. Watts'. Other female family members also enabled this research, as his daughter, Dr Margaret Williams, undertook locum work in his absence, and another daughter, Elizabeth Watts, designed the book's dustcover.[11] And when, in 1971, C.A.H. Watts delivered a talk on 'The Blue Plague' – which warned that far from having 'never had it so good', the British were beset with depressions – he did so alone, publishing the resulting article in the *Journal of the Royal College of General Practitioners* as a sole author the following year.[12] The ideas of this talk and article were expanded upon and extended for a lay audience in *Depression: The Blue Plague*, published in 1973. Here he once again acknowledged the support and assistance of his wife, who was, he wrote, 'a complete partner in this enterprise', but was 'too modest to admit to this role'.[13] Despite the longstanding collaboration that these acknowledgements imply, it was C.A.H., rather than Beatrice, who developed an esteemed publication record about psychiatry and general practice. Nonetheless, it is clear from them that Beatrice Watts had not relinquished an interest or expertise in childrearing, psychiatry, or medicine, and while her name is not on the cover of these later texts, her influence over the trajectory of the promotion of psychiatric care in general practice was expressed within them.

This chapter explores how the convergence of institutional, technological, and social trends between the late 1940s and 1960s encouraged general practice-based research into the psychological health of the family – and through this, encouraged an interest in mothers.[14] Ali Haggett has, for example, shown that while general practice was a key site for the emergence of male psychiatric illness, it was also a site that was shaped by gendered professional norms, and that male physicians were 'bound by the same nexus of constraints and expectations as their male patients'.[15] With regards to distress in women and mothers, British general practice was, of course, similarly informed by the cultural context in which it operated. This cultural context was one in which the family was of national significance. Like its precursor, the Second World War brought attention to the perceived value of children and to maternal health. This was reflected in the priority given to pregnant women and breastfeeding mothers in rationing, and by the measures introduced to shore up mothers' health, including making vitamins and milk accessible and available.[16] Afterwards, reconstruction efforts focused attention on the interlocking nexus of family stability and psychological wellbeing.[17] While the establishment of the National Marriage Guidance Council took place shortly before the war, attention to the psychotherapeutic role of the family mushroomed after the conflict; the origins of family therapy can be traced back to John Bowlby at the Tavistock in the late 1940s, for example, and the Institute of Family Psychiatry was established in 1950.[18] The postwar period saw the therapeutic emphasis move to relationships, and psychiatrists explored the potential of the family to be a site of intervention.[19] But general practitioners contended that they had privileged insights into the family within its natural environment and that this promised important insights into its health.

This chapter considers the impulses that encouraged interest in unhappy motherhood within general practices in the early decades of the welfare state. It establishes the early interest in mothers' mental health among a community of medical professionals with whom mothers were especially liable to be in regular contact. Moreover, anxiety about the pressures on the welfare state created a new need to understand 'milder' forms of distress that could be managed outside the hospital. An emphasis on research encouraged general practitioners to examine the communities they worked in, while the proliferation of antidepressant medications furnished general practitioners with treatment options that avoided the separation of the mother and infant. As this chapter argues, professional anxiety within general practice interacted with pharmacological developments and wider cultural agendas to encourage new research around early motherhood.

Childbirth, general practitioners, and the NHS

Numerous historians have explored the ways that medical specialisms have vied to assert their authority, power, and knowledge within maternity care.[20] While the NHS brought marked benefits to expectant women and mothers, its early years were a period of confusion and tension in services for pregnancy and childbirth.

Pregnant women found themselves at the juncture of several different services and specialisms, with midwives, general practitioners, and obstetricians all part of the maternity infrastructure. General practitioners, who were independently contracted within the tripartite system, were incentivised to have oversight of pregnant women: the NHS operated an obstetric list, on which the majority of general practitioners were listed (in 1957 there were around 19,340 general practitioners in England and Wales, of whom 14,400 were general practitioner obstetricians) – which paid general practitioners on it for their maternity services a slightly higher rate than those not.[21] There was, therefore, a financial reward for maternity work. In particular, general practitioners argued for the advantages of antenatal clinics within their practices. This allowed them, they said, to follow up regular absconders from pre-arranged appointments and facilitated regular observations by one person so changes could more readily be identified, an 'advantage over the hospital clinic'.[22] Nonetheless, services for pregnant women were manifold. In 1961, a general practitioner in Ayrshire, Scotland, identified a 'maternity welfare maze' while setting out the services available in his area. This comprised a consultant obstetric service, located in the maternity section of Ayrshire Central Hospital, with 112 beds, which provided consultant antenatal clinics, beds for booked and emergency births, and antenatal classes; three general practitioner maternity hospital units, with 84 beds between them, which were staffed by a matron, midwives, nurses, and general practitioners; a district nursing service, where midwives were available for home confinements and visited mothers and babies in the postnatal period; and a laboratory service. The services functioned well together, he said, but relied on close communication between teams. Ayrshire exceeded the national target of 70 per cent of all births to be hospital-based that was set out in the Cranbrook Report of 1959: in 1959 over 80 per cent of births in the area took place in hospital settings.[23] But the location of birth varied by practice and place, as did general practitioners' proficiency. This was acknowledged by general practitioners themselves. One general practitioner, having surveyed the outcomes of his obstetric practice in Warrington, England between the end of the 1940s and the early 1960s, observed that on occasion, 'enthusiasm has outstripped skill and good judgment'. Nonetheless, he concluded that the general practitioner had an important role in obstetrics, 'providing he takes trouble to know what he is and should be doing, to organize his practice efficiently, and to know the rules which he must keep if mothers and their babies are to remain safe in his care'.[24]

However, as labour increasingly moved to hospital settings, obstetrics in general practice, and particularly general practice maternity units, fell into decline.[25] The location of birth experienced a wholesale revolution in postwar Britain: before the Second World War, the majority of women gave birth at home; just a few decades later, by the mid-1970s, over 95 per cent of births took place in hospitals.[26] This shift was a product of changed medical and social attitudes to childbirth and was actively encouraged by professional bodies and government reports on the grounds of increased safety.[27] As births moved into hospitals, they became increasingly medicalised; the use of forceps, inductions, and caesareans increased.[28] The mothers that general practitioners saw in their clinics were, by the 1970s, increasingly likely to have experienced a birth that was hospital-based, medicalised, and interfered with.

How did mothers feel about their birth experiences within the new NHS? It is notable that just two years after its inauguration, a critical first-hand description of hospital birth was published; *National Baby* by Sarah Campion – the pen name of Mary Rose Coulton – set out the rigidity of the service's approach to pregnant and labouring women, and the authority it bestowed upon medical professionals at the expense of the patient.[29] Oral histories suggest that Campion's experience was not isolated and that women's experiences of hospital-based childbirth from the 1940s to the 1970s were liable to be impersonal, inhumane, and sometimes traumatic.[30] This reflects what mothers told sociological researchers. One 1960s study of 709 mothers of children under one in Nottingham, England, led by sociologists John and Elizabeth Newson, concluded that hospitals were the primary detrimental influence on women's attitudes to childbirth. 'Too often we heard complaints of the impersonal atmosphere of the labour ward, of a sense of the conveyor-belt, and, especially, of being left alone, sometimes for two or three hours, during the first stage of labour', they wrote.[31]

This verdict was echoed elsewhere. In 1965, Phyllis Mary Fleury received a prize from the British Medical Association for a survey of maternity care which found that birthing mothers were not infrequently made to feel rushed, peripheral, or troublesome. Many of the mothers in her survey reported being untended, lonely, and afraid during hospital labours.[32] This discontent endured. In the 1980s women told studies that their preferences had not been respected and that they had been disempowered during hospital births, with staff shortages and shift changes exacerbating their stress and loneliness. By contrast, women reflected favourably on general practitioner maternity units in community hospitals, staffed by midwives and general practitioners.[33] By the late 1980s, though, the number of general practitioner maternity units had drastically diminished.[34] These smaller units and home births had given way to hospitals, and the mothers encountered by general practitioners were likely to have had a medicalised and interventionist experience of childbirth.

Mothers had mixed views of general practitioners. A 1961 study found that mothers were widely appreciative of the health service and that general practitioners were held in particularly high regard: nearly 90 per cent were satisfied with the kind of attention the family received, and around 70 per cent had neither changed nor wished to change their doctor.[35] In both the 1970s and the 1980s, mothers continued to favour the antenatal care provided by their general practitioner over that provided in hospitals.[36] A 1980s study found that 16 per cent of new mothers had found their doctor to be the 'best' person to talk to about their pregnancy.[37] This satisfaction with antenatal general practice care, however, sharply contrasts with unhappy mothers' accounts of their postnatal care. Mothers' accounts of feeling dismissed, belittled, and misunderstood by general practitioners are widespread across the archives. The sense that they were seen as troublesome was not baseless. Research in the 1970s found that general practitioners were more likely to see female patients as a source of greater trouble than their male counterparts.[38]

In some cases, the friction between mothers and doctors seems to have been exacerbated by the dissemination of medical terminology and by lay access to medical concepts. One of Vivienne Welburn's interviewees in the 1970s observed that

> GPs are pretty ignorant aren't they? Depression's a tricky thing for them to deal with, they don't know much about it, they're too overburdened to go on refresher courses they ought to go on. I went to

this GP just after we moved. He said, 'You've been reading things like *Reader's Digest* haven't you?' and I was very hurt. I was so low... I mean I think I said, 'I think I'm depressed' or something and therefore I had attempted self-diagnosis which is not allowed, it means you've been reading things like *Reader's Digest*.[39]

If some doctors resented what they saw as self-diagnosis, others doubted the urgency of what mothers told them. Another mother told Welburn, for example, that her very young second child cried for an entire month. Exhausted and desperate, she went to her doctor who told her it was likely colic and would probably stop in three months. 'It was as if she'd hit me in the face', she said, 'I sat there and thought, "three months! I don't know how to get through to tomorrow morning!"'. That evening she resolved to take her life. While this intention was not realised, her testimony reflects the perilous consequences of not being taken seriously.[40] Given these experiences, it is unsurprising that during and after the 1960s dissatisfaction with general practitioners was one of the major impetuses for the establishment of alternative forms of care, including self-help groups and mother-baby networks.[41] The lack of knowledge and interest that women reported, however, was in contrast to the push to make general practitioners more insightful about the scale of the psychological afflictions in their practice populations. This push – towards research and an interest in psychiatric complaints – was stimulated by a confluence of factors made apparent by the establishment of the NHS.

General practitioners, the NHS, and the drive for research

The potential implications of the NHS were approached with trepidation by those within general practice. The majority of general practitioners opposed the service shortly before its launch, and some older general practitioners retired rather than work within the new system.[42] If the NHS was not welcomed among general practitioners, neither was it universally embraced; indeed, some general practitioners actively organised against the service.[43] General practitioners felt hard done by in comparison to their hospital-based colleagues and were preoccupied with financial complaints in its early years.[44] In March 1950 the *British Medical Journal* declared general practice to be at a 'crossroads': the general practitioner had been 'elbowed out of the hospital, finds himself more isolated than ever before from his colleagues in specialist and consulting practice, is plagued with paper work, and sees little prospect of obtaining those pleasant conditions of work so alluringly offered to him by the propagandists for the National Health Service'. Despite 'a wide range of exact diagnostic techniques and an armoury of powerful drugs', the general practitioner was floundering. He needed to recover his position as a 'family doctor', the journal urged, and avail himself of the new drugs and approaches that made home care possible.[45] At a 1956 meeting, C.A.H. Watts welcomed increased opportunities for general practitioners to discuss their psychotherapeutic practice, connecting this to their diminished standing: 'During the last 50 years practitioners have tended to rely on their tools and neglect their prestige', he indicated.[46]

Concern about the status of general practice was not easily or rapidly ameliorated.[47] A number of reports into the profession – some more critical than others – were commissioned and published across the 1950s and 1960s.[48] While in the mid-1960s, parliamentarians were at pains to emphasise the continuing importance of the general practitioner as the 'the individual's first line of defence against ill health', general practitioners felt that they were marginalised and neglected.[49] As one 1964 article lamented, general practice 'wallowed in its own drab inefficiency'.[50] One general practitioner rued that while 'in theory it is one of three equal pillars of the Health Service; in practice, at every point of contact with the other services, its inferior status is emphasised'.[51] This concern about the state of general practice was an impetus to fortify professional esteem.

For those interested in shoring up general practice's future, research was seen as an important means of asserting prestige.[52] The College of General Practitioners, established in 1952 (and which received a royal charter in 1967), was interested in general practitioner research from its beginnings.[53] A Research Committee was one of the four committees established by the College in January 1953.[54] A year after the College was founded, the Research Register contained 127 names; within five years this grew to over 550 names.[55] The emphasis on research, though, was not without its critics. According to some sceptics in the 1960s, the new college's leaders 'represented a metropolitan type of general practice' that found less traction after the establishment of the NHS, while the stress on the academic side of general practice and 'aloofness' from the political elements of medical care had diminished its potential influence; the research it produced was occasionally 'doubtful'. An 'anxiety state' had developed within the field; the quagmire was a result of 'negligence and misplaced effort'.[56] Others pointed to the lack of resources, facilities, and expert networks that might hamper general practitioners' research.[57] Research was not a panacea to general practitioners' discontent. In 1967, an article in the *British Medical Journal* rued that many general practitioners seemed to find their work uninteresting, and – in a profession beset by grumbling – were increasingly prone to emigrate.[58] Despite these criticisms, research was sometimes seen to be a tool to achieve professional fulfilment. In 1954, general practitioner John Fry encouraged research not only to advance medical knowledge but also to help general practitioners maintain 'interest in his work'.[59] The 1963 Gillie Report – which formulated recommendations around general practice – also encouraged general practitioners to undertake operational and clinical research.[60] It was broadly welcomed in medical journals. 'Participation in research', summarised the *British Medical Journal*, 'is a valuable antidote to the lack of stimuli to intellectual activity in present conditions of practice'.[61] Fry, who played a key role in establishing the General Practice Research Club, reiterated his support, suggesting that general practitioners had enviable access to patient information.[62] By the 1960s, then, new motivations for and a supportive infrastructure around research had emerged.

Mental health, women, and the general practitioner

While the NHS's establishment made the need to understand public health more urgent, interest in the mental pathologies of the population had deeper roots.[63] In interwar Britain, for example, the management of emotions was emphasised, ideas about psychology shaped politics and public policy, and branches of social work that concerned mental health professionalised and formalised their training.[64] The war, when it arrived, heightened attention to the idea that psychological tools could boost morale. Within this rubric, individual psychological health underpinned national well-being. General practitioners took notice of this trend.[65] Afterwards, the foundation of the NHS provided a stimulus for research into psychological problems. Within the NHS 'the planning of medical education, of general practice, of psychiatry, and particularly of community services, demands a clearer picture of the size and nature of the problem of psychiatric illness than is now available', wrote general practitioner and researcher Anthony Ryle in the 1960s.[66] Unsurprisingly, it affected the location of treatment, too. In the 1960s a visiting American psychiatrist noted that the NHS had several implications for mental healthcare in Britain: it improved the status of psychiatry based in psychiatric hospitals and encouraged experiments in treatment, he wrote, but it had curtailed the growth of psychiatry outside hospital walls. There, the general practitioner remained the primary provider of care.[67] In practice, mental health occupied a difficult position within the new structure, and the parity encouraged between physical and mental health provision in the Mental Health Act of 1959 never materialised.[68] Nonetheless, the establishment of the NHS, a growing awareness of the prevalence of milder psychological complaints, and later on, deinstitutionalisation, helped to position general practitioners at the forefront of mental health care. Or, as one Staffordshire-based general practitioner put it in 1959, patients with neuroses 'form the bulk of our daily work'.[69]

Some general practitioners were less than enthused by this. No doubt some of this feeling was a residue from a period when there were fewer treatment options for psychological complaints. Even C.A.H. Watts, a leading proponent of general practitioners' ability to address psychiatric problems within the community, admitted that when he first qualified in the 1930s his 'heart sank' at the prospect of 'another frustrating and possibly lengthy interview' with a psychiatric patient in his general practice.[70] When, in the 1940s, he returned from the medical corps and resumed medical practice he was 'amazed' by the number of depressed patients he saw, and it was only when his understanding of psychiatric problems increased and treatment options multiplied that his enthusiasm for psychological cases picked up.[71] Psychiatrist G.M. Carstairs observed in 1951 that it was remarkable that, given over 10 per cent of all patients presented with psychological needs, some general practitioners continued to distance themselves from psychiatric approaches. 'It is as if one were to deny the existence of microbes, or to dismiss penicillin as new-fangled nonsense', he chastised.[72] But these holdouts were buffeted by calls for greater interest in psychological complaints by those who agreed that general practice was, as Watts put it, 'an ideal laboratory for... observation and study'.[73] General practitioners could examine 'normal variations' while undertaking 'observational research', a general practitioner wrote in the *British Medical Journal* in 1957.[74] Research in the *Scottish Medical Journal* noted that general practitioners could combine knowledge of social contexts with clinical data.[75] The very factors that aided their research – intimate knowledge and sustained relationships – also positioned them as an appropriate source of care. Michael Balint, famous for his consideration of the clinical dynamic set forth in his 1957 book, *The Doctor, His Patient and the Illness*, championed the general practitioner as a psychotherapeutic agent.[76] There was, he wrote in the *British Medical Journal*,

> a vast field of research accessible, above all, to the general practitioner. It is he who knows intimately the patient's previous history, and it is he to whom the patient first turns with his fears, pains, or worries... It is the general practitioner– of all doctors – who can most easily get hold of and piece together the various bits of information about a patient, so that the picture should make sense. Moreover, his relationship with the patient is, as a rule, lasting, not ephemeral like that of a specialist.[77]

Others similarly underlined the value of general practitioners' contribution to mental healthcare.[78] Prominent psychiatrist William Sargant, for example, hailed C.A.H. Watts's 1966 study, *Depressive Disorders in the Community*, as 'one of the best books' to tackle the subject of depression because of the scale and range of cases that Watts was drawn into contact with. Watts saw, Sargant wrote, how patients actually lived, and in turn his book demonstrated how much psychiatrists had to learn from general practitioners.[79]

Observing this trend, professional organisations established sites for the discussion of psychological work within general practice.

The Royal College of General Practitioners directed early energy towards mental health research, establishing the Working Party on Psychiatry and the General Practitioner in the late 1950s.[80] Furthermore, the General Practice Research Unit (GPRU) was established at the Institute of Psychiatry in London in 1958, with a remit to study 'by epidemiological methods, of the causes, nature, course, extent, and distribution of extra-mural mental disorder in the setting of general practice where, under the conditions of the British National Health Service, information is obtainable about the health of the bulk of the population'.[81] The studies, headed by psychiatrists Michael Shepherd and Brian Cooper, were predicated on two ideas: that the general practitioner was at the crux of mental health care and that the prevalence of mental disorders was underestimated.[82] Their work showed that women outnumbered men in cases of psychiatric disorders in general practice and that women were more likely to be prescribed sedatives and tranquilisers and/or antidepressants.[83] General practice was a fruitful place for this research, the studies underlined, as it provided 'badly needed information about all the minor forms of morbidity which, though not for the most part severe enough to warrant hospital or specialist attention, nevertheless represent a heavy burden on the community in terms of distress and loss of working efficiency'.[84] By the 1980s the unit was argued to have 'demonstrated for the first time that most mental disorder escapes detection by the formal mental health services and that it is the primary care physician, not the psychiatric specialist, who assumes the major burden of responsibility for the care of mental disorder'.[85]

Of course, making milder forms of mental distress visible would be rather less useful should there then be no recourse for treatment. The postwar period saw a radical expansion of drugs that claimed to address psychological disorders. The most notable additions arrived in 1957, when iproniazid and imipramine came onto the British market, supplementing amphetamines and stimulants, as well as physical treatments, as potential remedies for depression. The availability of new antidepressant drugs at the end of the 1950s, as C.A.H. Watts said, enabled new approaches and drew new attention to milder depressions. Studies of mild depressions in the community now had potentially potent implications, and were no longer limited to being of mere 'academic interest'.[86] The early results of the use of imipramine in particular were 'most gratifying', he recalled, those 'were exciting days'.[87]

But some of his excitement was shortlived, as pharmacological interventions into anxiety, another psychological complaint frequently encountered in his general practice, proved less satisfactory.[88] Watts was not alone in finding that his enthusiasm for drugs was tempered as conflicting reports about their efficacy emerged.[89] Psychiatrists were anxious that manufacturers' efforts to encourage general practitioners to prescribe antidepressants might result in symptoms being underestimated and patients inappropriately treated at home.[90] These concerns did not hinder the regularity with which they were prescribed. Indeed, the decline of psychiatric bed numbers from its peak of 150,000 in the mid-1950s has been attributed in part to the availability of pharmacological interventions.[91] By the mid-1950s, nearly a third of general practitioners thought that they were seen to be the suppliers of medicine rather than medical advice.[92] But some of this reliance on prescribing drugs – a 'mainstay' of general practitioners' approach to psychiatric cases – may have been due in part to a lack of confidence in treating mental disorders. One 1950s study reported that general practitioners found treating psychiatric patients comparatively irritating and unsatisfying, given their poor rates of improvement.[93] It was within this context that drugs quickly became a bastion of psychological treatment in communities. In 1964, an article in the *Lancet* commented that 'where once the family doctor had little but advice to give his patients, he now has at his disposal a wide range of effective drugs. Rarely is his counsel unaccompanied by a prescription'.[94] Research by the GPRU reflected these findings: most psychiatric patients who received advice also received a prescription.[95] By 1974, an article in the *British Journal of Psychiatry* concluded that 'the treatment of psychiatric disorders in general practice consists principally of prescribing drugs, with relatively little use of social agencies and psychotherapy'.[96]

Housewives were an important constituency for these new prescriptions. The cultural association between women and neuroses was well-established by the mid-century, having been influencially promoted in the interwar period, when 'suburban neurosis' among housewives was positioned as an undesirable but common outcome of wider social changes. At this point, while men's stress was tied to their employment, women's anxiety was seen to be tied to the home, and particularly to the houses in the new suburbs that proliferated in the 1930s.[97] The atomising conditions on these housing developments, which were suggested to be devoid of community amenities, generated the 'suburban neurosis' that afflicted lonely and under-stimulated young housewives, argued London-based doctor Stephen Taylor in 1938.[98] The term was taken up by newspapers, which sent journalists out to investigate the phenomenon and published earnest letters from members of the public concerned about its prevalence.[99] Doctors warned that outpatient departments were swollen by ranks of lonely wives.[100] The Second World War, when it came, was hailed by some newspapers as bringing some housewives respite. The *Yorkshire Evening Post*'s medical correspondent wrote in 1940 that the 'WAR HAS KILLED "SUBURBAN NEUROSIS" – Women Left Behind Have a Cry – and Make New Friends'. The young wife was 'happy in her new job, she is now too busy to be lonely, and in her little spare time she is now too tired to be depressed', the article celebrated.[101] But these wives would find themselves encouraged back into the home at the end of the war, and in the following years, the phenomenon of married women's 'suburban sadness' was further disseminated within popular culture: films, television shows, and novels picked up the theme, popularising the stock figure of the housewife grimly enduring suburban malaise.[102]

The stock figure no doubt mirrored the isolated women drawn to light by prominent social researchers in postwar Britain. Social surveys highlighted the atomised social environments and fractured kinship networks found in the suburban housing developments and within high-rise homes that grew after the war, drawing a sharp contrast with the apparent interconnectedness and sustaining interdependence of inner-city families. These surveys made much of the loosening of family ties that rendered young wives relatively isolated, confined to their comparatively plush new homes.[103] (The most influencial of these 1950s studies, by Michael Young and Peter Willmott, was particularly attentive to the apparent value of living close to 'Mum' for working-class wives, whereas Beatrice Watts, for her part, emphasised the value of independence for young families in her Butterworth prize essay, arguing that the 'escape from grannie denomination' was of marked benefit to mothers of young children.[104]) In the later 1950s the *Lancet* returned to the idea of 'suburban neurosis', worrying that lessons in urban and social planning had not been implemented.[105] However, when Taylor and his colleague Sidney Chave revisited the concept in the 1960s, they uncoupled the new suburbs and the experience of 'new town blues'.[106] By then, though, the association between neurosis and suburban wifedom was not so easily unpicked, and it continued to circulate in national and local newspapers.[107]

This association between women and psychological distress was borne out not just in culture but in statistics. Postwar general practice surveys and landmark studies found that women presented with anxiety and depression at a rate that outstripped men.[108] Explanations abounded, but the trend was significant. As Ann Oakley observed, women were more likely than men to visit the doctor; were more likely, when presenting with similar symptoms, to be diagnosed with a psychiatric and particularly a neurotic disorder; and were prescribed more mood-altering drugs than men.[109] Tranquillisers were the primary medical treatment for depressed mothers from the 1950s onwards.[110] Unlike inpatient treatment, drugs allowed mothers to remain at home. As social researcher Enid Mills reported in 1962, hospitalising a psychologically distressed wife was a last resort for many families, for 'the routine of their home depends on them so much – especially if they have children – that the greatest efforts will be made to enable them to remain there'.[111] One study of prescriptions issued by general practitioners from March 1974 to March 1975 found that psychotropic (mood-altering) drugs accounted for nearly one in five of all prescriptions and that women were prescribed them at a greater rate than men across all age groups.[112] In the mid-1970s sociological work underlined the prominent role that tranquillisers and other psychotropic drugs had assumed in general practice. Patients expected to be prescribed pills, general practitioners told researchers, and some patients even demanded them, telling doctors that 'I've got to have them. I can't cope. The children are getting on my nerves'.[113]

It was against this changing social, therapeutic, and institutional background that general practitioners' research into mothers' mental health was conducted. One pioneering example of this was Anthony Ryle, whose work *Neurosis in the Ordinary Family: A Psychiatric Survey* (1967) formed an important part of the wave of studies on psychiatric distress in general practice populations.

Ryle's findings were towards the lower end of those who attempted to estimate the prevalence of psychological problems in the community.[114] Whereas the Wattses had worried that 30 per cent of their practice population in Ibstock presented with psychological symptoms, Ryle found that between 5 and 10 per cent of his community in Kentish Town, then a 'neither clean nor beautiful' part of North London, had signs of psychiatric morbidity.[115]

Anthony Ryle and the *ordinary family*

Anthony (Tony) Ryle was born in 1927 and qualified as a doctor a year after the inception of the NHS, for which his father, John Ryle – the first professor of social medicine and Director of the Institute of Social Medicine at the University of Oxford – was a prominent advocate. John Ryle was influenced by Richard Titmuss's argument that infant mortality was a policy failure, and in the early 1940s, he proposed the establishment of a national health service that would improve maternal and infant health.[116] Anthony Ryle would, in turn, be informed by his family's progressive political values, and was a great admirer of the values that the NHS embodied. His mother, Miriam Ryle (née Power Scully), helped to shape his perceptions of the family. She was not, according to Anthony Ryle's childhood diaries, particularly healthy, and seems to have experienced some depression in his youth.[117] Miriam embodied the limited opportunities granted to energetic women; Ryle reflected in the 1990s that she 'could have run General Motors with her energy, and she hadn't got anything to run'.[118]

Even before he published his work on the family and mental health, Ryle was interested in mothers' wellbeing. In 1955 he fiercely defended the need to prepare pregnant women for childbirth in a letter to the *British Medical Journal*. Working with pregnant women to prepare them for labour – in a way that might diminish fear and anxiety – was far from an indulgence, he argued. Rather, it was 'humanely and medically desirable', with potentially positive implications for infant and maternal health.[119] This was a theme that he returned to in 1969, when he suggested that pregnant women should have opportunities to 'express and explore her feelings', noting 'how few [hospitals] provide opportunities for women to discuss their feelings about mothering or means for them to enlarge their emotional confidence and competence'.[120]

Although he would subsequently become well-known as a psychotherapist, Ryle's early work was as a general practitioner. Working at the Caversham Centre in Kentish Town, North London – which had a predominantly working-class practice community – Ryle stressed the particular advantages of general practitioner-led research for understanding the social aspects of health.[121] He also advocated for greater intervention into families, arguing that general practitioners should 'be a real family doctor in the field of psychiatry'. Of course, this would have workload implications, as 'increased provision of services leads to increased demand'.[122] In 1961 his study of disturbance and pregnancy was published in the *British Journal of Psychiatry*. This argued that psychiatric disturbance in mothers had been underestimated, as only a minority of cases resulted in hospital admissions, and that these admissions were influenced by social, economic, and cultural factors as well as medical need.[123] Ryle used the patient records of 137 women who had between them experienced 313 full-term pregnancies. According to Ryle's criteria, there were twenty-three episodes of illness associated with these pregnancies: ten occurred in the first three months after delivery; five occurred from three to twelve months after delivery; and eight took place during the pregnancy itself. He argued that childbearing 'operated as a psychodynamic factor' but suggested that childbirth was not the direct cause of depression. As the cases Ryle discussed show, though, repeated pregnancies threw women into social and economic crises. One twenty-five-year-old woman had five children and lived in a 'dark, damp basement' he wrote. She had mild spells of depression, worsening when her youngest was two. She attempted to take her own life when her contraception failed. Following psychiatric advice, this young woman was sterilised and the pregnancy was ended; her depression did not return.[124]

Neurosis in the Ordinary Family, Ryle's subsequent study, which began as his MD thesis, surveyed 112 families and was carried out by a team of three researchers: Ryle; D.A. Pond, a psychiatrist; and Madge Hamilton, a psychiatric social worker.[125] It found that the remembrance of the 'emotional tone' of the home exerted an influence over the development of neurotic symptoms and advocated a 'family-centred' treatment approach to psychiatric problems.[126]

However, he rejected John Bowlby's maternal deprivation thesis, from which 'unjustifiable conclusions were often drawn'.[127] Ryle's work also reflected women's increasing uptake of part-time paid work, a trend he observed as having minimal impact on their mental health.[128] These themes were also picked up in a further, more famous research project that was also drawn in part from the Caversham Centre's practice list: sociologist Hannah Gavron's study *The Captive Wife: Conflicts of Housebound Mothers*, published in 1966. Gavron's work was a precursor to the self-consciously feminist sociological research into domesticity, mothering, and the family that burgeoned in the 1970s.[129]

Neurosis in the Ordinary Family was widely reviewed in medical journals, and its findings were cautiously welcomed alongside other studies of psychiatric distress in practice populations.[130] Like these other studies, it reflected the wider trends at work in postwar general practice: the emphasis on the family; the perceived importance of understanding 'mild' psychological disturbance; and the conviction that general practitioners had distinctive advantages when undertaking community-based research. However, general practitioners like Ryle were not alone in conducting investigations into mothers' experiences. As Ryle did, they worked in teams that brought together a constellation of perspectives on the family. The very vantage point and type of expertise that general practitioners underlined as advantageous to their work would, in fact, be contested by mothers themselves, who looked outside, or alongside, medical frameworks as they sought to understand and address their unhappiness.

Conclusion

In 1957, the literary critic and cultural theorist Richard Hoggart painted a gloomy picture of the lives of working-class mothers. While Hoggart wrote about working-class women with sympathy and warmth, he did not shy away from the many costs that mothering exacted from them. Younger mothers faced repeated childbearing with resignation, while physical complaints accumulated in their middle age. At this point, they felt there was 'little time for "doctoring,"' he wrote. Doctors, in turn, were pessimistic, as working-class middle-aged housewives 'look after themselves badly, work too long or hard, do not know how to relax, take insufficient sleep, have a badly balanced diet'.[131] While Hoggart's overstretched mother may have had little time for her doctor, general practitioners in the mid-century were encouraged to have an interest in her. These general practitioners had a financial incentive to undertake obstetrical work and operated within a social climate that placed the home and the emotionally attentive mother at the heart of its vision for the future.[132] As C.A.H. and Beatrice Watts commented in 1952, 'a happy home life is the best antidote to most neuroses. The general practitioner is in a unique position to assist in the construction of such homes... in this way he is going far in the direction of prophylactic psychiatry'.[133] In turn, the findings of general practitioner-led studies into the health of the family – such as those done by Anthony Ryle – revealed distress in 'ordinary' mothers. For psychiatrists and general practitioners, mothers promised a doubly satisfactory outcome, resolving one patient and preventing the creation of another.

The stimulus to have an interest in mothers and a new impetus towards conducting research, however, did not result in a surge of satisfaction with postnatal care among new mothers, an increasing majority of whom were giving birth in hospitals. Indeed, dissatisfaction with general practitioners appears to have been fairly widespread among distressed mothers, and concomitant services did not hold back on reflecting the perception that general practitioners varied in their approaches to unhappy mothers. While some doctors were sympathetic, others were insufficiently understanding of or knowledgeable about mothers' distress.[134] General practitioners may well have felt ill-equipped to diagnose postnatal depression. John Cox, a founding member of the Marcé Society for Perinatal Mental Health, established in 1980, recalled that the publication of a short article about his work to develop a new screening tool for postnatal depression (a tool that would become the Edinburgh Postnatal Depression Scale) created a stir. Within months he had received hundreds of letters and cards from general practitioners, he remembered. Postnatal depression was an issue that was 'worrying' general practitioners, he said, who were 'aware of the issues' but lacked the ability to identify or treat it.[135] General practitioners, then, encountered unhappy mothers within their clinics, contributed to their medical visibility, but often fell short of addressing unhappy motherhood.

A pregnant woman in a general practitioners' waiting room in the mid-1970s, though, would no doubt be relieved to find that her doctor was not her sole medical source of postnatal advice. She may have picked up a copy of *New Baby*, published by the Health Visitors' Association and distributed for free, and here would have read that some new mothers needed emotional support.[136] She would then have been visited at home by a health visitor – a nurse or midwife with additional training in public health and who held a particular responsibility for mothers and young children – soon after childbirth. While district midwives had responsibility for maternal and infant welfare immediately after birth, it was health visitors who worked with mothers once the very earliest days of motherhood had passed. If the general practice setting was a medical site in which mothers raised their distress, health visitors formed an important bridge between this medical domain and mothers' social and domestic worlds. C.A.H. Watts – who advocated for general practitioners' role in psychiatric care – championed the importance of health visitors in the 1970s. In his book that targeted a public readership, *The Blue Plague*, Watts repeated social researchers' concerns that new mothers in high rise flats too often found themselves 'marooned' and 'very much alone'. In this context, health visitors could play an important preventive and supportive role. Like general practitioners, health visitors had privileged insights and access to personal stories, he said. 'People are more confident and ready to talk in their own homes', Watts explained, 'and in the informal atmosphere of the home the health visitor is in an excellent position to uncover the mild depression which frequently follows childbirth'. Moreover, health visitors could liaise with other medical and state services, connecting families to further sources of support.[137] Others, outside the medical professions, concurred that health visitors could play a foundational role in supporting new mothers. It was health visitors – who did not have responsibility for treatment but played a key role in advice and support – who, according to Vivienne Welburn, were in the best position to detect and oversee depressed mothers.[138]

But while health visitors brought unhappy mothers into general practices, their work went beyond this and into the creation and dissemination of social measures. In this, they put into action ideas that had long circulated about how to address lonely women's unhappiness and isolation: in 1938 Stephen Taylor reproached the 'rotten little houses' of the interwar period and urged the creation of new social clubs to prevent suburban neurosis in sequestered housewives; in 1958, the *Lancet*, returning to suburban neurosis, advised that social planning lay at the heart of preventative psychiatry.[139] In postwar Britain health visitors, among others, acted on calls for the creation of new networks and social sites for isolated mothers. They, of course, could not recreate the inner-city kinship ties admired by social researchers. But they could help to create new communities based not on blood but on shared experience. It is here, then, that we begin to see a shift between types of expertise about mothers' experiences: the professional and the medical, and the lived, social, and experiential.

Notes

1 C.A.H. Watts and B.M. Watts, *Psychiatry in General Practice* (Devon, 1994 [1952]), 1–13.
2 Rhodri Hayward, *The Transformation of the Psyche in British Primary Care, 1870–1970* (London, 2015), 34.
3 'Marriages', *Evening Chronicle*, 24 April 1937; The General Council of Medical Education and Registration of the United Kingdom, *The Medical Register for 1936* (London), 53.
4 Beatrice M. Watts, 'The Influence of Home Conditions During the First Five Years of Life on the Physical and Mental Health of Children', *Research Newsletter*, os-4 (11), 1956, 63, 63–75, 65.
5 Ibid., 71–75.
6 Mary Ann Elston, 'Medicine: Half Our Future Doctors?', in *Careers of Professional Women*, eds Rosalie Silverstone and Audrey Ward (London, 2022 [1980]), 99–139, 99.
7 Ibid., 126–127.
8 Mary Ann C. Elston, 'Women Doctors in the British Health Services: A Sociological Study of Their Careers and Opportunities', Unpublished Doctoral Thesis, University of Leeds, Leeds, 1986, 382–383.
9 Morag C. Timbury and Maria A. Ratzer, 'Glasgow Medical Women 1951–4: Their Contribution and Attitude to Medical Work', *British Medical Journal*, 2, 5653, 1969, 372–374. and A.W. Ward, 'Careers of Medical Women', *British Medical Journal (Clinical Research Edn)*, 284, 6308, 1982, 31–33.

10 Elston, *Women Doctors*, 405; Ward, 'Careers', 32.
11 C.A.H. Watts, *Depressive Disorders in the Community* (Bristol, 1966), iv.
12 C.A.H. Watts, 'The Blue Plague' *The Journal of the Royal College of General Practitioners*, 22, 117, 1972, 233–239.
13 C.A.H. Watts, *Depression: The Blue Plague* (London, 1973), 10.
14 For wider histories of the NHS see Charles Webster, *The Health Services Since the War, Volume II: Government and Healthcare: The National Health Service 1958-79* (London, 1996); Geoffrey Rivett, *From Cradle to Grave: Fifty Years of the NHS* (London, 1998); Rudolf Klein, *The New Politics of the NHS: From Creation to Reinvention* (London, 2013); Andrew Seaton, *Our NHS: A History of Britain's Best Loved Institution* (New Haven, CT, 2023); Jennifer Crane, '"Save Our NHS": Activism, Information-Based Expertise and the "New Times" of the 1980s', *Contemporary British History*, 33, 1, 2019, 52–74; Roberta Bivins, *Contagious Communities: Medicine, Migration, and the NHS in Post War Britain* (Oxford, 2015).For more on the history of general practice, see Hayward, *Transformation of the Psyche*; Julian M. Simpson, *Migrant Architects of the NHS: South Asian Doctors and the Reinvention of General Practice, 1940s–1980s* (Manchester, 2018); Anne Digby, *The Evolution of British General Practice, 1850–1948* (Oxford, 1999).
15 Ali Haggett, *A History of Male Psychological Disorders in Britain, 1945-1980* (Basingstoke, 2015), 22.
16 Angela Davis, 'Wartime Women Giving Birth: Narratives of Pregnancy and Childbirth, Britain c. 1939-1960', *Studies in History and Philosophy of Science Part C: Studies in History and Philosophy of Biological and Biomedical Sciences*, 47, B, 2014, 257–266, 258.
17 Mark Jackson (ed.), 'Stress in Post-War Britain: An Introduction', in *Stress in Post-War Britain, 1945–85* (New York, 2015), 1–15, 2.
18 Bebe Speed, 'Family Therapy's Origins in the UK and Ireland – Date Chart', *Context*, 115, June 2011, 4–12.
19 Teri Chettiar, "More than a Contract': The Emergence of a State-Supported Marriage Welfare Service and the Politics of Emotional Life in Post-1945 Britain', *Journal of British Studies*, 55, 3, 2016, 566–591; and Teri Chettiar, 'Democratizing Mental Health: Motherhood, Therapeutic Community and the Emergence of the Psychiatric Family at the Cassel Hospital in Post-Second World War Britain', *History of the Human Sciences*, 25, 5, 2012, 107–122.
20 See, for example, Hilary Marland and Anne Marie Rafferty (eds), *Midwives, Society and Childbirth: Debates and Controversies in the Modern Period* (London, 1997); Anne Borsay and Billie Hunter

(eds), *Nursing and Midwifery in Britain since 1700* (Basingstoke, 2012); Joanna Bourke, 'Becoming the "Natural" Mother in Britain and North America: Power, Emotions and the Labour of Childbirth Between 1947 and 1967', *Past & Present*, 246, 15, 2020, 92–114; Gwenith Siobhan Cross, '"A Midwife at Every Confinement": Midwifery and Medicalized Childbirth in Ontario and Britain, 1920–1950', *Canadian Bulletin of Medical History*, 31, 2, 2014, 139–159.
21 'Report of the Maternity Services Committee' (London, 1959), 52.
22 P. O'Brien, 'Obstetrics in a General Practice, 1949-1963', *The Journal of the College of General Practitioners*, 8, 3, 1964, 281–303, 284.
23 J.S.K. Stevenson, 'Maternity Work in a General-Practitioner Unit', *British Medical Journal*, 1, 5240, 1961, 1673–1676, 1673.
24 O'Brien, 'Obstetrics', 302.
25 George Godber, 'The Effect of Specialisation on Maternity Services', *The Lancet*, 281, 7290, 1963, 1061–1066.
26 Angela Davis, 'Choice, Policy and Practice in Maternity Care since 1948', *History & Policy*, 30 May 2013, https://www.historyandpolicy.org/policy-papers/papers/choice-policy-and-practice-in-maternity-care-since-1948. Accessed 6 August 2024.
27 Royal College of Obstetricians and Gynaecologists, *Report on a National Maternity Service* (London: RCOG, 1944) and Royal College of Obstetricians and Gynaecologists, *Report on an Obstetric Service Under the NHS* (London: RCOG, 1954).
28 Tania McIntosh, *A Social History of Maternity and Childbirth: Key Themes in Maternity Care* (London, 2012), chapter 5.
29 Sarah Campion, *National Baby* (London, 1950), London, British Library, W35/2539.
30 Davis, *Modern Motherhood*, 84–111.
31 John Newson and Elizabeth Newson, *Patterns of Infant Care in an Urban Community* (Harmondsworth, 1976 [1963]), 25.
32 P.M. Fleury, *Maternity Care: Mothers' Experiences of Childbirth* (London, 1967), 46–47.
33 Catherine Boyd and Lea Sellers, *The British Way of Birth* (London, 1982), 76–81.
34 Irvine Loudon, 'General Practitioners and Obstetrics: A Brief History', *Journal of the Royal Society of Medicine*, 101, 11, 2008, 531–535.
35 Political and Economic Planning, *Family Needs and the Social Services* (London, 1961), 98–101.
36 Sheila Kitzinger, 'Women's Experiences of Birth at Home', in *The Place of Birth*, eds Sheila Kitzinger and John Davis (Oxford, 1978), 135–156, 148–149; Boyd and Sellers, *The British Way of Birth* 29, and Ann Oakley, *Becoming a Mother* (Oxford, 1979), 280.

37 Boyd and Sellers, *The British Way of Birth*, 224.
38 Gerry V. Stimson, 'General Practitioners, "Trouble" and Types of Patients', *The Sociological Review*, 22, 1_suppl, 1974, 43–60, 47.
39 Vivienne Welburn, *Postnatal Depression* (Glasgow, 1980), 109–10.
40 *Ibid.*, 112–113.
41 Cynthia Illingworth, 'The Emotional State of Mothers in the First Three Months after the Birth of a Baby', *Health Visitor*, 62, 2, November 1989, 340–342.
42 Digby, *The Evolution of British General Practice*, 333; Simpson, *Migrant Architects*, 35.
43 Andrew Seaton, 'Against the "Sacred Cow": NHS Opposition and the Fellowship for Freedom in Medicine, 1948–72', *Twentieth Century British History*, 26, 3, 2015, 424–449.
44 Charles Webster, *The Health Services Since the War, Vol. 1: Problems of Health Care: The National Health Service before 1957* (London, 1988), 356.
45 'The G.P. at the Crossroads', *British Medical Journal*, 1, 4655, 1950, 709–712.
46 'Psychotherapy and the General Practitioner', *British Medical Journal*, 2, 4986, 1956, 235–236.
47 Charles Webster, *The National Health Service: A Political History* (Oxford, 1998), 51.
48 See, for example, Stephen Taylor, *Good General Practice: A Report of a Survey* (London, 1954) and Stephen Hadfield, 'A Field Survey of General Practice, 1951–2', *British Medical Journal*, 2, 683, 1953, 684–706; J.S. Collings, 'General Practice in England Today: A Reconnaissance', *The Lancet*, 255, 6604, 555.
49 The Family Doctor, HC Deb 22 January 1964 vol 687 cc1230–42.
50 'Depression', *Medical Care*, 2, 4, 1964, 195–196.
51 Ian McWhinney, 'The Primary Physician in a Comprehensive Health Service: Further Reflections after a Visit to the United States', *The Lancet*, 289, 7481, 1967, 91–96, 93.
52 General Practice, Report of a W.H.O. Expert Committee, World Health Organization: Technical Report Series, No. 267. Geneva (London, 1964), 18.
53 Denis Pereira Gray, 'History of the Royal College of General Practitioners – The First 40 Years', *British Journal of General Practice*, 42, 354, 1992, 29–35, 33; Denis Pereira Gray, *Forty Years On: The Story of the First 40 Years of the Royal College of General Practitioners* (London, 1992), 18.
54 Gray, *Forty Years On*, 49; RCGP, ACE G18-3; ACE G18-2; ACE G18-1.

55 RCGP, ACE G4-2, 'The College of General Practitioners, Research Committee of the Council, 11 June 1957; 'College of General Practitioners', *British Medical Journal*, 2, 5055, 1957, 1233–1235, 1234.
56 'Depression', *Medical Care*, 195.
57 'Use of Medical Records', *British Medical Journal*, 1, 4816, 1953, 941; Mary E. Yuill, 'Medical Research and General Practice', *British Medical Journal*, 2, 4356, 1944, 26.
58 Andrew Smith, 'Future of British Medicine: The Possibilities', *British Medical Journal*, 2, 5548, 1967, 369–370.
59 'Research in General Practice', *British Medical Journal*, 2, 4896, 1954, 1100–1101.
60 *The Field of Work of the Family Doctor: Report of the Sub-Committee* (London, 1963), 23.
61 'Future Scope of General Practice. Medical Advisory Committee's Report', *British Medical Journal*, 2, 5361, 1963, 861–863, 862.
62 'Records In General Practice', *British Medical Journal*, 2, 5352, 1963, 309; Roger Jones and Peter Fitton, 'General Practice Research: Deaths and Entrances', *British Journal of General Practice*, 48, 426, 1998, 873; Robin C. Fraser, 'Research Methods in General Practice: A Report on a Course at the College', *Journal of the Royal College of General Practitioners*, 17, 83, 1969, 385–387.
63 Marshall Marinker, '"What is Wrong" and "How We Know It": Changing Concepts of Illness in General Practice', in *General Practice Under the National Health Service: 1948–1997*, eds I. Loudon, J. Horder, and C. Webster (Oxford, 1998), 5–91, 82.
64 Lucy Noakes, *Dying for the Nation: Death, Grief and Bereavement in Second World War Britain* (Manchester, 2020), 51. Hayward, *Transformation of the Psyche*, 63; Noel Timms, *Psychiatric Social Work in Great Britain (1939-1962)* (London, 1964), 21.
65 Marguerite Stewart, 'Psychology in General Practice', Unpublished Doctoral Thesis, University of Edinburgh, 1940, http://hdl.handle.net/1842/34101.
66 Anthony Ryle, *Neurosis in the Ordinary Family: A Psychiatric Survey* (London, 1967), 14.
67 C. Knight Aldrich, 'Psychiatric Consultation in General Practice', *The Lancet*, 285, 7389, 1965, 805–808.
68 Charles Webster, 'Psychiatry and the Early National Health Service: The Role of the Mental Health Standing Advisory Committee', in *150 Years of British Psychiatry, 1841–1991*, eds German E. Berrios and Hugh Freeman (London, 1991), 103–116.
69 G. Kagan, 'Psychoneuroses in General Practice', *Practitioner*, 182, 1090, 1959, 489–500, 489.

70 C.A.H. Watts, *Depressive Disorders in the Community* (Bristol, 1966), 1–2.
71 C.A.H. Watts, 'Perspective: Looking Back at Psychiatry in General Practice', *Bulletin of the Royal College of Psychiatrists*, 10, 1986, 162–165, 163.
72 G.M. Carstairs, 'Incidence of Psychiatric Cases in General Practice', *Edinburgh Medical Journal*, 58, 2, 1951, 72–81, 80.
73 C.A.H. Watts, 'The Incidence and Prognosis of Endogenous Depression', *British Medical Journal*, 1, 4980, 1956, 1392–1397, 1393.
74 John Hunt, 'The Renaissance of General Practice', *British Medical Journal*, 1, 5027, 1957, 1075–1082.
75 R.M. Mowbray, et al., 'The General Practitioner's Attitude to Psychiatry', *Scottish Medical Journal*, 6, 7, 1961, 314–321.
76 For more on Balint, see Shaul Bar-Haim, *The Maternalists: Psychoanalysts, Motherhood, and the British Welfare State* (Philadelphia, PA, 2021) and Shaul Bar-Haim, '"The Drug Doctor": Michael Balint and the Revival of General Practice in Postwar Britain', *History Workshop Journal*, 86, 2018, 114–132.
77 Michael Balint, 'Psychotherapy and the General Practitioner: I', *British Medical Journal*, 1, 5011, 1957, 156–158, 158.
78 See, for example, Ferguson Rodger, 'The Management of the Neuroses in General Practice', *Glasgow Medical Journal*, 32, 2, 1951, 48–49, 48.
79 William Sargant, review of *Depressive Disorders in the Community* by C.A.H. Watts, *World Medicine*, August 1966, n/p.
80 ACE G12-1, Psychiatry and the General Practitioner Working Party, 1956–1958, Box 35. Royal College of General Practitioners, London.
81 Greg Wilkinson, 'The General Practice Research Unit at the Institute of Psychiatry', *Psychological Medicine*, 19, 1989, 787–790, 787.
82 Michael Shepherd, et al., 'Minor Mental Illness in London: Some Aspects of a General Practice Survey', *British Medical Journal*, 2, 1964, 1359–1363, 1359.
83 Shepherd, et al., *Psychiatric Illness in General Practice*, 153, 164.
84 H.B. Kedward and B. Cooper, 'Neurotic Disorders in Urban Practice: A Three-Year Follow-Up', *The Journal of the College of General Practitioners*, 12, 2, 1966, 148–163, 148.
85 Michael Shepherd, 'Preface to the Second Edition', in *Psychiatric Illness in General Practice*, eds. M. Shepherd, B. Cooper, A. C. Brown and G. W. Kalton. New material by M. Shepherd and A. W. Clare. 2nd edn. (Oxford, 1981 [1966]), vii.
86 Watts, *Depressive Disorders in the Community*, 6.

87 Watts, 'Looking Back at *Psychiatry in General Practice*', 164.
88 Ibid.
89 'Drugs for Depression', *British Medical Journal*, 2, 5408, 1964, 522–523.
90 Brian Ackner, 'Imipramine and "Reactive" Depression', *British Medical Journal*, 1, 5185, 1960, 1570.
91 Brian Cooper, 'British Psychiatry and its Discontents', *Journal of the Royal Society of Medicine*, 103, 10, 2010, 397–402. The causal link between the pharmacological revolution and the beginnings demise of the asylum is contested. See Anne Rogers and David Pilgrim, *Mental Health Policy in Britain: A Critical Introduction* (Basingstoke: Macmillan, 1996), 67.
92 'Some Changes in General Practice Since 1948', *British Medical Journal*, 2, 4838, 1953, 722.
93 K. Rawnsley and J.B. Loudon, 'The Attitudes of General Practitioners to Psychiatry', *The Sociological Review*, 5, 1_suppl, 1957, 49–60.
94 'Prescribing in General Practice', *The Lancet*, 283, 7337, 1964, 803–804, 803.
95 Shepherd, et al., *Psychiatric Illness in General Practice*, 154.
96 D.A.W. Johnson, 'A Study of the Use of Antidepressant Medication in General Practice', *The British Journal of Psychiatry*, 125, 2, 1974, 186–192, 186.
97 For more on the wider gendering of stress, see Jill Kirby, *Feeling the Strain: A Cultural History of Stress in Twentieth-Century Britain* (Manchester, 2019), 75.
98 Stephen Taylor, 'The Suburban Neurosis', *The Lancet*, 231, 5978, 1938, 759–762. For more on this, see Hayward, 'Desperate Housewives and Model Amoebae', 42–62.
99 'Suburban Neurosis', *Sheffield Independent*, 11 June 1938; 'Suburban Neurosis: Wives Who Have Too Little to Do', *Nottingham Evening Post*, 9 February 1939; 'Suburban Neurosis', *Herts and Essex Observer*, 17 September 1938.
100 'Problem of the Lonely Wives', *Dundee Evening Telegraph and Post*, 8 June 1938.
101 'WAR HAS KILLED "SUBURBAN NEUROSIS" – Women Left Behind Have a Cry – and Make New Friends', *Yorkshire Evening Post*, 3 May 1940. Capitalisation in original.
102 Mark Clapson, *Invincible Green Suburbs, Brave New Towns: Social Change and Urban Dispersal in Postwar England* (Manchester, 1998), 122.
103 The most influencial of these studies was by Michael Young and Peter Willmott of the Institute of Community Studies. See Michael Young

and Peter Willmott *Family and Kinship in East London* (London, 2007 [1957]).
104 Watts, 'The Influence of Home Conditions', 74; Young and Willmott, *Family and Kinship*, chapter 3.
105 'Suburban Neurosis Up to Date', *The Lancet*, 271, 7012, 1958, 146–147.
106 Stephen Taylor and Sidney Chave, *Mental Health and Environment* (London, 1964).
107 'Inquiry into "Suburban Neurosis" Suggested – Many Young Wives Affected', *The Scotsman*, 22 March 1963; 'How Some Merseyside Housewives Found a Cure for… Suburban Neurosis', *Liverpool Echo*, 5 December 1967; 'Changing Role of Women in Modern Society', *Birmingham Post*, 3 December 1962.
108 For a discussion of rates of neurosis in female patients and general practice, see Robert Kellner, 'Neurotic Symptoms in Women: Attendances in a General Practice', *British Journal of Psychiatry*, 112, 1966, 75–77 and W. Lawton Tonge, et al., 'Prevalence of Neurosis in Women', *British Journal of Preventive and Social Medicine*, 15, 4, 1961, 177–179. For a major study see J.K. Wing and Anthea Hailey, *Evaluating a Community Psychiatric Service: The Camberwell Register, 1964–71* (London, 1972), 87.
109 Ann Oakley, 'Women and Health Policy', in *Women's Welfare Women's Rights*, ed. Jane Lewis (London and Sydney, 1983), 103–129, 105. For a discussion of gender and diagnosis, see Joan Busfield, *Men, Women and Madness: Understanding Gender and Mental Disorder* (Basingstoke, 1996), 16–18.
110 John Eddy and John Owen, *Obstetrics and Gynaecology in General Practice* (London, 1987), 181.
111 Enid Mills, *Living With Mental Illness: A Study in East London* (London, 1962), 76.
112 D.C. Skegg, R. Doll, and J. Perry, 'Use of Medicines in General Practice', *British Medical Journal*, 18, 1, 6076, 1977, 1561–1563.
113 Marie R. Huang, 'Issues in General Practitioner Authority in the National Health Service', in *The Sociology of the NHS*, ed. Margaret Stacey. Monograph 22. (Keele, 1976), 23–42, 29.
114 See Hayward, *Transformation of the Psyche*, 89.
115 Hayward, *Transformation of the Psyche*, 83. Comments on Kentish Town in Anthony Ryle and Madge Hamilton, 'Neurosis in Fifty Married Couples: Assessed from General Practice Records, Interviews by a Psychiatric Social Worker and the Use of the Cornell Medical Index', *Journal of Mental Science*, 108, 1962, 265–273, 265.

116 John Stewart, 'The "New Era in Medicine": John Ryle and the Promotion of Social Medicine', *Medical History*, 67, 3, 2023, 247–265.
117 Anthony Ryle, *Diary from the Edge, 1940–1944: A Wartime Adolescence* (London, 2014), 241.
118 Anthony Ryle, [interview with] *Transcript of an Interview Conducted by Dr. M.J. Bevan with Anthony Ryle*, "An Oral History of General Practice c. 1935–1952' (Oxford, 1995). Wellcome Archives, London, GP 29/1/61.
119 Anthony Ryle, 'Whither Natural Childbirth?', *British Medical Journal*, 1, 4915, 1955, 725.
120 Anthony Ryle, 'Personal View', *British Medical Journal*, 1, 5647, 1969, 840.
121 Anthony Ryle, 'The Neuroses in a General Practice Population', *The Journal of the College of General Practitioners*, 3, 3, 1960, 313–328; For further comments on this see F.M. Martin, J.H. Brotherston, and S.P. Chave, 'Incidence of Neurosis in a New Housing Estate', *British Journal of Preventative Social Medicine*, 11, 4, 1957, 196–202; Michael Shepherd, et al., 'Psychiatric Morbidity in an Urban Group Practice [Abridged]', *Proceedings of the Royal Society of Medicine*, 52, 4, 1959, 269–274.
122 Ryle, *Neurosis in the Ordinary Family*, 140.
123 Anthony Ryle, 'The Psychological Disturbances Associated with 345 Pregnancies in 137 Women', *British Journal of Psychiatry*, 107: 447, 1961, 279–286, 279.
124 *Ibid.*, 281–285.
125 Ryle, *Neurosis in the Ordinary Family*, 13–14.
126 *Ibid.*, 118–129.
127 *Ibid.*, 16.
128 *Ibid.*, 40.
129 Hannah Gavron, *The Captive Wife: Conflicts of Housebound Mothers* (Harmondsworth, 1976 [1966]).
130 Ryle, *Neurosis in the Ordinary Family*, 19, 133; J.G. Howells, 'Neurosis in the Ordinary Family [Review]', *Health Education Journal*, 27, 2, 1968, 105; Brian Kirman, 'Neurosis in London', *British Medical Journal*, 1, 5586, 1968, 233–234; M. Barker, 'Reviewed Work(s): Neurosis in the Ordinary Family, Mind and Medicine Monographs by Anthony Ryle', *British Journal of Psychiatric Social Work*, 9, 4, 1968, 212–213.
131 Richard Hoggart, *The Uses of Literacy* (London, 1957), 42–43.
132 Chettiar, 'Democratizing', 107–122; Elizabeth Badinter, *Mother Love: Myth and Reality: Motherhood in Modern History* (New York, 1981).

133 Watts and Watts, *Psychiatry in General Practice*, 197–198.
134 See, for example, Illingworth, 'Emotional State of Mothers', 340–342.
135 John Cox and Katherine Wisner, 'Recollections on the Early Days of the Marcé Society for Perinatal Mental Health from Professor John Cox', *Archives of Women's Mental Health*, 19, 2016, 197–200, 198.
136 Health Visitors' Association, *New Baby*, 1975, quoted in Catherine Ballard and Hilary Hackett, 'My World Became the Size of the Baby', in *Spare Rib Reader*, ed. Marsha Rowe (Middlesex, 1982 [first printed *Spare Rib*, June 1976]), 384–393, 391.
137 Watts, *The Blue Plague*, 101–103.
138 Vivienne Welburn, *Postnatal Depression* (Glasgow, 1980), 192.
139 Taylor, 'The Suburban Neurosis', 762; *The Lancet*, 'Suburban Neurosis Up to Date', 147.

2

Health visitors and the worlds of new mothers

José Bryce had her first child, a daughter, in November 1975.[1] It was not an easy labour: the epidural failed, but the medical staff kept trying; the hospital artificially accelerated the birth; she haemorrhaged; her daughter was delivered with forceps; and she was given a painful episiotomy. The weeks that followed were a struggle. Reeling from the recent death of her father, she would close the curtains to her house in Kensington, London, to avoid visitors. But help arrived via her 'grand' health visitor, who realised that after performing the necessary routines of mothering – feeding, nappy changing, soothing – Bryce would creep away from her baby and cry. This would not do, her health visitor decided: they would get her some antidepressants. She also urged Bryce to keep her baby physically close. It worked; things started to improve. In Bryce's narrative, the health visitor was instrumental in helping her manage this difficult, emotionally fraught period of baby rearing: she saw her distress, accompanied her to get help, and offered bracing support. Bryce recalled it as a turning point: 'from then on I managed to cope. 'Cos I wasn't coping before'.[2]

Bryce's experience highlights the important role of health visitors in recognising mothers' distress in postwar Britain. Unlike most other health professionals, health visitors' work is primarily preventative, advisory, and consultative, and is not based on clinical treatment – instead, they refer to other agencies, promote positive health behaviours, and interact with healthy populations.[3] Families with young children and babies are central to their work. As this chapter demonstrates, across the country, mothers in postwar Britain disclosed their feelings of sadness, loneliness, and discontent to health visitors. Such disclosures met a range of responses. Not all health visitors helped mothers to 'cope'; some interactions exacerbated mothers' feelings of inadequacy. Interactions were shaped by authority and class: some health visitors were, no doubt, part of the 'rather shadowy impalpable "them"' that Richard Hoggart recalled from his youth in a working-class area of Leeds.[4] But other health visitors, like Bryce's, saw beyond new mothers' closed curtains into the intimate emotional landscape of the home. I argue that postwar health visitors developed – to borrow Ross McKibbin's phrase – a 'sharp eye for the texture of private life'.[5] In the 1980s, these eyes bore witness to the political basis of mothers' private problems, and health visitors were one of the constituencies that resisted efforts to retrench the welfare state.[6]

This chapter, then, reflects the arguments of those who have moved histories of the social work professions beyond conversations about their role in control and surveillance.[7] It looks at how health visitors informed the experience of unhappy motherhood, and, in turn, how health visitors' interactions with unhappy mothers shaped their professional practice and political consciousness. This chapter draws on sociological studies to explore how mothers experienced and navigated health visits. It also uses research produced by and for health visitors, including *Health Visitor*, the journal of the Health Visitors' Association, the profession's union.[8] This journal underscores health visitors' professional preoccupations, research interests, and negotiations of mothers' worlds, as well as demonstrating the political concerns of the profession.

This ability to access the value systems of practitioners is particularly important in a field that has been associated with moralisation. Certainly, professionals in allied fields have found the lack of attentiveness to their 'on-the-ground' experiences frustrating. For example, feminist social worker and sociologist Sue Wise found the framing of social work as a form of control at odds with her labour. Wise argued that

> Continual reiterations of 'social work is the long arm of the state' tells us *nothing* of what this job entails for the average social worker, nothing about what kinds of people and problems you have to work with, nothing concerning what kinds of powers you actually have and even less about how it is experienced by the client on the receiving end of it.[9]

Such a critique is a useful reminder to consider the broader political alignments of health visitors in arguments about their social role. Health visitors have attracted less historiographical attention than some of their peers, but like other professions, they were active in responding to the shifting political and economic climate of postwar Britain. *Health Visitor* underlines the ways that in the 1980s health visitors saw mothers' struggles as a product not of individual choices but as a result of the wider political and economic landscape. This chapter therefore makes three arguments: that health visitors have helped to shape mothers' articulations, experiences, and responses to unhappiness; that in the 1980s, health visitors organised to resist the Thatcherite social and economic agenda; and that health visitors have played an important role in creating community resources around motherhood, acting as a bridge between the medical sphere and mothers' social worlds.

While it is not the thrust of this chapter, it is worth observing here that health visitors have played an under-recognised role in advancing medical awareness of postnatal depression. Psychiatrist Brice Pitt's seminal 1968 study of postnatal depression was prompted by a health visitor.[10] Pitt subsequently described health visitors as an 'ideal consultant to the newly delivered woman with doubts and fears (which means practically every woman who has just come home with a new baby)'.[11] Jenifer Holden, who in the 1980s worked with psychiatrists John Cox and Ruth Sagovsky to develop the Edinburgh Postnatal Depression Scale – a widely used screening tool – was a qualified health visitor.[12] Health visitors subsequently played a crucial role in the validation of this tool.[13] At the end of the 1980s, Cox, Sagovsky, and Holden argued that specially trained health visitors could play an important role in helping mothers recover from postnatal depression. One mother reflected to them that 'I could get everything in the open with her, and after a few weeks I really felt I was getting rid of the depression; it was actually coming away from me'.[14] This mother was not alone in seeing the health visitor as a significant figure.

Health visitors feature widely, if unobtrusively, in mothers' accounts of distress. Their part was sometimes as a 'walk-on' character, their role a bit part on a wider stage. But for some mothers, they played a fondly remembered role in the period of adjustment to a new baby; for others, health visitors are an anonymous stumbling block, perceived as an unwelcome, middle-class arbitrator of working-class motherhood. The health visitor is a figure who has been invested with a number of conflicting meanings: friend, confidant, supporter, irritant, disappointment, spy.

The total sum of these interactions is enormous.[15] One 1969 study found that in London alone 24,000 people a day received a service from a health visitor, 850 of whom were unsupported mothers, 1,150 were expectant mothers, and 7,550 were mothers and babies: this latter group thus made up just over 30 per cent of the people served.[16] The annual report submitted by the medical officer for the London borough of Haringey in 1972 reported that despite understaffing, nearly 42,000 home visits had been made by health visitors, 1,974 of which were to pregnant women, 10,509 to mothers of children under one year old, and 21,189 of which were to children aged between one and five years old.[17] An early 1980s survey found that 96 per cent of new mothers reported that they had been seen by a health visitor.[18] This chapter establishes health visitors as a profession that, allied with mothers, raised the visibility of unhappy motherhood in postwar Britain.

Health visiting, history, and the family

As José Bryce's description of her health visitor as 'grand' suggests, mothers' interactions with health visitors were shaped by class. This has its roots in the profession's history. The emergence of health visiting in Manchester and Salford in the 1860s took place in a period of increasing concern about public health.[19] This anxiety was profoundly classed and gendered. In the later nineteenth century, working-class mothers were seen to be culpable for the spread of ill health and disease.[20] The final decades of the nineteenth century and the start of the twentieth century also witnessed middle-class ideas about a 'proper childhood' gain traction.[21] Although working-class women were employed as health visitors in Manchester from 1867, upper-class women remained heavily involved with the administration of the service.[22] These factors converged to have an enduring effect on the perception of the service.[23] It is little surprise, then, that working-class families did not always trust health visitors.[24]

Like the allied fields of nursing and social work, the story of health visiting is one of increasing professionalisation.[25] Health visitors are now registered nurses or midwives with additional training in public health nursing, but a nursing background was not obligatory at the profession's beginnings. Instead, the origins of health visiting lie in sanitary inspection, and in 1896, the Women Sanitary Inspectors' Association was established. In 1915, the name was changed to the Women Sanitary Inspectors' and Health Visitors' Association.[26] At its beginnings health visiting required no formal training – the first course was set up in 1892 – though by the early 1900s an increasing number of local authorities were employing health visitors, a trend that was confirmed after the 1907 Notification of Births Act.[27] So it was in 1909 that the Local Government Board first set out the statutory qualifications that health visitors should hold.[28] Health visiting received a boost in 1917 during National Baby Week when the film *Motherhood* depicted a health visitor playing a crucial role in the redemption of a young working-class mother.[29] In 1918, the Maternity and Child Welfare Act broadened the responsibilities of local authorities around maternity and child welfare.[30] That year the Women Sanitary Inspectors' and Health Visitors' Association registered as a trade union affiliated with the National Union of Women Workers and the National and Local Government Officers' Association. Shortly after this, regulations prescribed a two-year training course for health visitors, or one-year training for graduates, nurses, or experienced health visitors.[31] Ideas about the importance of innate feminine qualities endured, however, and in 1919, the *British Medical Journal* warned that professional training should not place too much emphasis on training because health visitors' 'greatest qualification should be the possession of womanly sympathy and consideration'.[32]

Despite this increasing professionalisation, there was concern that the work was widely misunderstood. As C. Phyllis Armitage's *Health Visiting: The New Profession* lamented in 1927, the public had a 'hazy notion that the health visitor is a person who runs a crèche, or knocks at the doors of the houses in her district and asks, without having been invited, whether she may see the baby'. Health visiting was, she underlined, of far greater significance than this.[33] At this point, mothers' emotional health was not a major concern for health visitors, although Armitage suggested that the anxious mother 'should not allow her mothering to take the form of ceaseless worrying'.[34] In the 1930s, the development of social medicine helped to reinforce the importance of health visiting.[35] Home visits continued to make up the bulk of the health visitor's work, but they also met mothers and babies in maternity and child welfare centres and worked in schools.[36]

In 1946, the National Health Service Act instructed local health authorities to provide a health visitor service and expand the remit of their responsibilities to encompass a wider spectrum of people needing health care.[37] Despite this expansion, mothers remained central to health visitors' practice.[38] Nonetheless, in light of these shifting professional, structural, and social conditions, the Ministry of Health convened a review of health visiting in the 1950s. It first met in 1953 under the chairmanship of Sir W. Jameson. The committee met twenty-two times in London but also ventured outside the city, undertaking numerous visits to other parts of the country. As part of its research the working party solicited diaries from health visitors in England, Wales, and Scotland. The cases are searing, and show the depth of engagement health visitors had with families. The diary of one Welsh mental health liaison health visitor noted a case that had been referred to her following a maternity and child welfare visit. The mother was forty-seven and a mother of eight. She had been depressed since the birth of her youngest child five months earlier. Ill health had been rampant: during her last pregnancy, all the children had whooping cough, and since the youngest's arrival, three children had had glandular fever; the baby had bronchial pneumonia, and the mother had influenza. But those were not the family's only problems. They owed money to the City Treasurer for the home help service, and the mother worried about the cost of clothing required for one of her sons to attend grammar school. The health visitor referred them for financial help, helped to apply for financial support for school clothing, and arranged postnatal appointments for the mother and vaccination appointments for the baby.[39] The role of the health visitor, then, bridged the general practice and the home; it involved both medical and social care and practical help. Health visitors saw and supported mothers in their social, economic, and familial contexts. But there were too few of them: when the Jameson Committee reported in 1956 it estimated a need for 11,500 qualified health visitors, compared with the existing 8,000 full-time equivalent health visitors, nearly one-third of whom were 'acting health visitors' who lacked qualifications. These untrained health visitors were not, as was pointed out in a parliamentary discussion of health visiting, evenly distributed around the country, and were instead more prevalent in Scotland than in other parts of Britain. To address this, the Report estimated that an additional 3,500 qualified health visitors were needed. This push towards professionalisation and standardisation was shared with other related professions. The Younghusband Report, which investigated social work, similarly reflected these themes when it published in 1959, and recommended the further recruitment and training of social workers.[40] Within this nexus of interconnecting and occasionally intersecting health and welfare services, the Jameson Report underlined that the health visitors' role was preventative and advisory, 'a truly medico-social worker... playing a full part in both preventative medicine and social action'.[41]

By 1960, it was felt by prominent health visitors that 'medical and social problems are changing', and a didactic approach to guidance was falling out of favour.[42] This perhaps reflected the nascent shift towards the recognition of the value of lived experience, as well as heralding a changing attitude to authority that would become apparent towards the end of the decade. Health visiting work was changing too, as in the 1960s health visitors were increasingly attached to general practices and their responsibilities were broadened to include care for the elderly and the unwell.[43] In a day-to-day sense, though, health visiting continued to place mothers and infants at the heart of its activity.[44] Indeed, the emphasis on the mother-child relationship was given as a justification for keeping the profession heavily feminised; in 1960, a leading health visiting tutor answered the question 'Is there a place for male health visitors?' with a resounding no.[45] The enduring importance of work with mothers was reflected in *Health Visitor*, which published research that explored, for example, the use of screening questionnaires for postnatal depression, the establishment of parenting groups, and mothers' postpartum emotional experiences.[46]

Mothers' experiences of health visitors

What mothers felt about health visiting has, however, been largely lacking in histories of health visiting, an omission notable because in the postwar years there were increased efforts to understand families' interactions with state services.[47] It is notable that health visitors sometimes played a critical, if under-recognised, role in the production of these studies: health visitors, for example, conducted interviews with nearly 14,000 women who had children in a particular week of 1946. The results of these interviews formed the basis of the study *Maternity in Great Britain: A Survey of Social and Economic Aspects of Pregnancy and Childbirth*, commissioned by a Joint Committee of the Royal College of Obstetricians, Gynaecologists and the Population Investigation Committee and published in 1948.[48] Elsewhere, health visitors were one of the objects rather than the agents of study. For example, a 1961 study by the research organisation Political and Economic Planning investigated families' views of welfare services, finding that the majority of families had interacted with health visitors, and most mothers were satisfied with the help they received. This was particularly the case for meetings held at welfare clinics; home visits attracted more ire, with women reporting that they were visited at an inconvenient time and their visitor was 'nosey', a 'busybody', or that 'she was not much help'.[49] Other studies in the 1960s found that public feelings were generally positive about social services, although some confusion remained about their various remits.[50]

More recently, sociological research has helped to make mothers' experiences of health visitors visible. One mother, reinterviewed as part of Wiggins' and Oakley's *Looking Back at Becoming a Mother* project, recalled that following the birth of her daughter in the winter of 1975, she set about trying to prepare for Christmas festivities. It was too much, she recalled, and it exhausted her. She found herself feeling disconsolate and depressed, wondering what she had done. The feeling diminished as a routine set in, feeding became established, and her 'lovely' health visitor visited. She was 'fantastic, she was so wonderful and so kind', the mother recalled. 'She sort of just blew the problems away, you know, like "nothing to worry about and do this and do that, and she'll be fine and don't you worry"'. The health visitor visited often, and the mother felt well supported. The health visitor entered her family lore:

> oh she made it so light-hearted rather than this great worry and tragedy thing that I can't cope, I can't make this baby sleep, I don't know what to do, you know. I've fed her, I've done her burp, you know, I've changed her, everything and she's still crying and crying and crying, you know. And Mrs [...] just said 'oh it's time for you to go to bye-bye's' and it stuck, you know.[51]

While not all health visitors shaped family in-jokes, health visitors sometimes weighed in about family life in ways that reflected changing social norms. Or, seen another way, health visitors have helped to embed and promulgate social trends. As one mother reflected in 1980, 'I was depressed and lonely and the Health Visitor thought it would be a good idea [sending her child to nursery]. I've definitely benefited, I'd be lost without it. I can't stand being indoors, I must have some freedom. After all, you are a person, you are not just a mum'.[52] This health visitor's recommendation may have been influenced by the increasing acceptance that childcare held benefits for both mothers and children. Indeed, one 1980s textbook on psychology for nurses and health visitors underlined the dangers of being 'house-bound' for women, advocating for paid work as a means to mitigate against it:

> A crucial consideration is the recent finding of an extremely high incidence of depression among house-bound women... With no outlet such as a job, tied to the house by the presence of several dependent children, a large proportion of mothers (especially among the working class) become isolated and hence depressed. Mothers, on the other hand, who do go out to work are far less likely to suffer from depression, anxiety and feelings of low self-esteem.[53]

For other mothers, though, advice to seek paid employment was less fruitful. A mother wrote in a 1988 information booklet about postnatal depression that, desperately lonely following the birth of her baby, her general practitioner advised pills, and her health visitor suggested getting a job: neither recommendation helped.[54]

It was not just the advice itself but the basis of expertise that mothers questioned. In particular, expertise was doubted when it was seen to emerge from abstract knowledge rather than personal experience. Elizabeth Farrell told Oakley in the 1970s that 'you've got to have been through having children yourself to understand what it means and entails'. Another mother, 29-year-old Jane Tarrant, told Oakley that one health visitor was 'very sweet, but she's not even married'. This made her doubt the depth of her understanding, explaining that:

> I know it sounds wrong to say it, but it *must* be different. I think that the health visitor who's had her own child she was *so* much more sympathetic... You can read anything in a book but then I feel they're just trotting advice out of a book. They haven't *actually* had to deal with a baby themselves.[55]

Younger mothers echoed this. In one 1984 study, teenage mothers told researchers that health visitors lacked hands-on experience: one 17-year-old mother commented that 'They have never had babies so they don't know'; a 19-year-old mother said, 'she's in her late 50s and never had any children of her own'; and an 18-year-old single mother explained that 'They've never had children of their own and so they haven't any experience to help you with any baby problems'.[56] Vivienne Welburn argued that health visitors were vital to identifying and supporting depressed mothers but commented that some cases were not picked up because health visitors were not necessarily mothers themselves and did not see that some mothers had 'smiling depressions'.[57] As Oakley identified, mothers implied that 'experience breeds sympathy'. However, the conflict was not, she suggested, between 'the expert and the non-expert' but between those who held different *kinds* of expertise.[58]

Of course, taxonomies of expertise obscure the overlaps of the types of knowledge held by individuals. Some health visitors had academic knowledge, professional insight, *and* lived experience. Ellen George, a 29-year-old ex-health visitor, was interviewed in the 1970s as part of Oakley's *Becoming a Mother* study. George felt 'desperate' and depressed after the birth of her daughter. Her professional experience was of little help: 'I mean I've done all this academically, which I don't think helps at all', she reflected. Instead, her academic knowledge made her 'worried about breaking down'. Her general practitioner prescribed Valium, 'which didn't make any difference', and, while her husband was reluctant to acknowledge the severity of the situation, she eventually received help from a social worker friend, who told George that she understood how she was feeling because of her first-hand experience. Her friend directed George to reach out to a general practitioner, who prescribed a different antidepressant, and put her in touch with her sister-in-law, 'who'd also been very depressed... She was really fantastic, and she described the whole thing, she'd had practically the same experience'. George was told to make sure she always had someone with her, and so, with the help of a neighbour, her husband, a friend, and the antidepressant (a prescription that made her feel less depressed but still 'pretty ghastly'), she started to feel better.[59] George's story is a reminder that professional insight into distress is not necessarily an inoculation against the experience of it. It also underlines that postwar women's social networks came through to provide support at times of crisis, asserting the value of experiential expertise as a complement to medical knowledge.

Other health visitors also drew on their own experiences to enhance medical knowledge. In 1983, health visitor and single mother Veronica Selwyn Smith warned in a nursing journal that, in her experience, financial struggles and loneliness were the primary problems that single mothers faced. Despite her anxiety about being a lone mother, she had a positive experience with her own health visitor, but others had to navigate more fraught relationships.[60]

Negotiation, class, community

Mothers' relationships with health visitors were neither compliant nor deferential but were subject to personal negotiation and individual dissent. Indeed, psychology researchers John and Elizabeth Newson found in their 1960s study of childrearing in Nottingham that health visitors and university researchers were given different answers to the same questions. They attributed this to mothers' desire to please – or at least not aggravate – health visitors.[61] Their study, which conducted over 700 interviews with mothers of children under one year old, explored a wide range of topics relating to approaches and experiences of childcare. The interviews sought to establish a 'permissive' atmosphere and relied upon interviewers having a 'pleasant manner and a certain skill in persuading cooperation'. Health visitors were perfect for the role, the Newsons felt, as they had in many cases already established relationships with the families and were an experienced, well-trained workforce. Indeed, the full project was only made possible when health visitors were brought on board as interviewers. However, this brought complications. Health visitors, in their usual role, gave childrearing advice and wore uniforms, and were thus likely seen to represent 'an alien authority and part of the "Them" which is officialdom': this could affect mothers' responses. But this prior relationship with the service could do more than inhibit open disclosure. Health visitors identified in advance families with whom they had a tricky relationship, in which they were tolerated with 'polite hostility' or their work actively thwarted; here, the project sent an alternative interviewer to the household.[62] Elsewhere, another 1960s study found that social workers, as a broad sweep of employees, were generally assumed to be middle-class.[63] Mothers' interactions with health visitors, then, were shaped by the asymmetry of authority and frequently by class.

Struggling working-class mothers did not always welcome the health visitor. One mother told Oakley and Wiggins that she had a 'horrendous' childbirth in the 1970s and in the early weeks of mothering, she felt depressed and cheated, as the disjuncture between the reality of mothering and its more romanticised expectations became clear. Despite these struggles, her health visitor was not welcome. She used to 'hate' the health visitor coming, she explained:

> Because they were like really middle class, especially here, and you just felt like you had to tidy all the house up and be spick and span and sit there and I just always felt they were judging me... I'm from a very working class background and I just thought... get the house tidy.[64]

This fear of judgement was not without basis. State-authorised bodies were able to exercise various forms of social control over working-class families in Britain, and working-class mothers were particular targets of social workers' intervention. Pat Starkey has, for example, argued that the '"problem mother" provided an ideal vehicle for the deflection of blame' during and immediately after the Second World War.[65] As Starkey says, the particular construction of the 'problem family' that was prevalent in the 1940s was soon displaced by other configurations of concern, but no doubt the suspicion lingered that professions allied with social work were visiting in a moralising capacity. Misgivings around health visitors were clearly well-established. In the 1970s, psychiatrist Brice Pitt, addressing a lay readership, encouraged mothers not to view health visitors as 'a snoop or a busybody, but as an expert and a friend'.[66]

Other differences arose within this period, particularly when the febrile activist climate of the 1970s took root. Recalling her early years in the feminist movement, working-class mother Rose Brennan recounts joining a consciousness-raising group in 1972 and finding it a 'haven of support', drawing a contrast with her 'distraught' health visitor, to whom she was a 'puzzle':

> Why did I insist on crying? Didn't I have two delightful babies, a husband who didn't beat me, a house and enough money? In my own confusion I pretended that my daughter was a 'difficult feeder'. Health visitors understand that sort of problem.[67]

Thus, mothers actively negotiated disclosure. In some cases, distressed mothers told authorities what they thought they wanted to be told; in other cases, women adhered to narratives that eased challenging conversations. Other mothers evaded disclosure when their relationships with health visitors felt superficial, or when staff shortages meant that relationships could not develop to become sufficiently trusting.[68] This evasion would have been little surprise to health visitors themselves. They knew mothers looked to other sources of knowledge. In 1988, *Health Visitor* explained that a survey of 400 women, either pregnant or with children under two, found that health visitors were held in high esteem, but that family, friends, and books were seen by some mothers as more informative on particular areas of babycare.[69]

It was not just class that shaped relational dynamics. In the 1980s, health visitors were sometimes less than sympathetic to the structural racism experienced by mothers of colour, and liable to believe racist stereotypes about childrearing. At the same time, Black health visitors reported that white parents sometimes snubbed them as sources of expertise.[70] Other mothers, perhaps responding to the proliferation of social scientific interest in women, objected to 'continuous data collection' when health visitors surveyed them about their emotional wellbeing. Where mothers did participate in surveys, health visitors could observe the disjuncture between what was visible and what was conveyed on questionnaires: one health visitor reported back to a researcher that a mother who gave 'near perfect answers' did so with 'tears streaming down her face'.[71]

However, where relationships were effective – no doubt shaped by time, availability, and personality of individual health visitors, and by a myriad of other exigencies – unhappy mothers stressed health visitors' importance. Teresa, a Bristol-based mother, told a 1981 survey of new mothers that her health visitor was 'the most cheering and encouraging friend'.[72] Sylvia, from Glasgow, responded to the same survey that she was 'still very depressed' but was receiving help from her doctor after a 'long talk' with her husband and health visitor.[73] In 1986, Jean, a mother based in North Wales, told a local newspaper about her overwhelming anxiety after the birth of her third child. Initially reluctant to talk to her health visitor – worried that her child might be taken away from her – she finally opened up:

> She came round and explained what was happening to me. She hadn't wanted to tell me what was wrong before as she thought it was up to me to let her know. She had been keeping a close eye on me though, and by visiting so often I had begun to trust her. She explained to my husband what was happening and got me some expert help and treatment from the doctor and hospital… If you do have any sort of post-natal depression, you can get over it – but a lot of self-help is needed and confidence in those who are willing to help.

Mothers who empathised with Jean were urged to contact a local branch of MIND, the national mental health charity.[74]

By the 1980s, a number of charities and organisations that claimed expertise in postnatal depression operated across Britain, and affiliated local groups for struggling mothers were widely dispersed. These groups frequently publicised health visitors as a source of support. For example, in the late 1980s, a depressed mother explained in a booklet published by the self-help group, the Meet-a-Mum Association (MAMA), that her health visitor had played a critical role in connecting her to medical care.[75] Another mother remembered in the same booklet that her health visitor 'seemed to understand how I was feeling. This was the beginning of the long, slow road to recovery'.[76] In turn, health visitors spread the word about self-help groups in their communities. One mother, exhausted, lonely, and depressed at the routine nature of life with a baby, called her health visitor, who came round 'straight away and was very helpful. She explained that the feelings I had were natural for a mother. I was not alone'. The health visitor recommended MAMA, where the mother made valuable new connections.[77]

Other health visitors played a role in establishing groups.[78] Newpin (New Parent Infant Network), for example, was established in south London in 1982 by a group of health professionals with the aim of improving mothers' mental health and, through this, lessening the incidence of child abuse. Newpin offered a drop-in and self-referral advice centre and ran therapeutic support groups, including a personal development programme.[79] Its first co-ordinator was Anne Jenkins, a former health visitor. Social workers and health visitors could refer parents to the project. Although it was lauded as a 'lifeline' by a *Horizon* broadcast on BBC2 in 1989, by which time around 500 mothers had passed through the project and further Newpins had opened, its financial survival was in doubt.[80] Other projects ran on a smaller scale and relied on peer support. One health visitor wrote in *Health Visitor* in January 1983 about their experience of founding a support group for depressed and anxious young mothers. The group was, she said, a 'safety valve through which [the mothers] can let off feelings of despair, frustration and hopelessness before these become intolerable'.[81] A few months later, the journal returned to the theme in an article that explored health visitors' establishment of three local groups, two of which targeted new mothers. There was, they said:

> a need to help first-time mothers come to terms with their feelings and, by expressing them, understand them more fully. In sharing these emotions with other mothers, they realize that a varied range of feelings are quite normal and acceptable and that learning to live with a baby often takes time.

The piloting of the postnatal group was successful, the health visitors noted, although they lamented that some of the more isolated mothers they had invited had not taken up the offer. However, 'perhaps the greatest achievement of a group of this kind is to stimulate the beginnings of social contact and friendships for these first-time mothers, who need to feel they are not alone in their new and sometimes joyful, sometimes anxious situation'.[82] The importance of mothers' social networks was affirmed in a similar project detailed in the issue. This group, organised by a health visitor and a psychiatric social worker in inner London, was joined by a small group of self-referred middle- and working-class mothers. The mothers admitted that their pre-baby lives seemed 'uncluttered' in comparison with the realities of life with a small child and that they were 'surprised and worried over their unexpected feelings of anger and inability to find solutions to problems. They were tired, tied down and lonely'. Once again, a key outcome of the group was lasting social connections and a community of fellow new mothers.[83] Some health visitors sought to address some of the time and energy that linking new mothers to groups – and keeping women abreast of local developments – could absorb. In the 1980s, a former health visitor, Rita Bell, helped to establish a magazine to promote health education and to connect women to nearby mothers' groups, the *Hailsham Mums' Newsline*. Edited by a health visitor, the magazine was distributed for free to women at new birth visits, at clinics, and to mothers who moved into the area. It received a 'staggering' response, Bell noted, with demand for the first issue so great that an additional 50 copies had to be printed following the initial run of 150.[84] But health visitors did not only espouse the value of parenting support groups in their own professional journals. In 1983, health visitor and researcher Deborah Hennessy provided a how-to guide for nurses on forming parent support groups. Here she noted that their emergence had been driven by recent 'rapid, stressful' social changes.[85]

Politics, the New Right, and radical health visiting in the 1980s

Hennessy was not alone in identifying that social structures were changing. In the 1980s, the social contract that underpinned community ties was fraying. During this period, health visitors saw first-hand the effects of rising levels of deprivation, inequality, and poverty among vulnerable families. Health visitors argued that structural inequalities, rather than individual failings, were the cause of families' struggles, in direct contradiction to the prevailing political winds, and they wrote sympathetically of their plight. A health visitor who established a group for 'at risk' families in a deprived part of Cheshire in 1981 wrote the following in *Health Visitor*:

> Many of the families in this area have low incomes and inadequate housing and face a daily struggle to provide their children with essential food and clothing. Often, most of the parents' energy is used in attempting to cope with an impossible lack of facilities.[86]

These families were among those who suffered the most from New Right economics – with its focus on individualism, wealth creation, and repudiation of active redistribution – that prevailed under Margaret Thatcher's premiership from 1979 to 1990.[87] Contemporary observers described Thatcherism as an 'attack' on the welfare state and drew a 'stark' picture of its consequences.[88] There was, for example, a 7 per cent reduction in state expenditure on social assistance in the decade that followed 1979, and the link between welfare benefits and inflation was severed.[89] Poor mothers gained little from Thatcher's rhetorical commendation of the family as the bulwark of national life. This ideology of the family positioned the nuclear, heterosexual two-parent family as vital to the maintenance of the social fabric.[90]

Part of this ideology rested upon ideas about the intrinsic privacy or self-containment of the family. Thus, in the 1980s, health visitors' work took place against a background of increasingly contentious conversations about state intervention in families. Ferdinand Mount, who played a crucial role in the development of the Conservative Party's 1983 election manifesto, wrote in *The Subversive Family* (1982) that what was 'always affronting, offensive and distressing' was the imposition of the public official into private spaces. The health visitor was no exception. She was, he wrote, 'the most helpful of all public visitors'. But new mothers

> cannot help being continuously aware that she is there as an inspector as well as an adviser. Her eye roams the room and the baby for

evidence of dirt, neglect, even brutality. This kindly, middle-aged body has at her ultimate disposal a Stalinist array of powers... these powers are miles away from her mind as she dandles the baby and boosts the mother's confidence by praising and encouraging her; and yet that potential hostility inherent in her inquisitorial role never ceases to mark the relationship with unease which may flare into resentment at a tactless word.[91]

As Jane Lewis observed, though, some on the Left also saw health visitors as unwelcome outriders of middle-class values into working-class families. Both Left and Right, she said, overstated the capacity of working-class families to resist hardship and ignored their willingness to accept help – albeit on their terms.[92]

Within this context, health visitors were vocal about the effects of state cost-cutting. *Health Visitor*'s editorial in March 1983 wrote scathingly about rising rates of deprivation, unemployment, and poverty. It asked:

> Why then, when so many families are still caught up in 'the cycle of deprivation' regardless of which party is in power, are health visitors still caught up in an ongoing debate about whether being 'political' – in the sense of bringing about some social change in these conditions – means bringing party politics into their work? Why is there this curious reluctance to acknowledge that a whole series of official inquiries and research reports have emanated from successive governments for at least 20 years, each showing that all is not well with our welfare state.

Both parties had paid 'lip service' to reports while failing to implement their recommendations, the editorial observed, asking, 'Is it really so difficult for the health visitors who are concerned about the social conditions in the community in which they work to stop equating "political action" with party politics...?'[93] The same issue published an article explaining the role of the treasurer in the NHS. This article was commissioned, the journal explained, on the basis that:

> In a time of financial cutbacks, the finance officer assumes a more than usually powerful role in the NHS. If health visitors and their managers are to speak on equal terms with finance officers and be effective in fighting for their corner, they must learn to understand

the basic principles of NHS finance and planning... Health visitors cannot afford to be either politically or financially naïve.[94]

The following year, the editorial of *Health Visitor* acknowledged increasing politicisation: across the preceding decade, there had been an 'increasing emphasis on the necessity for health visitors to become "politically aware"', it explained.[95] Professional organisations reflected a heightened awareness of the impact of political decisions on children and families. In the 1980s, the Council for the Education and Training of Health Visitors wrote that:

> Equally disadvantageous to children and their families is the deprivation suffered from living in the decaying, declining inner areas of our large cities. To encourage and stimulate an awareness of health needs, to motivate individuals and families to improve their own conditions, to take community action for better housing, schools, play areas and health services by teaching the value of health, must be a priority of health visitors and others.[96]

The emphasis was placed on encouraging the improvement of conditions through community action alongside amending individual behaviours. In 1989, a study of new mothers published in *Health Visitor* painted a stark picture of the differences in amenities available to young families in more and less affluent areas. One health visitor told the study that the 'real answer' to mothers' unhappiness was 'a reasonable income, decent housing and proximity to an extended family'.[97] Neither did health visitors hold much truck with politically expedient moral panics. Health visitors would not believe the 'popular Conservative myth' that young single women were becoming mothers simply to leapfrog the council housing queue, *Health Visitor* stressed.[98]

The establishment of the Radical Health Visitors Group (RHVG) was one manifestation of this consciousness. The idea for the group emerged at a one-day research seminar in 1980, but word spread quickly: around fifty people turned up at the first meeting, drawn there by limited advertising and word-of-mouth promotion. The group emerged from 'discontent, as most radical groups are', founding member Jean Spray noted. Health visitors bore witness to the damaging consequences of political and social policies, Spray argued, and as a result were 'a frustrated, isolated and increasingly crisis-ridden group of workers'. The group sought to advocate on the local and global issues that affected its members, including feminism, racism within the health service, and baby deaths in poorer regions.[99] Members had wider political commitments, too; Spray, for example, wrote an article in the *Socialist Organiser* about the impact of Conservative health cuts and the battle to prevent the closure of a local hospital.[100]

The RHVG took a while to find its feet, but following a series of initial meetings, the group became what Spray calls a 'politically conscious organisation'. The group, led by a core membership of six to twelve people, firmed up its infrastructure, advertised monthly meetings, and set up a newsletter. Though the core group was run from London, groups ran across the country, and these groups came together to run workshops, where discussions explored the challenges that health visitors encountered when their work led them to make interventions that were perceived as 'political'. Its meetings were promoted in *Health Visitor*. The RHVG was never large – peaking at 120 subscribed members – but it arrived at a crucial moment: workers within the NHS were increasingly politicised, the effects of financial cuts within the service were taking hold, and health was becoming an important topic within the labour and women's movements. Nonetheless, Spray recalls a 'touching but depressing level of political naivety in the wider membership'. The group folded after half a decade, the core organisers too run down to organise it. Despite this short lifespan, the group should be seen as emblematic of the self-consciously politicised nature of some health visiting work in the 1980s.[101] Although the group dissipated, at the end of the 1980s, some of the RHVG members joined the Public Health Alliance, which brought together those who shared an interest in inequalities and public health.[102]

Within the mainstream of health visiting, too, shifts were occurring. At the end of the 1980s, the extent of the HVA's financial problems became clear, and it became evident that a merger with another union was on the cards. Its general secretary, Shirley Goodwin, resigned.[103] Seeking to shake off its 'scrappy' image, the HVA sought to carve out a more corporate identity; it was a 'new look for a new decade', the journal announced.[104] Nonetheless, alongside other trade unions, its political work continued.[105] In the late 1980s and early 1990s, the Association moved against government cuts and warned of privatisation in the NHS ('something nasty this way comes', it explained about the National Health Service and Community Care Bill in 1990), condemned government policies that it warned would be harmful to children, women, and families, defended women's health and women's work at trade union meetings, and called for other unions to come together to oppose government plans.[106] It also provided spaces in which mothers' unhappiness was framed in social and political terms. In 1990, two representatives from Newpin told *Health Visitor* that postnatal depression could be caused by isolation and poor social and medical support, condemning the medicalisation of childbirth and the dehumanisation of pregnant women. More honest conversations about motherhood, midwife-led care, and greater social support were needed, they argued.[107] Fortunately, by the end of the 1980s, Newpin was far from alone as a site of support and guidance for new parents.

Conclusion

Health visitors were one of the professional communities on the frontline of postnatal care in postwar Britain. Health visitors, within distressed mothers' narratives, are often anonymous and instrumental. Even where the health visitor was obstructive, unhelpful, or unsupportive, they feature in mothers' stories. But they also feature in glowing terms, hailed as a source of support and sympathy. Whether perceived as sympathetic or judgemental, health visits were a service that was problematised, negotiated, and shaped by both adult agents in the dyad. Mothers were not coerced into disclosure but made conscious, thoughtful appraisals of the relationship and adjusted their discussion of their emotional lives in response to this; health visitors were not exclusively coercive, condemning agents, but were often conscious of the political drivers of deprivation and how this impacted mothers.

In the 1980s, their professional body was, like other unions in the welfare sector, concerned about the consequences of cuts and retrenchment. Within this context, their work on the frontline of postnatal care was rarely felt to be secure, and in the 1980s, health visitors worried that their position was vulnerable within the looming NHS reforms. Some put this anxiety wryly. In 1988, Ann Saeger wrote ten commandments for health visitors, recommending that they be sung at the start of the day, like a hymn. The first of these was that 'Thou shalt love the NHS, especially thou shalt revere thy beloved health authority and thou shalt keep thy fingers crossed that at the next re-organisation, as part of the economy drive, health visitors will not be axed'. The final commandment reflected the fact that health visitors – an almost exclusively female workforce – faced the same pressures as other women workers in the late 1980s. 'Thou shalt endeavour to go home in a cheerful mood, listen to and solve all domestic problems, cook the dinner, washup, do washing, ironing and vacuuming and still be attractive. Thou shalt never fall onto thy sofa, say "God, I've had a lousy day" and reach for a stiff gin'.[108] Little wonder that studies in the late 1980s found health visitors to be a stressed group of workers.[109]

More generally, health visitors bore witness to social, economic, and cultural change, and in everyday interactions, they communicated this to mothers: normalising, for example, mothers undertaking paid work and taking up childcare provision, and encouraging groups that tackled social atomisation. Richard Titmuss argued in the 1960s that the social services came about 'apologetically', a recognition that capitalism and industrialisation had left some basic needs unmet.[110] One of the needs that health visitors hoped to address was loneliness, promoting self-help groups for new mothers. The development of self-help groups, as Chapter 3 shows, had far-reaching implications. It marked a substantive shift in the location of expertise around struggling motherhood towards experiential expertise claimed by mothers themselves. Health visitors, therefore, bridged not only the clinic and the home but also the types of knowledge that circulated about mothers' emotional experiences.

Notes

1 I am using the pseudonyms that were used in the original *Becoming a Mother* study and in its resulting publications, *Women Confined* (1980) and *Becoming a Mother* ([1979] 1980), as Oakley has done in publications that have recently emerged from the *Looking Back*

on *Becoming a Mother* project. See, for example, Ann Oakley, 'A Small Sociology of Maternal Memory', *The Sociological Review*, 64, 3, 2016, 533–549.
2 Meg Wiggins, *Looking Back on Becoming a Mother: Longitudinal Perspectives on Maternity Care and the Transition to Motherhood* [Data Collection] (Colchester: Economic and Social Research Council, 2013), https://doi.org/10.5255/UKDA-SN-850818, Grant Reference ES/J006343/, M07, 13–14.
3 Judith Wagorn, 'Health Visiting', *Nursing: The Add-on Journal of Clinical Nursing*, 2, 2, June 1982, 54.
4 Richard Hoggart, 'The Welfare State Appearance and Reality', *Social Work*, 17, 1, 1960, 13–17, 13.
5 Ross McKibbin, 'Social Class and Social Observation in Edwardian England', *Transactions of the Royal Historical Society*, 28, 1978, 175–199, 178.
6 At the close of the 1980s, for example, the Health Visitors' Association explicitly condemned the government for its silencing of work linking unhealthy diets to poverty. 'HEA Refuses to Publish Report Linking Unhealthy Diet to Poverty', *Health Visitor*, 62, 12, December 1989, 359.
7 Selina Todd, 'Family Welfare and Social Work in Post-War England, c.1948–c.1970', *The English Historical Review*, 129, 537, 2014, 362–387; John Welshman, 'The Social History of Social Work: The Issue of the 'Problem Family', 1940–70', *The British Journal of Social Work*, 29, 3, 1999, 457–476.
8 Jennifer Smith, 'Illustrations from the Wellcome Institute Library: The Archive of the Health Visitors' Association in the Contemporary Medical Archives Centre', *Medical History*, 39, 3, 1995, 358–367. See, for example, Madeleine Simms and Christopher Smith, 'Teenage Mothers: Some Views on Health Visitors', *Health Visitor*, 57, 9, 1984, 269–270; Kedar N. Dwivedi, 'Mother-Baby Psychotherapy', *Health Visitor*, 57, 10, 1984, 306–307; Sydney Brandon, 'Depression after Childbirth', *Health Visitor*, 56, 1, 1983, 13–15.
9 Sue Wise, 'Becoming a Feminist Social Worker', in *Feminist Praxis. Research, Theory and Epistemology in Feminist Sociology*, ed. Liz Stanley (London and New York, 1990), 236–249, 239.
10 Brice Pitt, '"Atypical" Depression Following Childbirth', *British Journal of Psychiatry*, 114, 1968, 1325–1335, 1326.
11 Brice Pitt, *Enjoying Motherhood: How to Have a Happy Pregnancy* (London, 1978), 114.
12 John Cox, Jeni Holden, and Ruth Sagovsky, 'Detection of Postnatal Depression: Development of the Ten Item Edinburgh Postnatal Depression Scale', *British Journal of Psychiatry*, 150, 1987, 782–786.

13 *Ibid.*, 783.
14 Jenifer Holden, Ruth Sagovsky, and John Cox, 'Counselling in a General Practice Setting: Controlled Study of Health Visitor Intervention in Treatment of Postnatal Depression', *British Medical Journal*, 298, 6668, 1989, 223–226.
15 John Welshman, 'Family Visitors or Social Workers? Health Visiting and Public Health in England and Wales 1890–1974', *International History of Nursing Journal*, 2, 4, 1997, 5–22, 7.
16 Tyrrell Marris, *The Work of Health Visitors in London: A Survey, 1969*. Greater London Council Research Department of Planning and Transportation, County Hall, London. Research Report No. 12 (London: Greater London Council, 1971), 5–6. London, Wellcome Archive, K51004.
17 Report of the Medical Officer of Health for Haringey (London, 1972), 43. https://wellcomecollection.org/works/q2n7ay26.
18 Catherine Boyd and Lea Sellers, *The British Way of Birth* (London, 1982), 237.
19 G.M. Owen, 'Health Visiting', in *Nursing, Midwifery and Health Visiting Since 1900*, eds Peta Allan and Moya Jolley (London, 1982), 92–105.
20 Kate Billingham, Jane Morrell, and Clive Billingham, 'Reflections on the History of Health Visiting', *British Journal of Community Health Nursing*, 1, 7, 1996, 386–392, 387; Carol Dyhouse, 'Working-Class Mothers and Infant Mortality in England, 1895–1914', *Journal of Social History*, 12, 2, 1978, 248–267; Jane Lewis, *The Politics of Motherhood: Child and Maternal Welfare in England, 1900–1939* (London, 1980). For more on infant welfare see Hilary Marland, 'A Pioneer in Infant Welfare: The Huddersfield Scheme 1903–1920', *Social History of Medicine*, 6, 1, 1993, 25–50; Jane Lewis, 'The Social History of Social Policy: Infant Welfare in Edwardian England', *Journal of Social Policy*, 9, 4, 1980, 463–486.
21 Harry Hendrick, *Children, Childhood and English Society, 1880–1990* (Cambridge, 1997), 9–15.
22 Vanessa Heggie, 'Health Visiting and District Nursing in Victorian Manchester; Divergent and Convergent Vocations', *Women's History Review*, 20, 3, 2011, 403–422, 407–408.
23 Robert Dingwall, Anne Marie Rafferty, and Charles Webster, *An Introduction to the Social History of Nursing* (London, 1988), 192.
24 Robert Dingwall, 'Collectivism, Regionalism and Feminism: Health Visiting and British Social Policy 1850–1975', *Journal of Social Policy*, 6, 3, 1977, 291–315.

25 For more on professionalisation in nursing, see chapters in Anne Borsay and Billie Hunter (eds), *Nursing and Midwifery in Britain since 1700* (Basingstoke, 2012). For more on social work, see John Welshman, 'The Social History of Social Work: The Issue of the 'Problem Family', 1940–70', *The British Journal of Social Work*, 29, 3, 1999, 457–476.
26 Enid Eve (ed.), 'Introduction', in *Manual for Health Visitors and Infant Welfare Workers* (New York, 1921), 1–16, 2.
27 Notification of Births Act (1907).
28 Margaret McEwan, *Health Visiting: A Textbook for Health Visitor Students*. 2nd ed. (London, 1957), 22.
29 Linda Bryder, 'Mobilising Mothers: The 1917 National Baby Week', *Medical History*, 63, 1, 2019, 2–23, 13.
30 The Maternity and Child Welfare Act 1918.
31 Amanda Kelsey, 'The Making of Health Visitors: An Historical Perspective, Part 1', *International History of Nursing Journal*, 5, 3, 2000, 44–50.
32 'Health Visitors', *British Medical Journal*, 2, 3070, 1919, 572.
33 C. Phyllis Armitage, *Health Visiting: The New Profession* (London, 1927), preface.
34 *Ibid.*, 178–179.
35 Council for the Education and Training of Health Visitors, *An Investigation into the Principles of Health Visiting* (London, 1982 [1980]), 13.
36 *Health Visiting as a Career* (London: Joint Consultative Committee of Institutions Approved by the Minister of Health for the Training of Health Visitors, and of Organisations of Health Visitors, 1939), 1. London, British Library, YD.2005a.1665.
37 National Health Service Act 1946, London: HMSO, Part III, 24. I. For more on this, see Kelsey, 'The Making of Health Visitors'.
38 Llywelyn Roberts, I.G. Davies, and Beryl D. Corner, *Textbook for Health Visitors* (London, 1951), 159.
39 Department of Health, *An Inquiry into Health Visiting: Report of a Working Party on the Field of Work, Training, and Recruitment of Health Visitors* (London, 1956), 88.
40 HEALTH VISITORS AND SOCIAL WORKERS TRAINING BILL, HC Debate, 24 November 1961 vol 649 cc1684-775.
41 An Inquiry into Health Visiting, 116.
42 N.C. Daniells, 'Meeting the Challenge of Change', *Royal Society of Health Journal*, 80, 4, 1960, 356–359, 356.
43 This shift was contested in medical journals' research and letter pages. See, for example, Joyce M. Akester and A.N. Macphail, 'Health

Visiting and General Practice', *The Lancet*, 284, 7356, 1964, 405–408; John Fry, J.B. Dillane, M.M. Connolly, and E.V. Kuenssberg, 'Health Visiting and General Practice', *The Lancet*, 284, 7358, 1964, 526–527; R. Ann Abel, *Nursing Attachments to General Practice: Staff Implications for Schemes for Attachment of Local Health Authority Staff (Health Visitors and Home Nurses) to General Practice*, Study No. 1. Department of Health and Social Security Social Science Research Unit (London, 1969). London, Wellcome Archive, K50675.

44 Welshman, 'Family Visitors or Social Workers?', 18–19; Report of the Committee on Local Authority and Allied Personal Social Services, CMND. 3703 (London: HMSO, 1968), 291.

45 G.M. Francis, 'The Health Visitor of the Future', *Royal Society of Health Journal*, 80, 4, 1960, 354–356, 354.

46 See, for example, in just one issue, Cynthia Illingworth, 'The Emotional State of Mothers in the First Three Months after the Birth of a Baby', *Health Visitor*, 62, 2, November 1989, 340–342; Agnes McConville, 'Setting Up a Parenting Group', *Health Visitor*, 62, 2, November 1989, 338–339; Monica Briscoe, 'The Detection of Emotional Disorders in the Post Natal Period by Health Visitors', *Health Visitor*, 62, 2, November 1989, 336–337; Lisa Curtice, 'Talking About How Difficult We Find It', *Health Visitor*, 62, 11, November 1989, 343.

47 Billingham, Morrell, and Billingham, 'Reflections', 390.

48 *Maternity in Great Britain. A Survey of Social and Economic Aspects of Pregnancy and Childbirth*. Joint Committee of the Royal College of Obstetricians and Gynaecologists and the Population Investigation Committee (London and New York, 1948).

49 Political and Economic Planning, *Family Needs and the Social Services* (London, 1961), 123–125.

50 Noel Timms, 'Knowledge, Opinion and the Social Services', *The Sociological Review*, 9, 3, 1961, 361–365.

51 Wiggins, *Looking Back on Becoming a Mother*, M16, 14–15.

52 Martin Hughes et al., *Nurseries Now: A Fair Deal for Parents and Children* (Harmondsworth, 1980), 12.

53 H.R. Schaffer, 'Social Development in Early Childhood', in *Psychology for Nurses and Health Visitors*, ed. John Hall (London and Basingstoke, 1988 [1982]), 165–181, 171.

54 Meet-a-Mum Association, *Behind the Painted Smile: An Insight into Postnatal Depression* (London, 1988), 23. London, British Library, 95/03037.

55 Oakley, *Becoming a Mother*, 306–307. Italics in original.

56 Madeleine Simms and Christopher Smith, 'Teenage Mothers: Some Views on Health Visitors', *Health Visitor*, 57, 9, 1984, 269–270.

57 Welburn, *Postnatal Depression*, 192.
58 Oakley, *Becoming a Mother*, 306.
59 *Ibid.*, 144–146.
60 Veronica Selwyn Smith, 'Single Parents – A Personal View', *Nursing: The Add-on Journal of Clinical Nursing*, 2, 20, December 1983, 578.
61 John Newson and Elizabeth Newson, *Patterns of Infant Care in an Urban Community* (Harmondsworth, 1974 [1963]), 272–273.
62 Newson and Newson, *Patterns of Infant Care*, 268–269.
63 Noel Timms, 'The Public and the Social Worker: Results of a Pilot Research Project', *Social Work*, 19, 1, 1962, 3–7.
64 Wiggins, *Looking Back on Becoming a Mother*, M45, 1–17.
65 Pat Starkey, 'The Feckless Mother: Women, Poverty and Social Workers in Wartime and Post-War England', *Women's History Review*, 9:3, 539–557.
66 Pitt, *Enjoying Motherhood*, 114.
67 Rose Brennan, 'You've Come a Long Way', in *'68, '78, '88: From Women's Liberation to Feminism*, ed. Amanda Sebestyen (Dorset, 1988), 240–243, 241.
68 Jane Robinson, *An Evaluation of Health Visiting* (London, 1982), 80.
69 'What Mothers Think of You', *Health Visitor*, 61, 9, September 1988, 262.
70 Marie-Claude Foster, 'Health Visitors' Perspectives on Working in a Multiethnic Society', *Health Visitor*, 6, 9, September 1988, 275–278.
71 Illingworth, 'Emotional State of Mothers', 340.
72 Boyd and Sellers, *The British Way of Birth*, 185.
73 *Ibid.*, 185–186.
74 'How Your Baby Can Drive you to Distraction: Birth Brought Jean Close to Suicide', *North Wales Weekly News*, 10 July 1986.
75 Meet-a-Mum Association, *Behind the Painted Smile: An Insight into Postnatal Depression* (London, 1988), 21–22. London, British Library, 95/03037.
76 *Ibid.*, 27.
77 *Ibid.*, 24.
78 Vari Drennan (ed.), 'Changing Health Visiting Practice', in *Health Visitors and Groups: Politics and Practice* (Oxford, 1988), 1–30, 16.
79 Myra Gurr and Anne Hansen, 'NEWPIN: An Opportunity for Positive Change', *Psychiatric Bulletin*, 21, 8, 1997, 480–482.
80 'A Lifeline for New Parents', *The Scotsman*, 19 June 1989; A.D. Cox et al., 'Evaluation of a Home Visiting and Befriending Scheme for Young Mothers. Newpin', *Journal of the Royal Society of Medicine*, 84, 4, 1991, 217–220.
81 Jane McKears, 'Group Support for Young Mothers', *Health Visitor*, 56, 1, 1983, 16.

82 Valerie Moulds et al., 'Innovations by a Primary Health Care Team 2. A Postnatal Group for First-Time Mothers', *Health Visitor*, 56, 8, 1983, 296–297.
83 Phoebe Thomas and Ann Sullivan, 'A Mothers' and Babies' Group in a Family Health Clinic', *Health Visitor*, 56, 8, 1983, 299–300.
84 Rita Bell, 'Hailsham Mums' Newsline', *Health Visitor*, 62, 2, February 1989, 59–60.
85 Deborah Hennessy, 'Parent Support Groups', *Nursing: The Add-on Journal of Clinical Nursing*, 2, 19, November 1983, 552–554, 552.
86 Shirley Palfreeman, 'Mother and Toddler Groups Among 'At Risk' Families', *Health Visitor*, 55, 9, 1982, 455–459.
87 Felix Römer, 'Poverty, Inequality Statistics and Knowledge Politics Under Thatcher', *The English Historical Review*, 137, 585, 2022, 513–551, 518.
88 Ian Gough, 'Thatcherism and the Welfare State', in *The Politics of Thatcherism*, eds Stuart Hall and Martin Jacques (London, 1983), 148–168.
89 A. Scott-Samuel et al., 'The Impact of Thatcherism on Health and Well-Being in Britain', *International Journal of Health Services*, 44:1, 2014, 53–71, 55.
90 Gillian Pascall, 'Women and the Family in the British Welfare State: The Thatcher/Major Legacy', *Social Policy & Administration*, 31, 1997, 290–305.
91 Ferdinand Mount, *The Subversive Family* (London, 1982), 174.
92 Lewis, 'Anxieties about the Family', 48.
93 Editorial, 'The Politics of Poverty', *Health Visitor*, 56, 3, 1983, 81.
94 Gerald Vinten, '1. Who Holds the Purse Strings?', *Health Visitor*, 56, 3, 1983, 94–96.
95 Editorial, 'Professional Practice in Perspective', *Health Visitor*, 57, 10, 1984, 289.
96 Council for the Education and Training of Health Visitors, *An Investigation*, 36.
97 Illingworth, 'Emotional State of Mothers', 341.
98 'Housing and Support Needs for Young Single Mothers', *Health Visitor*, 62, 11, November 1989, 326.
99 'Baby Deaths "Too High"', *Huddersfield Daily Examiner*, 28 May 1982; 'Racism and Health Visiting', *Health Visitor*, 57, 10, October 1984, 291.
100 Jean Spray, 'Brent Feels the Brunt', *Socialist Organiser*, 119, 10 February 1983, 8.

101 Jean Spray, 'The Radical Health Visitors Group', in *Health Visitors and Groups: Policy and Practice*, ed. Vari Drennan (Oxford, 1988), 108–113.
102 V.A. Berridge, D.A. Christie, and E.M. Tansey (eds), 'Public Health in the 1980s and 1990s: Decline and Rise', in *Wellcome Witnesses to Twentieth Century Medicine*, vol. 26 (London, 2006), 20–21.
103 Despite some reservations among its membership, in 1992, the union merged with the Manufacturing, Science and Finance Union. See 'Shades of Opinion: Members' Thoughts on Merger Partners', *Health Visitor*, 62, 11, November 1989, 329–330.
104 Editorial, 'A New Look for a New Decade', *Health Visitor*, 62, December 1989, 357.
105 'HVA At Scarborough: Professional Power Dissected', *Health Visitor*, 62, 12, December 1989, 366.
106 'Child Benefit Frozen Again', *Health Visitor*, 62, 12, December 1989, 358; 'Women "Hit Hardest" by NHS Reform', *Health Visitor*, 62, 12, December 1989, 362; 'Conference: TUC Women on the Alert', *Health Visitor*, 63, 5, May 1990, 151; 'Market Forces the Pace', *Health Visitor*, 63, 1, January 1990, 1; 'HVA Slams White Paper Proposals', *Health Visitor*, 62, 5, May 1989, 141–142; 'Unity Call in Fight against White Paper', *Health Visitor*, 62, 11, November 1989, 327.
107 'Post Natal Depression: Does It Exist?', *Health Visitor*, 63, 5, May 1990, 154–155.
108 Ann Saeger, 'The Ten Commandments for Health Visitors', *Health Visitor*, 61, 1, January 1988, 15.
109 Michael A. West, Avril Jones, and Yvonne Savage, 'Stress in Health Visiting: A Quantitative Assessment', *Health Visitor*, 61, 9, September 1988, 269–271.
110 Richard Titmuss, 'The Limits of the Welfare State', *New Left Review*, 1, 27, September–October 1964, 28–37, 29.

3

Expertise and experience: mothers' self-help

In 1978, journalist Esther Rantzen presented a BBC *Man Alive* documentary about postnatal depression, 'Baby Blues to Breakdown'. The *Man Alive* series drew a wide viewership and was known for addressing some of the moment's most pressing issues, but Rantzen could not have anticipated the 'deluge' of letters that this particular programme would provoke.[1] Mothers, it seemed, were keen to articulate their experiences and to connect with others who had shared the same struggles. Rantzen understood: she had been – unexpectedly, frighteningly – depressed following the birth of her first child. Neither was she one to sit back. The letters provided the impetus for the national spread of the Meet-a-Mum Association (MAMA), encouraged by Rantzen with the support of *Woman* magazine the following year.[2] MAMA aimed to bring new mothers together in small self-help groups to diminish depression, share experiences, and reduce loneliness.[3]

The association grew rapidly. Groups were soon to be found across the country, spanning from northern Scotland to South Wales. Local newspapers announced new groups and promoted existing ones, and in so doing acknowledged the breadth of maternal emotion, and gave voice to what mothers saw as the social circumstances that could give rise to maternal unhappiness. In 1979, the *Aberdeen Evening Express* covered the establishment of a local group and sympathetically explained, 'boredom and loneliness can often breed depression when a woman finds herself tied to the house with a small baby constantly making demands as her only companion for much of the day'.[4] In 1984, the founder of a group in South Wales told the local newspaper that new mothers struggled to disclose their distress:

They feel somehow that they will let themselves down by admitting that they feel depressed when they have a brand new, beautiful baby. They feel there's something missing within themselves. It's only when they start talking to other women with young babies that they realise that other people have exactly the same feelings at some time or another.[5]

By the late 1990s, MAMA had over seventy groups, and had published booklets, leaflets, and hosted a series of study days about postnatal depression, bringing together mothers with lived experience, medical practitioners, and researchers to share their expertise and perspectives.[6]

Rantzen was not finished, however, and in 1981, she appealed to pregnant viewers of the consumer programme *That's Life* to share their experiences of maternity care. The response to the survey was remarkable: in all, it gathered 6,000 responses.[7] The survey resulted in a two-part television programme, *That's Life – Having a Baby*, broadcast the following year, and a book, *The British Way of Birth*.[8] The book gave voice to some less palatable maternal feelings. Julia, for example, who was admitted to a mother-and-baby unit for psychological support, wrote that she felt, 'Terrible. I felt as if there was no point in living. I did not enjoy the baby at all'. Other women struggled with the isolation and relentless demands of early motherhood. Linda explained that, 'I used to be a person in my own right. Now all I am is somebody (or something) to feed, wash and change her'.[9] These explanations of experience were complemented by statistics. Of the 5,721 women who answered the survey's question about postnatal depression, 2,668 women reported feeling it 'a little', and 181 'a lot'. Moreover, these distressed mothers were not reliant on medical care, and many reported turning to a sources of support that were informal and non-medical; half of them identified mothers with shared experiences, or a friend or family member, as the best person to talk to.[10]

BBC documentaries; the development of MAMA groups; the thousands of mothers who responded to the *That's Life* survey; and the publication of a book that gave space to mothers' firsthand experiences: together these highlight three arguments that run through this chapter. First, I argue that mothers asserted agency in setting up groups that sought to address some of the social and political issues that exacerbated their emotional struggles: they understood postnatal depression and unhappy motherhood to benefit from *social* solutions. Second, I show that mothers' groups undertook political as well as emotional activism. Third, this chapter argues that mothers – some prominent, like Esther Rantzen, but many thousands more who lived 'ordinary' lives – drew upon their experiences, and indeed their ordinariness, to assert non-medical forms of authority around unhappy motherhood. As Claire Langhamer has shown, the category of 'ordinariness' performed political, affective and social work in the postwar years, and was both socially coveted and sociologically interrogated. It was also gendered, for as Langhamer explains, women were both more likely to feel themselves to be ordinary and were more likely to be perceived as ordinary. Moreover, the housewife embodied ordinariness *par excellence*.[11] While Langhamer focuses on the years immediately following the Second World War, 'ordinariness' retained its imaginative and rhetorical tug in the decades that followed. This ordinariness was frequently implicit, surfacing through shared cultural codes. Sometimes, though, it was made explicit, as when in 1989 one mother explained to the *Lincolnshire Standard* that the National Childbirth Trust (NCT) branch she was a part of was not full of 'weirdos or snobs' but was instead 'ordinary mothers who enjoy being part of a club and meeting other people with young children'.[12] Ordinariness was thus a bulwark against stigma and a defence against caricature. While the groups that mothers formed at the grassroots and promoted through local newspapers sometimes gave platforms to medical experts, they also contested, negotiated, and supplemented this with experiential knowledge. This chapter examines some of the ways that mothers used experiential knowledge to solidify new communities and share understandings about their experiences.

This chapter, therefore, explores some of the grassroots groups set up to address the challenges of motherhood and mothering. The organisations explored in this chapter, though distinct from one another, were created in a postwar world in which, as Lynn Abrams has written, women were discussing their feelings and undertaking a 're-imagining of the self' in quietly revolutionary ways.[13] Some of these, like the NCT, have been explored by historians before; others are less familiar.[14] In looking at these familiar and these less well-known groups, this chapter contributes to a wider historiographical project that examines women's self-help groups and housewives' associations as sites of growth and self-expression in postwar Britain.[15] These groups were, as Caitríona Beaumont says, 'multilayered' sites for the expression and the development of women's experiential expertise.[16] The groups explored in this chapter addressed a spectrum of negative maternal emotion, running from the mild and transient to the more serious and enduring. Some of these communities, like MAMA and the Association for Post-Natal Illness (APNI), specifically mobilised around postnatal depression; others were looser emotional coalitions, bringing women together to address a wider breadth of feelings, problems, and experiences. Other groups focused in particular on the practical and emotional struggles experienced by unmarried mothers.[17] The groups that worked explicitly around postnatal depression tended to build relationships with medical experts, whereas those that addressed a wider spectrum of distress adopted social approaches. The leaders of these organisations came from across the political spectrum and had a range of views on the feminist politics of the 1970s and 1980s. It is notable, though, that shared experience is the common thread through the various networks. These groups highlight the civic work done by distressed mothers in building support systems and community groups, as well as organising social action. This chapter is particularly attentive to the ways that unhappy mothers mobilised local newspapers as a communications infrastructure that both incidentally and deliberately emphasised their ordinariness. Further, this chapter turns to social survey responses from members of grassroots groups to examine how mothers explained their own discontent. These mothers used the opportunity presented by social science surveys to present a political as well as personal subjectivity, articulating the emotional struggles of new motherhood as products of the changing postwar world.

Self-help and the contradictions of the postwar world

While it has a longer history, self-help as a strategy and as a structure proliferated in Britain following the 1960s. This decade was, as the erstwhile editor of the *Guardian* newspaper's Women's

Page observed, the 'Do-It-Yourself Decade'.[18] Newspapers played an important role in the creation of this self-help culture. It was via *The Guardian*'s letter page, for example, that in 1960 women laid the groundwork for what would soon become the National Housewives Register (initially named the Housebound Wives Register, it changed its name in 1966, and then in 1987 it renamed itself the National Women's Register).[19] These groups were increasingly endorsed as important non-professional sources of social support. In 1978, the World Health Organisation's (WHO) Alma Ata Declaration emphasised individual, family, and community responsibility for health, prompting the European Regional Office of the WHO to stress the role of self-help groups in health promotion.[20] Backing for self-help also developed at a national level. In 1979, the Conservative Party Manifesto – as part of a broader ideology of state retrenchment from welfare provision – encouraged self-help groups, arguing that 'in the community, we must do more to help people to help themselves, and families to look after their own'.[21] The emphasis on self-help took place in 'the Lean Years' for the NHS.[22] The expansion of mothers' self-help groups should thus be read against a political backdrop that was increasingly oriented towards options that operated outside state-funded services. In some cases, mothers were explicit about the breach in state services that they were attempting to fill. In 1982, a mother involved in setting up a MAMA branch in the Scottish town of Peterhead told the *Aberdeen Evening Express* that her initial general practitioner had 36,000 patients on their list; a feeling that her care had been inadequate was a stimulus for establishing a branch of the self-help group.[23] However, while some groups saw themselves as meeting needs that welfare services could not, others were established in part to lobby the state for these needs.

By the end of the 1980s, self-help groups were widespread: in 1986, Stephen Lock, editor of the *British Medical Journal*, argued that self-help organisations constituted a 'fourth estate' in medicine.[24] There was, however, some debate about what self-help actually was.[25] Lock argued for a 'composite' definition:

> a voluntary organisation, usually of peers, who have come together for mutual help and support, in satisfying a common need, overcoming

a common handicap or life disrupting problem, and bringing about desired social or personal change, or both.[26]

This sharing of common experience was particularly important for discussions of motherhood. In 1988, psychotherapist and psychiatrist Jane Price argued that 'the company of other women of all ages' was 'the single most healthy resource for young mothers', yet society was structured in such a way that this network was not allowed to develop.[27] Within this atomised society, the infrastructure of self-help and grassroots organisations created new sites of emotional disclosure and personal growth.[28] These self-help groups were a part of the development of 'cultures of telling' in the 1960s and 1970s, part of what Lynn Abrams has persuasively framed as an 'expressive revolution'.[29] This revolution brought mothers together in a number of national and local organisations. Some of these, like APNI, were specifically oriented around serious unhappiness; others, like the NCT, addressed postnatal depression and milder forms of maternal unhappiness within a broader remit of interests; others, like Mothers in Action and the Working Association of Mothers (WAM), used mothers' struggles as evidence for the need to address structural social issues. But the groups had more than emotion in common. Despite their different aims, these diverse groups adopted similar approaches: they emphasised the value of mothers' networks and built communities, and through this, they acknowledged mothers' expertise that was derived from experience.

The NCT: experience and expertise

One source of support that was available to pregnant women and new mothers from 1956 was the NCT (initially titled the Natural Childbirth Association, it renamed itself in 1961). Established by Prunella Briance in response to the stillbirth of her daughter following a gravely mishandled hospital birth, the NCT began as an advertisement in the personal column of *The Times* newspaper on 4 May 1956: 'A natural childbirth association is to be formed for the promotion and better understanding of the Dick-Read System', the advertisement stated, referencing the advocate of fear-free, natural childbirth, obstetrician Grantly Dick-Read.[30] In 1957 the NCT held its first meeting, and in 1959 it hosted its first antenatal class. From there the organisation grew rapidly; by the early 1960s, it had established a formal structure, secured charitable status, and set up a central office, while at the grassroots level organisers had set about founding local branches. As Jenny Kitzinger has observed, the wider climate of the 1960s was conducive to the organisation's growth: anti-establishment feeling, intensifying consumer power, and increased emphasis on bodily rights created a climate amenable to its development. By 1968, its income had risen twelvefold from the start of the decade, reaching around £12,000 a year. Nearly two decades later, membership reached 40,000, with 320 branches supported by sixteen salaried staff members.[31] As this balance of membership to salaried staff and to lay teacher-led branches implies, though, the organisation rested heavily on the involvement and time of non-professional women. As Kitzinger notes, the centrality of lay teachers was not by design: they were originally seen as a temporary resource to be utilised until a sufficient number of medical antenatal teachers were trained in natural childbirth techniques. This never transpired, and lay leadership was soon seen to have benefits, with teachers represented as relatable and accessible to expectant women.[32] Its lay teachers were among the most ardent proponents of natural childbirth. In 1957, readers of the *Kent Messenger* were told by an advocate of the approach, Pamela Rice, that she had been prompted to research natural childbirth by her contrasting experience of two labours; one 'glorious' and one that made her feel that she was 'just another baby-producing machine'. The newspaper evidently expected some resistance to the piece, though, framing it as a 'challenging article by a Kent farmer's wife'.[33]

Some of this resistance came from health professionals, with whom the organisation mediated a relationship that was occasionally marred by mutual suspicion. Health professionals were liable to distrust what they saw as quackery, and women seeking natural childbirth in the late 1950s reported being dismissed as naive by midwives and doctors. In 1958, Lydia McCully, a teacher in Dumbarton, Scotland, was actively discouraged from pursuing the natural childbirth that she desired. Not easily dissuaded, she condemned what she saw as the 'slaphappy indifference to the emotional side of childbirth' in hospitals.[34] Despite the distrust of its approaches within hospitals, the NCT sought to cultivate close links with health professionals in the 1960s and supported the idea that doctors were the experts.[35] Although his methods and arguments were controversial within the medical community, it is notable that obstetrician and medical professional Grantly Dick-Read was the organisation's first president. That the NCT and mainstream medical practice could be amenable to one another was similarly underlined in newspaper coverage of the organisation and its grassroots groups. Area organiser Celia Booth set out her modest aspirations to the *Eastbourne Herald Chronicle*, reflecting that 'we don't want to tread on medical ground, but only to help. We hope that when inquiries are made, doctors who may be too busy to give detailed explanations will bear the association in mind'.[36] In a neighbouring area of the south coast, the *Worthing Herald* stressed the professional and personal qualifications of the local NCT antenatal teacher, Pat Pillow. Pillow was a mother of four, a nurse, and a certified midwife, the newspaper explained, and the NCT itself included doctors, midwives, and physiotherapists as well as parents.[37] The support of these professionals lent the organisation legitimacy it implied.

Despite the organisation's deference to medical professionals, its founder's conservative political sympathies (Briance was no natural political radical), and its fairly mainstream positioning, the NCT's interest in childbirth directly and obliquely challenged established norms. The 1959 Cranbrook Report and then the 1970 Peel Report both advanced the idea that hospitals were the appropriate site for childbirth, and encouraged an ever greater proportion of births to take place within their walls. But the 1950s to the 1980s were also the 'heyday' for the natural childbirth movement, and in the 1970s the feminist movement challenged the gendered dynamics of medical authority.[38] Thus questions about medicalisation, intervention, and pain management within childbirth became contentious and political issues in postwar Britain.[39] While seeking to emphasise its respectability and deference to doctors' expertise, the NCT's role in advocating for low-intervention and well-informed childbirths brought to the surface troubled issues around power, medical authority, and mothers' agency.[40] Given this, it is unsurprising that in the 1970s the organisation did not find easy alliances; as observed by Vivienne Welburn, the NCT was seen in this decade as radical by conservative doctors and conservative by feminist activists.[41] Nonetheless, it was significant that while advocating for 'natural' childbirth, educating women about what to expect while giving birth, and pushing against the tides of medicalisation – adopting the general principle 'mothering is not a problem to be solved' – the NCT enabled the dissemination of non-professional forms of expertise. This was a conflicted area for it: the organisation sought to distance itself from 'gossip' about childbirth, but its grassroots practice stimulated the discussion of women's first-hand experiences.[42]

It was within this vexed context that in the 1980s women reported mixed experiences of its antenatal classes. While some women found them inspiring and empowering, other women, perhaps intuiting the distrust between the NCT and the health service, found themselves dreading a hospital birth. As one woman reported to the *British Way of Birth* survey, NCT classes 'gave you much more confidence in your own ability and helped you realise that you must stand up for what you want for your baby – within reason. However, sadly it made me feel that the hospital could be more of an enemy than a friend and I dreaded my labour'. But the NCT was not alone in offering antenatal courses; the NHS, too, invited pregnant women to attend classes. The lay expertise of the NCT may have compared favourably to the professional expertise offered in these. One mother told the *British Way of Birth* survey that her NHS classes 'would have been better if they had been given by women who had experienced childbirth and not by middle-aged spinsters'. Others also favoured the NCT classes, reflecting that its classes had 'a more informal attitude and encouraged more discussion'. But the NHS classes had a major advantage over the NCT classes – access to real babies, and tours of relevant hospital units.[43]

It was in postnatal care that experiential expertise came into its own. Members emphasised the value of mothers leaning on one another for support. One particular advocate was Margaret Dennis, a member of the organisation's Oxford Post-Natal Support Group. Dennis had experienced severe postnatal depression following the birth of her second baby and was keen to normalise the struggles of early parenthood, which she did in a short, bright pink handbook. She drew specific attention to postnatal depression, informing readers that concern about it was so widespread that expectant mothers might erroneously anticipate distress as a natural consequence of childbirth. Such anxieties were overblown, she suggested, for proportionally few women did experience postnatal depression, but it was nonetheless important to seek help if needed. This help could be medical, but a support group could be invaluable, she suggested, urging readers to

> talk about how you feel – if not to your husband or to an existing friend, then to someone in your local Support Group... Do remember you are not alone: probably there is another new mother living quite near you who feels just the same, and just as guilty. Sharing feelings like these can put them into perspective; and you may help someone else by confessing these thoughts to her.[44]

Other women agreed, and postnatal branches proliferated. By the mid-1970s, it was felt within NCT headquarters that these branch-level support groups required co-ordination and in 1977 a postnatal co-ordinator was recruited. The need for new guidelines, initially published as the *Guidelines for Postnatal Support*, stimulated the formation of a Postnatal Working Party in 1979. The success of the working party resulted in the establishment of the Postnatal Committee.[45] In the 1980s the organisation recognised that its postnatal provision had moved towards 'mothers befriending other mothers' in branch-level support groups. These aimed to 'break isolation, knowing that it's ok to talk babies or not talk babies with someone who understands from recent experience'.[46]

Three years after its establishment, the Postnatal Committee oversaw the publication of its pamphlet *Mothers Talking about Postnatal Depression*, which aimed to reassure those close to new mothers that although postnatal depression was not wholly unusual, it was not to be readily expected. It should, however, be taken seriously, it urged. The pamphlet explained that the symptoms of distress were numerous and varied, and that mothers might successfully hide their feelings from their families, doctors, and health visitors. Introducing the pamphlet, the Postnatal Committee's chair, Liz Waumsley suggested that the impetus for the booklet came from a demand for more information about postnatal depression among those 'involved in the care and support of new mothers and their families', and emphasised the value of mothers' own testimonies.

While some of the booklet might seem 'harrowing', she warned, 'all those who contributed the personal accounts did so because they felt that they would be helpful for other people to read'.⁴⁷ The pamphlet was largely given over to women's testimony, allowing the women to, as Hilary Marland has observed, describe in their own words their experiences and explanations.⁴⁸

Other NCT publications likewise created platforms for mothers to share their experiences and challenges; for instance, in the 1980s, the NCT released a booklet on disabled mothers' experiences featuring the voices of several disabled women, whose accounts were often moving, including one mother with polio who reflected that

> coming home, that was devastating... neither of us knew what to do with her and the fact that she cried an awful lot and I was so tired... Everything just seemed to be a very long dark tunnel that I couldn't see any way out of.

Another disabled mother reported that 'I felt dreadful; and I couldn't cope... I wouldn't go through it again for anything'.⁴⁹ In its creation, though, the booklet reflected the broader social shift toward self-expression in postwar Britain and highlighted the therapeutic benefits of having these experiences recognized, noting that the interviews themselves had been construed as valuable by the self-selected respondents.⁵⁰ Mothers, then, embraced opportunities to share their struggles, and were seen to find the process of expressing their experiences validating and useful.

Where were these struggling mothers to go for support? Dr Desmond Bardon, psychiatric advisor to the NCT (and a member of the Association for Improvements in the Maternity Services, and the Association of Radical Midwives),⁵¹ was pessimistic about state-led care and argued that social support had an important role to play. 'I know that women must support each other in these anxious situations', he wrote, for 'Health is only marginally in the gift of doctors'.⁵² The 'pooled opinion of a number of experienced women who can offer love and all sorts of support to a depressed mother may be much safer for her than the fashionable or deep-seated prejudices of either a well-meaning or hostile professional', he explained.⁵³ Mothers seemed to agree. The mothers in *Mothers Talking* were particularly critical of their general practitioners. 'Hilary' reported that she had 'come to realise, quite surprisingly, that general practitioners seem to know little about postnatal depression and sometimes cannot even recognise the illness, let alone prescribe effective treatment'.[54] 'Carol' visited her general practitioner feeling exhausted and ill, and was tested for any physical root causes but, when these tests proved fruitless, was told she was a 'puzzle', and that 'it would probably pass and that I should just plod on'.[55] Such complaints about interactions with health professionals were levied against overlapping backgrounds: an emphasis on self-help had emerged in the 1960s that facilitated the assertion and development of experiential expertise, and created new possibilities for self-advocacy and articulation outside the medical model; the expanding availability of antidepressants, as noted in Chapter 1, had led to a sense that a prescription was a likely outcome of a meeting with a health professional; the feminist critique of medicine as a bastion of patriarchal power, developed during the 1970s, had disseminated new critical approaches to the profession. Moreover, at this point in the 1980s, it was widely apparent that the NHS was experiencing intersecting financial pressures, and while the public still held the service in great affection, by the close of the decade the strain on the NHS was such that political mood around it was 'thoroughly gloomy'.[56]

It was in this context – one in which medical expertise and provision was often found to fall short, and that the ethos of 'self-help' was rising – that mothering groups and mother-to-mother supportive contacts flourished. Such an approach was endorsed by the NCT. Attending a mother-and-baby group could help a mother 'escape from her own four walls, and could ease her loneliness and benefit her children', advised *Mothers Talking*. For unhappy mothers for whom group settings were inappropriate one-to-one support might instead be beneficial, the guide suggested, especially if the supporter had themselves experienced postnatal depression.[57] This emphasis on the value of shared understanding and experience was reiterated in mothers' testimony. One contributor to the pamphlet, Margaret, underlined that 'What I desperately needed was someone to talk to who had been through the same thing... Friends can be sympathetic but of no real practical help if they haven't had depression as they just can't understand'.[58] Another, Ann, reflected that 'I do wish I could have talked to someone who'd also experienced postnatal depression, without fear of being labelled'. Julia agreed, arguing that 'what I feel I really needed during that bad time, was just someone to talk to who understood that there was something wrong'.[59] Waumsley, who introduced *Mothers Talking*, discussed her own experiences of postnatal depression and the ways it helped her to support other mothers:

> It seems that someone like me, who has herself experienced it and can be an understanding and constructive listener, will often be welcomed in addition to existing friends and 'supporters'. Perhaps it is too much effort sometimes, or seems too boring, to describe to family and friends how you feel; and perhaps someone who knows without being told can help best during a particularly bad patch.

The value of this mother-to-mother postnatal support, Waumsley argued, was its non-professional nature. NCT postnatal support networks provided 'warm, friendly, caring and natural human relationships'.[60] It was 'loving, uncritical acceptance' and 'encouragement' that would help distressed mothers. 'More than anything', *Mothers Talking* suggested, 'she needs other people to "mother" her, and to listen to her'.[61] This warmth and receptiveness made postnatal groups useful for mothers whose experiences erred towards the milder ends of the emotional spectrum as well as those who identified with the label of postnatal depression. In 1986, for example, mothers on the outskirts of Glasgow, in East Kilbride (a new town, designated in 1945), were told by their local newspaper that the local NCT branch was a source of support for lonely and exhausted mothers who lacked support networks as well as those with postnatal depression.[62]

Despite the advocacy of the NCT and its branches some hesitancy about the utility of self-help in addressing unhappy motherhood remained. As Maggie Comport, advice columnist for *Chat* magazine, wrote in 1987, mothers' self-help groups were 'often seen as second-best to professional aid – appealing to only one class of woman, limited in usefulness to mild cases of [postnatal depression], a back-up for correct medical treatment, or a last resort... Sometimes groups are condemned outright as a load of meddling amateurs'.[63] While the NCT attempted to rebuff these critiques, the organisation was acutely aware that it had a predominantly middle-class membership and a reputation for eccentricity: at a

MAMA study day in the early 1990s, the chair of the Leighton Buzzard branch of the NCT attempted to distance the organisation from the stereotype of its members as 'over informed, middle class cranks who wear Laura Ashley frocks, drive 2CVs, eat vegeburgers and drink herbal tea at coffee mornings', and assured attendees that the organisation did not in fact recommend to expectant mothers that they should 'object violently to all forms of pain relief other than cubes of frozen grape juice, natural sponges and spirited renditions of *Ten Green Bottles* at the height of a contraction'.[64] But stereotypes are difficult to shift, and the financial cost of attending an NCT-run antenatal group embedded its association with the middle-classes. If ease of participation was limited by class, it was less constrained by geography. By the late 1980s, NCT postnatal groups could be found from Caerphilly in Wales to Newcastle, England, and beyond.[65]

The NCT had other limits, though. When journalists and women's magazine editors Deirdre Sanders and Jane Reed set out to investigate women's experiences in the 1980s, they heard from Rosalind, who found herself 'sitting in this two-up two-down place looking at the four walls going bananas, thinking I've got to get out, what am I going to do' after the birth of her daughter. Her local NCT branch was 'marvellous' but was 'not really stimulating'; it was re-entering paid work that made her feel 'so much better'.[66] The growth of mothers' self-help groups, then, was encouraged by deficiencies in medical support and driven by mothers' belief in the value of their lived experience. Nonetheless, they were sometimes the conduit to rather than the endpoint of respite from unhappiness.

Mothers in Action: politics, expertise, and self-organisation

So, too, did acknowledging the changing composition of families, as lone motherhood became increasingly visible and widespread following divorce law reform at the end of the 1960s. The NCT was not established to advocate for these families, and much of its literature was predicated on the assumption that families would primarily comprise of nuclear, married, heterosexual couples. But other organisations stepped into this breach and mothers established groups that raised the profile of the issues that closely pertained to their lives. The work of these broader organisations draws attention to three arguments made in this chapter. First, the acknowledgement of unhappiness and emotional wellbeing played out in discussions of living standards, mobilising emotions as evidence of the need for structural change. Second, mothers' organising was political activism. Third, expertise was derived from experience within these groups, demonstrating the value accorded to non-professional forms of knowledge.

One such example of an organisation was Mothers in Action, founded in 1967 by five 'unsupported' mothers. This language reflected the enduring power of the model of the nuclear family in which the man was the financial provider, but it also reflected the isolation that women mothering alone experienced. In 1968, its constitution set out the aim of the group as 'to press for the best possible status for unsupported mothers and their children', though by 1972, this was amended to 'one parent families regardless of race, religion or nationality'.[67] Despite this change – which ostensibly made the group inclusive to lone fathers – the group remained closely focused on the issues that affected lone mothers. Before it discontinued its membership structure in 1972, 'ordinary' membership of the pressure group was only open to unsupported mothers, which included single mothers, divorced and separated mothers, widowed mothers, and mothers whose husbands were unable to work, while 'associate' membership was open to any others.[68] It abolished its membership structure in order to retain its identity as a 'radical pressure group'.[69] Before this, the group had attracted over 200 members in the London area.[70] It aimed, it said, to 'represent the views of the consumer'.[71] The group was founded on three beliefs: that every mother had the right to keep her child and to raise them in 'decent conditions'; that mothers had the right to choose to work, and should not need to worry about the quality of childcare while doing so; and that unsupported mothers were 'ordinary women with ordinary children' and deserved social acceptance.[72] Its aims contained some overlap with Gingerbread, another organisation that worked to improve the situation of lone parents. Rather than working in competition, the two organisations attempted to come to a consensus about how their work could complement one another.[73]

One of Mothers in Action's early campaigns was a letter-writing campaign in 1968 around the shortage of day nurseries, an issue that would remain of enduring interest. Mothers in Action not only pointed to the flaws in the existing system – particularly highlighting the difficulties that it posed for low-income mothers and criticising the enduring influence of Bowlby's ideas about the impact of maternal deprivation – but also put forward a number of proposals to improve and address the lack of affordable, flexible, and good quality childcare for young children.[74] Those campaigning for state-provided childcare in the 1960s and 1970s faced an uphill battle, as there was limited political will to make progressive change to the status quo.[75] The organisation developed factsheets about the kinds of childcare available for children under five years old.[76]

Childcare was not the only area of agitation, however: the organisation campaigned in a number of areas to improve the lives of single mothers, proposing legal reforms, local authority-provided accommodation ('not in separate blocks!'), housing reform, residential jobs, longer nursery hours, provision of play centres for schoolchildren during holidays and after school, more education and training opportunities for single mothers, an unsupported mothers' allowance, and tax reform so that nurseries and childminders were not paid for from taxed income. The organisation also campaigned around pregnant women's and working mothers' rights.[77] In 1970, the organisation held a march to Downing Street on the issue of housing for lone mothers – even delivering a doll in a shoebox to the Minister for Housing to symbolise the plight of the homeless child – and in 1972, it revised its housing sheet to note that 'Housing, or lack of it, is probably the biggest single cause of human misery in our society', a misery that particularly afflicted unsupported mothers.[78] In 1974, it again drew up a plan for housing, noting the despondency that precarious or unsatisfactory housing created for single mothers.[79]

Mothers in Action gave members a platform to articulate their own experiences.[80] Shirley Frost, a founder of the organisation, called her invitation to address a conference organised by Oxfordshire Children's Department in September 1969 'something of a breakthrough'. 'An amateur with a captive audience of professionals is something of a rarity', she observed. But Frost was not an amateur on her own experience, and she eloquently set out her own situation. She was a single mother of a four-year-old son living on supplementary benefits. Frost's financial situation was precarious:

If I buy toys, clothes, stocking, magazines or cigarettes; visit the cinema, take my son on an outing, buy birthday presents, have my hair cut, my shoes mended and my clothes cleaned I either have to cut down on food or I get into debt. Because I haven't a refrigerator and I need food on a small scale I waste nearly as much as I eat... I would like you to see the letters I receive from mothers who are saddened because they cannot provide many things for their children which others have. This is where the sense of deprivation comes in.[81]

The following year, Frost drew upon her own experiences at a symposium organised by the National Council for the Unmarried Mother and her Child. 'I think I am right in saying that history is being made here today; to have a mother speaking to you from the platform is a new departure, though not an entirely unexpected one', she began, 'I think it is only right that you should hear from both the administrators and the consumers of social services'. The talk was based on 'my own experiences as a mother, my members' experiences, and publications of one sort or another', she explained. As such, it was 'neither exhaustive nor scientific but I hope it will stimulate thought and activity on this very contemporary problem – substitute care for children of all ages'. Frost was forthright: single mothers were taxpayers and should not be seen as a burden; the care of children was a social good; supporting single mothers was necessary because 'people are still the most valuable and precious commodity that we have'; people did not start off equal, so measuring individual contributions was pointless and punitive; and withholding support for single mothers – who, she said, shared the same concerns as other mothers, but in more acute ways – could only stem from a moral objection 'and as such will not be tolerated for very much longer'.[82] The campaigning work of Mothers in Action, while not oriented around unmarried mothers' feelings, was nonetheless based upon values that emphasised their full humanity.

The Working Association of Mothers, loneliness, class and feminism

WAM was founded in May 1969 by Diana Priestley, a mother of two young children. Until the birth of her first child, Priestley had 'an interesting and stimulating life' as a nurse and then within advertising for *New Society*; it was her own experience of the transition from paid work to full-time mothering that inspired Priestley to establish WAM, a self-help co-operative.[83] WAM set out to address the problems of housebound mothers through practical action, including playgroups, holiday play centres, a part-time employment agency for mothers, coffee mornings, a babysitting service, and discussion groups. WAM's archival documents contain a folder for sources of personal inspiration: this folder contains letters from Grahame Leman, a sympathetic management consultant, and a single book: Hannah Gavron's sociological study, *The Captive Wife*, suggesting that sociology helped to inspire self-help.

WAM began after the National Suggestions Centre (one of several organisations founded by sociologist and activist Michael Young) supported Priestley's idea of a co-operative of working mothers. After the idea was featured in the magazine *WHAT?*, press coverage arrived 'thick and fast'.[84] Coverage emphasised the association's moderate aims. *The Times*, for example, wrote that the hope of WAM was to 'release women to work part time and relieve them for a few hours to visit the dentist or the hairdresser, or prepare for a new career'.[85] The idea gained attention beyond the south of England, and regional and city newspapers helped to promote the association. The *Liverpool Echo* noted the creation of WAM as aspiring to 'help women escape from the mentally stultifying life of children and chores' but warned that it hoped it did not lead to 'BASH!', the Bedraggled Association of Suffering Husbands.[86] *The Birmingham Daily Post* affirmed that Priestley's idea had likely entered the minds of legions of mothers before her, all of whom might have suspected that 'united, women could give each other a break and maintain the individuality of the mother to the benefit of the family and that, divided, we fall under the 24-hour tyranny which produces isolation and destroys confidence'. Priestley disputed the idea that the housebound mother was the good mother, arguing that it was the quality of the relationship that was important. Informed and engaged mothers were more likely to be able to cope 'when you think you will go barmy', she said. Housework was not an effective distraction, for it 'can become an obsession... it should not be a day's job but something to do efficiently and fast. If you enjoy doing home-based things you are fortunate rather than virtuous'.[87] Similar ideas appeared in newspapers north of the border. In December 1969, Priestley was featured in the *Aberdeen Press and Journal*, which praised her approach as showing 'the calm of a born organiser and the enthusiasm of a liberated young mum'. Priestley told the paper that 'Mothers have a great deal to give to the community, if only they could get out and give it. Usually they can't get out, because there are no facilities for having their children looked after. The British haven't come to terms with what they mean by working mothers'. Paid work was not detrimental to the family, for 'when mothers suffer from the isolation of being housebound then their children suffer as well'.[88] It is important that mothers' freedoms were defended as beneficial for the whole family in these articles – a rhetorical device that explicitly feminist organisations would resist – but this mobilisation of children's wellbeing was nonetheless used to further women's aspirations towards greater liberty.

The major movement emphasising women's shared problems was, at this moment, women's liberation, but WAM kept its distance. Attendees at a meeting in 1969 were told that the group's aim was 'practical action and not militancy'[89] and a meeting of the Pinner Young Conservatives that it had no connection with women's liberation. Despite this emphasis on moderation, Priestley told the Conservative meeting that the co-operative's 'intention is to show that changing patterns in work, education, housing and family living have brought isolation and conflict to many women, and to find ways of re-integrating them into society'.[90] Priestley was aware that the need for such a group stemmed from breaches in state and social provision. In 1971, Priestley explained that WAM aimed to address 'some of the gaps left by our Social Services... I think the formation of groups of people who want to help each other and their community is an urgent necessity now when the state and local authorities cannot and/or will not provide this help'.[91] Where national policy was lacking, some local councils helped to support WAM's services: in Twickenham, for example, a holiday play centre was supported by a small grant from the council.[92] Leman was also aware of the ways in which WAM addressed needs that society might, in other contexts, meet. 'In a small village in the old days, all this and everything you do would have happened automatically', he wrote to her in 1970. 'What you are trying to do, in effect, is to re-create village conditions in the suburban desert'. Such an approach was not going to be without its risks, he warned; 'In doing this sort of thing, you are of course poaching on professional preserves and may frighten the pros'.[93]

It was, however, the self-help nature of WAM that positioned it as an object of national interest. In July 1969, Leman wrote to the features editor of the *Telegraph* weekly magazine to suggest a feature on WAM, suggesting that it 'might be given a unique slant by handling it primarily *as an example of self-help*'. Leman had become interested in self-help through his role as an executive of the National Council on Alcoholism and argued that '*most* social problems, from small things like dental caries to big things like mental illness, can be solved *only* by self-help, and *only* if [Her Majesty's Government], foundations, and charities stop trying to support only full-blast paternalist solutions and adopt the more cost-effective policy of subsidising professional help for self-help organisations'. On this 'larger theme of self-help versus paternalism', he wrote, 'I have a sort of private sense of mission about getting self-help taken more seriously than it is'.[94] Leman encountered little success with the *Telegraph Magazine*, but WAM did attain some national coverage via newspapers and a BBC interview, and yet more in local newspapers. This coverage did not inevitably lead to funding, however, and in August 1970, Leman warned Priestley that the 'problem of imprisoned young mums' was not likely to be seen as a 'very important one – relative to many other unsolved problems'. He urged her not to give up hope but to remember that the struggle was because she was trying to accomplish something.[95] WAM was indeed working on multiple fronts.

Just a few months after the co-operative's launch, Priestley's branch of WAM in Richmond had over 100 members on a register of women who wanted part-time work, and a branch in Harrow had gathered 60 women onto its register, a sign that, as Priestley said, 'WAM had succeeded in making women who felt isolated by their own family problems aware of the fact that their problems were shared by many other women'.[96] Soon groups operated across the country, and its newsletter reflected the many different practical, investigatory, and campaigning activities that these local groups undertook. The newsletter, *wam news*, also provided space for members to correspond about their experiences. In 1970, a mother wrote in, warmly endorsing the Workers' Educational

Association (WEA) as a way to 'rehabilitate' after having a baby: 'I was not a born mother and after a long love affair with an interesting and lucrative career, I couldn't cope with being an over-30 Mum'. Knowing no one in her local area, she felt 'lonely and cut off' – a situation remedied when her health visitor recommended a coffee morning, where she met an 'enterprising mum' who had established a WEA group, 'a social gathering with a purpose'.[97] The next issue's front page urged readers to 'dispense with the GUILT'. The article pointed to the multiple, contradictory ways that mothers were made to feel like failures and told readers that 'if you feel strongly about these issues then let's hear about it, here, on these pages'. This, the newsletter argued,

> is really what WAM is trying to do. We have to seek out attitudes which prevent women from having freedom of choice, as individuals, to use their talents or abilities in the way that they think is best for themselves and their families.[98]

WAM, then, was both action-focused – organising babysitting services, an employment agency, children's play groups, coffee mornings, and research reports into children's play facilities, among other activities – and also provided a site for mothers to explore the ways that they navigated mothering.[99] This activity brought the organisation to the attention of the Tavistock Institute of Human Relations.

In 1971, two representatives from the Tavistock – Patrick Quinn and Elliot Stern – attended a WAM meeting. The Tavistock was, they explained, 'especially interested in grass roots movements springing directly from community needs, how they develop and how they can influence policy'. Research was, they said, currently focusing on family needs and social planning – and it was here that WAM could potentially be involved in the research programme.[100] The outcome of this interest was a survey of members of WAM's Brighton branch.

This survey was far from the first social science study of women's understandings of their lives. Indeed, Helen McCarthy has pointed to the 1960s as a 'wider social-survey "moment" amongst graduate and professional women, who were increasingly enlisted in the production of new, social-scientific, knowledge about themselves'.[101]

This survey culture is a background against which mothers' responses to the Tavistock study should be read. As McCarthy observes, through 'attending to the particular kind of introspection and performance prompted by the social-scientific enquiry, we can explore this body of material as comprising an intimate archive of feeling'.[102] The mothers who responded with a self-conscious awareness of class, and their positioning of struggles as outcomes of social change rather than personal fallibilities, should thus be read as part of a culture of socially situated self-reflection among middle-class women that the survey itself played an active role in cultivating. Moreover, the survey offered an opportunity for self-construction. As McCarthy has argued, professional women's organisations were 'gripped by a peculiar kind of survey fever' in the early to mid-1960s: these surveys, she shows, 'purported to describe the realities of women's work and family lives, but the image they reflected prized personal characteristics such as determination, courage and ambition, alongside the capacity to organize, delegate and manage and discipline the feminine self'.[103] The survey here gave respondents the opportunity to demonstrate other personal attributes: social acumen, proactive personal agency, and self-understanding. The Tavistock WAM study, then, allowed mothers to articulate their emotional lives while also constructing a selfhood that stood as a bulwark against its vicissitudes. Put another way, the survey created an opportunity for member-mothers to observe the negative experiences that drove them into the group while underlining the proactive steps they had taken to mitigate them: this affirmed an enterprising management of self.

The survey sought to understand WAM's membership, what members wanted or gained from the group, and how membership might address individuals' needs. A common thread in the responses was the role of the association in addressing loneliness. As Fred Cooper has shown, loneliness was a widespread feature of broader postwar anxieties about life stages and living conditions, as well as a core constituent of particularly gendered anxieties among medical practitioners about the mental condition of housewives.[104] It was also a theme in sociological studies, described by Ann Oakley in 1974 as an 'occupational hazard for the modern housewife,' a conclusion that reinforced Hannah Gavron's earlier observation that social isolation was prevalent among young mothers.[105] Mothers' responses to the

WAM study demonstrate that this climate of anxiety had permeated their self-descriptions of their emotional experiences. Perhaps it had become an acceptable language within which distress and malaise could be expressed and action legitimised; perhaps it was the most accurate language that mothers could reach for to self-diagnose the conditions of raising young children. Undoubtedly, though, loneliness was a significant emotional frame for WAM members. One mother, for example, responded to the survey that she joined the Brighton group due to 'the feeling of loneliness on being in a strange area with a small child – I saw this as a way to get to know people'. Another responded that it was prompted by a 'Realisation of lack of contact locally', while another wrote that it was 'Birth of a second child accompanied by feeling of being confined to the home'; 'Loneliness', wrote another; 'Arrival of first child and subsequent isolation at home'; 'Just a feeling of isolation and being tied to the house'. Another offered a more extended analysis: 'We moved to this area 5 months ago, and after 3 months I didn't know anybody. Neighbours were unfriendly and with only a young baby for company I was lonely, depressed and bored. My husband read about WAM in the local paper and encouraged me to give it a try'. This sense of isolation rings through the responses: 'Being in a state of social and mental isolation, solely with young children', wrote one mother. Another mother explained that she had removed herself from paid employment, moved area, and struggled to find appropriate childcare, all of which led to loneliness: 'I had left work to have a baby and was living in a new neighbourhood. I was feeling very isolated and welcomed meeting other mothers and their children. Babysitters were hard to find and proved expensive'. This isolation caused practical as well as emotional problems: one mother could not even go to the dentist.[106] WAM members in Brighton were not alone in experiencing this loneliness; loneliness and boredom have also emerged as themes in oral histories with wider constituencies of working-class women.[107]

The benefits of WAM membership were multiple for these mothers, although most respondents reflected that social contact had been the most valuable part of joining the group. For some mothers, it had assisted a personal transformation: 'I felt more confident – part of the community. I was happier. It gave me more contact with people. I saw my problems more in perspective. The responsibility of child care was shared with others. Things happened during the week. Life was less inevitable and monotonous'.[108] Another mother wrote that she had 'met other young mothers who lived nearby. Got to know them well enough to call in for a chat. Lost feeling of isolation. Helped to feel part of the community'. Another mother wrote that 'it gave the reassurance that one's lack of human contact was more due to social situation than to some personal failing – which gave the confidence to change the situation'. Another mother wrote that it 'Provided a continuing structure of social introductions – and making WAM work extended one mentally and physically, putting the previously overwhelming child/domestic situation in a better personal balance. Also became thus less self-oriented, which is mentally healthier!' The effect on identity was as important: 'the friends I made were the first since I became a mother who were in just the same position as myself – graduate kitchen-sink mums. Therefore self respect and identity raised considerably'. Joining had made one woman 'feel a little less housebound, still a human being, and problems smaller because you find other women have similar views'.[109]

WAM was not representative of mothers as a whole – something that members acknowledged. Asked about the 'typical' WAM member, respondents to the Brighton survey repeatedly acknowledged the middle-class, and often progressive, orientation of the group ('well educated, left-wing politically, liberated socially', wrote one respondent), although some put forward more expansive definitions: 'A person with children in need of help', wrote in one woman. The middle-class domination of the group was not accepted uncritically by members, and several members suggested that it could be more effective if it were more inclusive of working-class mothers. 'I think it is too middle-class in approach to be of much use to people from working-class backgrounds', wrote one respondent to the survey. 'Members have a social conscience but very little understanding from experience of what it is like to be hard up'. Another respondent expressed a similar frustration: 'More publicity and canvassing to bring WAM to notice of needy mothers & not just vegetating middle class mums, often frustrated "domestic" graduates'.[110] This dominance of graduates was perhaps overstated. It is, of course, likely that there was some regional variation between the branches – the Brighton branch may well have had a greater preponderance of graduates, but of the 100 women who joined Diana Priestley's late 1960s register of those who wanted part-time work in Richmond, twenty-five were graduates.[111] This is roughly in line with the proportion of women entering higher education in the 1960s: as Carol Dyhouse has shown, the proportion of female students remained relatively stable until the late 1960s to early 1970s, at which point women slowly began to make up more than a quarter of the university student population.[112]

Caitríona Beaumont has argued for the uncoupling of the term 'women's movement' from its association with feminism, underlining that between the 1920s and the 1960s mainstream and conservative women's organisations – while endorsing domesticity as women's primary role – played an important role in shaping women's citizenship and political participation.[113] The mothers' organisations that were established in and following the late 1960s should be seen within the same frame. While some – by no means all – held explicitly feminist views, others offered political opportunities that contributed to a more broadly defined women's movement. Some WAM members were active in or were sympathetic to the feminist movement of the 1970s, but others undertook political action in ways that sought to improve women's lives without directly using the frameworks of women's liberation. Of course, some mothers joined WAM through a sense that the organisation complemented their politics. 'I became interested in positive action/co-operation among women after reading some WL [Women's Liberation] writings', wrote a member. She was not alone as a feminist WAM member in Brighton: at least four other survey members responded that they were also in women's liberation groups.[114]

Some political action was direct. WAM members, for example, agitated around issues that affected mothers and children. In May 1972, vans – into which mothers and toddlers were crammed – travelled to Westminster to join a 'toddlers' Demo' for better play and educational facilities for under-fives. The demonstration and petition, handed to Margaret Thatcher, then Minister for Education and Science, was organised by the National Campaign for Nursery Education and Renée Short MP.[115] Diana Priestley attended the march with her children. Upon arrival, 'the children fell into line as if they attended demonstrations frequently. Their faces took on a slightly stern look. Yes, it was definitely their demonstration – they looked with brotherly feeling at all the other children wearing badges and signs, and surged ahead with determination'. An elderly woman started a chant – 'more nursery schools NOW!' – that was taken up intermittently by the crowd; Joel, Priestley's toddler son, wearing a miner's helmet, joined in: 'he roared, as any true miner would. "MORE nursery schools NOW!"'. The petition was given to Thatcher as she hurried to a meeting she declared to be 'frightfully important'. The march disbanded. Toilets were not forthcoming, and Joel urinated between a Bentley and a Rolls Royce; Priestley's daughter, who also needed to wee, was held over a drain.

Reflecting on the day, Priestley rued that it had likely not achieved its aims:

> I sensed the barrier that had not been broken through. The barrier between those who accepted the need, in terms of theory and research, and brought the argument down to cash, and those who saw small children as individuals with startling originality and razor-edge minds so easily trammelled by conditioned adults. Crushed by long hours gazing at the world out of high windows; or by tidy mind-the-flowers gardens, keep-off-the-grass parks, don't-touch shops, be-quiet-someone's-asleep flats, you'll-dirty-your-nice-dress parties, I've-just-cleaned-that-floor mums.
>
> Would our brave new world of more nursery schools now fulfil our dreams of countless children playing and working together in light airy spacious carefree places built for them? Or would it turn sour, with inadequate buildings, overcrowded classes, long waiting lists [?][116]

The march did not achieve its aims: provision for under-fives and their parents continued to be under-resourced. Joel did, however, get the last line in *The Surrey Comet*'s newspaper coverage. Pictured on the front page, sitting alongside five serious toddlers bearing placards ('DON'T FORGET ME!' said one board) and handmade protest t-shirts, Joel told the paper that they were 'going to London for a demonstration. We're going to get some seesaws for the children who haven't got any'.[117] Neither WAM members, nor their children, should have their politics underestimated.

Mothers within WAM also took a global view of politics. Asked about the contemporary major problems facing women, one woman wrote that

Assuming that women today (and their families) are reasonably housed, fed, and so on, I would say that over-population, pollution and the arms race are the major problems. None of them stare us in the face at this moment, but they will, very soon. These problems face the whole world, of course, but Western women (i.e. excluding those in the Third World, who struggle to survive) have to learn to make themselves think about these complex and overwhelming problems and try to do something about them. When one has a home and a family, it's very easy to use them as an excuse not to face these problems, and of course we have all been conditioned to the idea that our leaders (usually men) know best.[118]

Perhaps unsurprisingly, though, given the context of the survey, the majority of respondents commented on the challenges that faced women while mothering young children. This, too, had political roots, however, and respondents pointed to both patriarchal norms and capitalist values as exacerbating mothers' problems. 'Lack of provision of Day nurseries and Creches… Bad pay. Discrimination against women: people's attitudes to working mothers & wives', commented one respondent. Others were franker in their assessment. 'MEN!' wrote one respondent, and

RECREATION (lack of) intelligent active women tied to a home and small children. Loneliness in the home. Overwork for those who do break lose [sic] because their husbands usually expect a perfect home, dinner and well behaved children after a day's work. Most men seen seem unable to share responsibilities or to accept the needs of a woman for self expression outside the home.[119]

Another reflected that she did not know if women faced greater challenges than in the past but suggested that perhaps

we are more aware of them and that follows for menkind as well – problems of society, alienation and other by-products of capitalism. Women at home can become very isolated and those going out to work face the problem of 'oles' and sometimes end up doing all house work and a 9–5 shift, and I think it's ofetn [sic] difficult – particularly for young girls to be acceptably 'permissive'.

While expectations around married women's paid work and independence had expanded, respondents noted, ideas about domestic responsibility had not kept pace. One respondent pointed to the 'generally accepted idea that a woman should be able to work so as not to lead a "cabbage like" existence, yet still keep home and family immaculate, and keep up hobbies and interests of her own'. Another respondent concurred:

> Coming to terms with the social changes. We are still torn between our conventional Housewife, Mother in the home outlook, and yet pressures economically are for her to go out and maingtin [sic] a 'happy' family as well. the women who does not work is often called a parasite by her husband and society. and yet for the women [sic] who works, her financial rewards hardly warrant the strain of a job. Also, facilities for children to be minded are non-existent.

While these responses point to sympathy with the drivers of the women's liberation movement, feminism was also seen as a cause of potential tensions for mothers. A respondent held the women's movement responsible for causing women additional anxiety: 'guilt feelings among "housewives" due to "Women's Lib" pressure to work', they wrote. While ideas about women's liberation were, then, sometimes raised sympathetically, these ideas could clash with both the under-resourcing of childcare and the belief in the potential rewards of childrearing.

Other mothers saw the major challenges that faced women as being due to changing social, cultural, and economic patterns. Geographical mobility, for example, was held responsible for mothers' isolation, while contradictory attitudes towards mothers' work resulted in emotional conflicts. 'A more mobile society means more newcomers to an area – a group that are automatically isolated and can easily remain so for a long time, especially mothers at home with pre-school children', wrote one survey respondent. 'The change in society's attitudes to (a) children (b) women's employment means that many mothers feel vaguely guilty about having children at all, and specifically, staying at home "cabbaging" rather than earning their own living – very difficult to do when children are very young', she continued. Another mother reflected that

> The trend seems to be that women move away from their home towns because of husband's job etc. they no longer have the support and

> help of their parents and family and feel isolated. The pressures, put on women today not to be cabbages, how their attitudes and behaviour can affect the children are sometimes overpowering. Contented 'stay at home knitting wives' tend to be made inferior.

Isolation was a major theme of the responses, with mothers pointing to a sense that their generation was unusually sequestered from intergenerational sources of help.

Some respondents worried that education and employment exacerbated the shock of becoming a mother. The major challenges facing contemporary women, one respondent wrote, were the 'Over-education for the simple everyday requirements of bringing up a family. Various pressures to make you feel guilty if you don't have a job'. Alongside the loneliness of unsupported childrearing, guilt underpinned many of the responses. One mother wondered

> Whether it is possible to combine being married and having children with a career/job.... how can she experience all 3 things without becoming totally frustrated with such a fragmented existence.[120]

The emotional costs of this fragmentation were widely repeated across the survey results. Driving the tension that many mothers reported were the conflicting cultural, social, and economic impulses to undertake paid work *and* full-time childcare. 'Too much pressure is put on women to go to work', argued one respondent. 'If a woman wants to stay at home she is considered a "cabbage"'.[121]

But women took up paid work for reasons other than the threat of cabbage-dom. Respondents stressed the need to contribute to the financial stability of the family, the self-respect facilitated by economic freedom, as well as its social and intellectual benefits. Some respondents gave answers that drew on the ideas of the women's liberation movement – one mother, for example, wrote that paid work 'provides her with a measure of economic independence. Economic dependence is the greatest single cause of women's inferior position in our society. This leads direct [sic] to her sexual exploitation within the marriage bond and... to conditioning for her role'. Others framed it as a product of the emphasis placed on wage-earning, even while underlining the contribution that women's unpaid domestic labour made to the economy. One response explained women's paid work as important:

Because this is the valuation which our present society places upon people, and because the labour of everyone should be recognised as having a value. I believe that every women [sic] should be paid to run a home and raise children, because it is work.[122]

This respondent's suggestion was supported by a broader national campaign for the recognition of women's domestic work. Feminist interest in women's household labour emerged first in the nineteenth and early twentieth centuries but gained increased salience in the postwar period. Although it made little headway and was controversial even within the feminist movement, the international campaign for Wages for Housework, which entered public circulation in Britain in 1972, was one of the key sites for debate about the recognition of women's household work. The feminist evaluation of household work was manifold and sometimes conflicting. 'On the one hand they sought to describe women's household work as insidious drudgery legible within a broader public context of exploitative patriarchal capitalism', Sarah Stoller has explained. But 'On the other hand they articulated the social value of caring and lamented both the existing and imagined consequences of its reduction to mere work'.[123] This respondent's suggestion to the WAM survey, then, should be seen within a broader context of the evaluation of the nature of domestic and caring labour.

While some of the mothers' organisations – WAM and Mothers in Action, for example – sought to address the *causes* of mothers' unhappiness – including the vexed relationship with paid and unpaid work – other organisations, such as the NCT and MAMA, addressed unhappy motherhood and postnatal depression more directly, and in ways that coupled lived and medical expertise.

The Association for Post-Natal Illness: medical knowledge and experiential networks

Another organisation that focused on postnatal depression and drew on clinical knowledge was the Association for Post-Natal Illness (APNI). Like other mothers' organisations, the idea emerged from personal experience. Established in 1979 by Clare Delpech, who had experienced postnatal depression, the organisation was prompted when Delpech read work by Merton Sandler.[124] Sandler was a proponent of the relationship between brain chemicals and depression and was instrumental in the development of psychopharmacology and early antidepressants. This complemented Delpech's curiosity about chemical pathology.[125] From the beginning, APNI had strong medical representation on its committee — Sandler was its first president — although day-to-day administration was led by mothers.[126] APNI supported depressed mothers through a telephone line, a peer-to-peer support service, and by responding to letters.[127] Volunteers needed to have recovered from their own experiences of postnatal depression so that they could act as 'living proof' that it was possible to recover from it.[128] It initially operated from Delpech's house, with the help of several volunteers, but in 1981 moved to a space provided in Queen Charlotte's Hospital, Sandler's base. Although the base moved away from the hospital three years later, this underlines the close relationship between the charity and the medical profession. The organisation was proactive in its work with medical professionals, sharing information about the development of the Edinburgh Postnatal Depression Scale with them.

Newspapers, particularly through women's pages and agony aunt columns, referred distressed readers to the organisation.[129] Sometimes distressed mothers' feelings reflected broader national threats: one mother who was referred to APNI by the *Sunday Mirror*'s agony aunt in the mid-1980s was haunted by anxieties about nuclear annihilation.[130] The following year, APNI was again cited as a source of support by the *Sunday Mirror*'s agony aunt, who reassured one suicidal mother of two that its members were 'all mums who have suffered as you are suffering now'.[131] Like MAMA, APNI had regional branches which used local newspapers to reach out to potential new members and to create networks of experiential knowledge.[132] As one mother who founded a group in Cornwall told her local newspaper in 1982:

> I hope that having been through the experience myself I can perhaps help others to get over it. I know that being able to chat to someone who has been through the same thing can be a big help, at least you know you are not the only one to have these feelings. Some doctors are not at all sympathetic and it can drag on for a long time for some people.[133]

This mother reminds us that work for unhappy mothers was a dispersed grassroots movement and that experiential expertise was a supplement, or even an alternative, to medical expertise. This local and national press recognition likely helped the organisation gain prominence: by 1989–1990, APNI received between 150 and 600 letters and 50 phone calls a week. Eleven years after its founding, it had 3,387 members.[134]

Mothering expertise and the local

A common thread between these diverse organisations was their use of local and national newspapers to share information about the establishment of new branches. This underlines that work around unhappy motherhood extended far beyond the metropole and indicates that we should look to small, suburban, town, and village-based grassroots groups for examples of maternal organising. It also suggests that the press, and in particular local newspapers, played a key role in making 'ordinary people' and the qualities of 'ordinariness' visible and, along with other sites, fixed value and authenticity onto their voices. As Claire Langhamer has underlined, in postwar Britain, 'Ordinariness was a powerful position from which to resist and to challenge authority, to assert rights and to make demands'.[135] The use of the local press implied that unhappiness afflicted 'ordinary' mothers; women that could be, and were, your neighbours.

Further, mothers used these local publications to underline their expertise. When, in 1985, Scottish mothers Anne Williams and Linda Shaw promoted a local APNI group, they drew to the fore the value of their first-hand experience: they were 'a group of women in Aberdeen who know all about [postnatal depression] because they have experienced it', the *Aberdeen Press and Journal* reported.[136] The article appeared alongside a warning for dog walkers in the nearby countryside, and a piece about the fundraising efforts of local nurses; such positioning emphasised the ordinariness of the distressed mothers and their rootedness in the local community. These mothers were not alone. The Association for Improvements in the Maternity Services (AIMS) was established in 1960 when

Sally Willington published a letter in a national newspaper, but mothers used local presses to spread the word about grassroots branches.[137] Irene Climie of East Ayrshire, Scotland, told her local paper in 1982 that her health visitor had recommended she contact the NCT, and that she was subsequently so convinced of the utility of mothers' groups that she became the postnatal contact for the Ayrshire NCT group and the local contact for APNI.[138] In 1987, Debbie Lloyd used her personal experience as a mother to appeal for volunteers for the local APNI helpline through the *Solihull News*.[139] After eight weeks of living in Northampton, mother-of-five Donna Beckwith established the town's first MAMA group, sharing her own experience of postnatal depression in the *Northampton Herald & Post*.[140] In Norfolk, Carolyn told her local paper that postnatal depression had laid her low; she subsequently established a branch of Depressives Associated.[141] Across Britain, then, local newspapers became a tool for the assertion of experiential maternal expertise and indirectly underlined the ways that distress could affect ordinary mothers.

These local newspapers stressed the social role played by postnatal support groups. In the late 1970s, Lynne Alderson explained in the *Reading Evening Post* that postnatal depression was common and widely recognised; meeting other mothers in the same situation through the local NCT branch could make it tolerable.[142] In the *Huddersfield Daily Examiner* – in an article next to the astrology column, an article about a new dress pattern for Christmas, and a piece about the freeze-marking of horses – the local NCT branch chair explained that 'For a woman who has worked out of the area where she lives and whose friends are mostly those people she worked with, she may find that she is alone with no social contacts'.[143] In the Scottish town of Linlithgow, Patricia Russell told the *West Lothian Courier* about the local branch of the NCT in 1986. Social support in the postnatal phase was critical, she said, for 'mothers used to working full-time often discovered that, with the birth of their child, they had to establish new friendships... NCT's post-natal sessions gives these mothers a chance to develop friendships and build up confidence through the help of more experienced parents'.[144] From Ayrshire to Aberdeen, to Bury, to Bristol, to Cornwall, to West Lothian: self-organised communities of experience asserted the value of their knowledge to build networks and used the humdrum platform of local newspapers to emphasise the ordinariness of unhappy motherhood.

Conclusion

Mothers established self-help and peer support groups across the postwar period. These groups operated across a variety of grassroots sites, extending maternal activism beyond the metropole. These local groups made use of humdrum communication organs – local newspapers, for example – to build networks, extend their reach, and draw attention to the 'ordinariness' of unhappy mothers. The groups underline distressed mothers' agency in postwar Britain: the experience of unhappy mothering – both severe and mild – served as a creative and political stimulus. While some of the groups, such as APNI, offered targeted support that drew on medical expertise around postnatal depression, others sought to alleviate some of the social factors that exacerbated mothers' unhappiness, such as loneliness or under-employment. These groups were part of the postwar rise of the culture of self-help that accelerated from the 1960s. But they had more vexed and varied relationships with other social changes. They had diverse responses to the feminist movement that gained momentum from the late 1960s to the end of the subsequent decade, for example. While some sought to distance themselves, others aligned themselves with its aims. Perhaps inevitably, some such groups were ephemeral, while other organisations have endured and flourished. The NCT, which continues to have a high national profile, for example, maintained its interest in postnatal experiences. In 1989, two Scottish representatives, Isobelle Mitchell and Morag Une, launched a quarterly newsletter.[145] In its first issue, the value of mothers' experiential expertise was reaffirmed:

> Any advice we may give is based on experience with our own children, not on training; assuming that those who have coped with some of the common difficulties which arise in early parenthood are the right people to support new parents faced with similar anxieties. We can't teach people how to be parents, but often our sympathetic 'befrienders' are seen as 'models', who have so far successfully

brought up their own children. The most important aspects of this 'support' are that it reinforces the parents' confidence in their ability to care for, and enjoy, their baby, and that it eases the feeling of isolation felt sometimes by new mothers at home alone with their babies.[146]

The organisation also continued to raise awareness of postnatal depression.[147] In the 1990s, the Postnatal Committee published guidelines for depression support groups and organised a national experience register in order to connect mothers with an advisor who had lived experience.[148] Experiential expertise, then, was valued within these mothers' movements. Moreover, mothers' groups were frequently political in their orientation, seeking not only to recognise mothers' unhappiness and distress but to address the social contexts from which these emotions emerged: isolation, boredom, and exclusion from public space. These organisations – at both a national and grassroots level – laboured to bring to light the challenges of motherhood. It is somewhat surprising, then, that in 1996 the Health Visitors' Association and the NCT held a joint conference in London titled *Postnatal Depression: Focus on a Neglected Issue*. Neither organisation had neglected the issue, and both worked with medical experts who researched the topic – and the foreword for the conference's papers affirmed that postnatal depression was 'an issue of major concern to NHS maternity and child health care services today'.[149] Neither did the conference languish in terms of the prestige of speakers or the number of attendees: it was chaired by prominent child psychologist and author Penelope Leach, whose bestselling *Your Baby and Child* was first published in 1977. Moreover, it was attended by over 450 NCT members and health professionals. Thus, the conference's title should be interpreted as a rhetorical flourish, rather than a *mea culpa:* this should be remembered so as to keep in mind the preceding three decades of emotional, social, and political work done at the grassroots by 'ordinary' mothers.

Notes

1 Katharina Dalton, *Depression after Childbirth: How to Recognise and Treat Postnatal Illness* (Oxford, 1989 [1980]), 3.

2 Esther Rantzen, 'Foreword', in *Depression after Childbirth: How to Recognise and Treat Postnatal Illness*, ed. Katharina Dalton (Oxford, 1989 [1980]), v–vi.
3 'That's Love, Esther', *Daily Mirror*, 19 June 1979.
4 'Mum's Best Friend is Another Mother', *Aberdeen Evening Express*, 10 October 1979.
5 'The Isolation of Mothers', *Glamorgan Gazette*, 16 February 1984.
6 Meet-A-Mum-Association, *Friendship and Support for All Mothers* (Surrey, 1996), 2. London, British Library, YK1996/a.18338; Meet-a-Mum Association, *Behind the Painted Smile: An Insight into Post-Natal Depression* (Warwick, 1988), 25. London, British Library, 95/03037; Meet-a-Mum Association, *Lifting the Veil of Silence: On Emotional Problems after Childbirth* (Warwick, 1993). London, British Library, 95/03034.
7 Catherine Boyd and Lea Sellers, *The British Way of Birth* (London, 1982), 1.
8 *Ibid.*, 3.
9 *Ibid.*, 180–189.
10 *Ibid.*, 234–235.
11 Claire Langhamer, 'Who the Hell Are Ordinary People?' Ordinariness as a Category of Historical Analysis', *Transactions of the Royal Historical Society*, 28, 2018, 175–195, 183.
12 'Don't Let Things Get You Down, Mum', *Lincolnshire Standard*, 11 May 1989.
13 Lynn Abrams, *Feminist Lives: Women, Feelings, & the Self in Post-War Britain* (Oxford, 2023), 5
14 For more on the NCT and postnatal depression, see Hilary Marland, "Drowned in a Sea of Inhumanity': Natural Childbirth, Postnatal Depression and the National Childbirth Trust, 1956–80s', *Social History of Medicine*, 2023, https://doi.org/10.1093/shm/hkad083.
15 For work that argues for the importance of women's self-help and self-organising, see Lynn Abrams, 'The Self and Self-Help: Women Pursuing Autonomy in Post-War Britain', *Transactions of the Royal Historical Society*, 29, 2019, 201–221, and Caitríona Beaumont, 'What Do Women Want? Housewives' Associations, Activism and Changing Representations of Women in the 1950s', *Women's History Review*, 26, 1, 2016, 147–162.
16 Caitríona Beaumont, 'The "Housewife as Expert": Re-thinking the Experiential Expertise and Welfare Activism of Housewives' Associations in England, 1960–1980', in *Everyday Welfare in Modern*

British History: Experience, Expertise and Activism, ed. Caitríona Beaumont, Eve Colpus and Ruth Davidson (Cham, 2024), 71–93, 73.

17 For more on the modern history of unmarried motherhood, see Pat Thane, 'Unmarried Motherhood in Twentieth-Century England', *Women's History Review*, 20, 2, 2011, 11–29. I have used a range of terms here – unmarried, lone, and single mothers – to avoid repetition, but it is worth noting that languages have shifted across the twentieth century.

18 Mary Stott, *Women Talking: An Anthology from the Guardian Women's Page, 1922–35, 1957–71* (London, 1987), 225.

19 Emine Saner, 'I Met Women who Wanted to Discuss Non-Baby Things' - How 60 Years of the National Women's Register Changed Lives', *The Guardian*, 27 February 2020.

20 Stephen Hatch and Teresa Hinton, *Self-Help in Practice* (Sheffield, 1986), 3.

21 Conservative Manifesto 1979. Retrieved from http://www.margarethatcher.org/document/110858 [Accessed 5 May 2023].

22 Brian Abel-Smith, *The National Health Service: The First Thirty Years* (Her Majesty's Stationery Office, 1978), 42–47.

23 'Community Action', *Aberdeen Evening Express*, 13 March 1982.

24 Stephen Lock, 'Self Help Groups: The Fourth Estate in Medicine?', *British Medical Journal*, 293, 6562, 1986, 1596–1600, 1596.

25 Tina Posner, 'The Development of Self Help Organizations: Dilemma and Ambiguities', in *Self Help and Social Welfare: England and West Germany*, eds S. Humble and J. Unell (London and New York, 1989), 51–61, 52.

26 Lock, 'Self Help Groups', 1596.

27 Jane Price, *Motherhood: What it Does to Your Mind* (London, Sydney and Wellington, 1990 [1988]), 140.

28 Abrams, 'The Self and Self-Help', 201.

29 Lynn Abrams, 'Heroes of Their Own Life Stories: Narrating the Female Self in the Feminist Age', *Cultural and Social History*, 16, 2, 2019, 205–224, 206–207.

30 Grantly Dick-Read's influential book *Natural Childbirth*, published in 1933, was followed in 1942 by *Revelation of Childbirth* (republished as *Childbirth Without Fear* in 1944). 'A Natural Childbirth Association', *The Times*, 4 May 1956.

31 Jenny Kitzinger, 'Strategies of the Early Childbirth Movement: A Case-Study of the National Childbirth Trust', in *The Politics of Maternity: Services for Childbearing Women in Twentieth-Century Britain*, eds Jo Garcia, Robert Kilpatrick, and Martin Richards (Oxford, 1990), 92–115, 93.

32 *Ibid.*, 102.
33 Pamela Rice, 'The Most Beautiful Experience of a Woman's Life', *Kent Messenger*, 8 March 1957.
34 'Lydia's Hubby Saw Her Baby Born', *Sunday Mail*, 26 January 1958.
35 Marland, 'Drowned in a Sea of Inhumanity', 4; Kitzinger, 'Strategies', 105.
36 'Woman's World: New Organiser', *Eastbourne Herald Chronicle*, 20 April 1957.
37 'She Prepares Mothers for Childbirth', *Worthing Herald*, 19 January 1968.
38 Marland, 'Drowned in a Sea of Inhumanity', 71.
39 'The Growing Interest in Natural Childbirth', *The Times*, 1 September 1966.
40 Kitzinger, 'Strategies', 104–105.
41 Vivienne Welburn, *Postnatal Depression* (Glasgow, 1980), 75.
42 Kitzinger, 'Strategies', 105.
43 Boyd and Sellers, *The British Way of Birth*, 53–55.
44 Margaret Dennis, *The First Few Weeks of Motherhood: Some Suggestions for New Mothers*. Oxford Post-Natal Support Group, The National Childbirth Trust, Handbook No. 2, December 1974. London, Wellcome Archives, SA/NCT/D/3/1.
45 Rosaleen Mansfield, An Historical Survey of Postnatal Support, also published in *New Generation*, September 1983, London, Wellcome Archives SA/NCT/D/3/1; Meeting of Postnatal Committee, 7 May 1980. London, Wellcome Archives SA/NCT/D/3/1.
46 Rosaleen Mansfield, 'An Historical Survey of Postnatal Support', also published in *New Generation*, September 1983. London, Wellcome Archives SA/NCT/D/3/1.
47 Liz Waumsley, 'Foreword', in *Mothers Talking about Postnatal Depression* (London, 1983), 0. London, Wellcome Archives, SA/NCT/A/7/1.
48 Marland, 'Drowned in a Sea of Inhumanity', 88.
49 National Childbirth Trust, *The Emotions and Experiences of Some Disabled Mothers* (London, 1984/1985), 19–20.
50 *Ibid.*, 6.
51 Desmond Bardon, 'Forewords', in Maggie Comport, *Towards Happy Motherhood: Understanding Postnatal Depression* (London, 1987), ix.
52 *Mothers Talking about Postnatal Depression* (London, 1983), 2–3. London, Wellcome Archives, SA/NCT/A/7/1, 29.
53 Bardon quoted in Maggie Comport, *Towards Happy Motherhood: Understanding Postnatal Depression* (London, 1987), 204.
54 *Mothers Talking about Postnatal Depression*, 5.

55 *Ibid.*, 6.
56 Roberta Bivins and Mathew Thomson, 'Anniversary fever? History and the culture of NHS celebration', *Modern British History*, 36, 1, 2025, hwae066, https://doi.org/10.1093/tcbh/hwae066, 5. It's notable that 'ordinary' people continued to value the NHS across the 1970s and 1980s in the face of these pressures. See Agnes Arnold-Forster, 'Ordinary People and the 1979 Royal Commission on the NHS', *Twentieth Century British History*, 34, 2, 2023, 275–298.
57 *Mothers Talking about Postnatal Depression*, 3.
58 *Ibid.*, 6.
59 *Ibid.*, 13.
60 Waumsley, 'Postnatal Support Now', Postnatal Pack: Resources for Co-ordinators and Supporters, NCT Postnatal Committee, 1987. London, Wellcome Archives, SA/NCT/D/3/3.
61 *Mothers Talking about Postnatal Depression*, 4.
62 'Post-natal Depression', *East Kilbride News*, 8 August 1986.
63 Maggie Comport, *Towards Happy Motherhood: Understanding Postnatal Depression* (London, 1987), 204.
64 Meet-a-Mum Association, *Go Forth and Multiply But… What is the Impact of a New Baby on the Family, a MAMA Study Day* (London, 1992), 20. London, British Library, YK/1996/a.20.
65 Waumsley, 'Postnatal Support Now'.
66 Deirdre Sanders and Jane Reed, *Kitchen Sink, or Swim? Women in the Eighties: The Choices* (Harmondsworth, 1982), 193–195.
67 Constitution, 28 September 1968 London, LSE Women's Library Archives, 5MIA/01; Constitution, 12 May 1972. London, LSE Women's Library Archives, 5MIA/01.
68 Mothers in Action, Penny Milsom, Unsupported Mothers on Social Security, September 1971. London, British Library, J/X0315/11; Constitution, London, LSE Women's Library Archives, 5MIA/01.
69 Press Statement, 'The Future of Mothers in Action', 1 March 1972. London, LSE Women's Library Archives, 5MIA/02/02.
70 Papers re. Margaret Deshmane Membership, 'To All London Members'. London, LSE Women's Library Archives, 5MIA/05/02.
71 Correspondence re. Membership/mailing List, 'Mothers in Action'. London, LSE Women's Library Archives, 5MIA/05/01.
72 Mothers in Action. London, British Library, J/X0315/11.
73 Minutes and Supporting Papers 1971. London, LSE Women's Library Archives, 5MIA/02/01.
74 Mothers in Action, Plan for Day Care (n/d), London, British Library, J/X0315/11.

75 Jane Lewis, 'The Failure to Expand Childcare Provision and to Develop a Comprehensive Childcare Policy in Britain during the 1960s and 1970s', *Twentieth Century British History*, 24, 2, 2013, 249–274.
76 Mothers in Action, Alternative Care for Children Under Five, May 1972. London, British Library, J/X0315/11 (11).
77 Mothers in Action, Plan for Pregnancy, London, British Library, J/X0315/11; Mothers in Action, Working Mothers' Charter: For the Benefit of Working Mothers and Their Children. London, British Library, J/X0315/11 (15).
78 Mothers in Action, Housing Sheet, May 1972. London, British Library, J/X0315/11 (4).
79 Mothers in Action, Plan for Housing, London, British Library, J/X0315/11.
80 See, for example, Mothers in Action, Penny Milsom, Unsupported Mothers on Social Security, Study Pamphlet No. 2, September 1971. London, British Library, J/X0315/11 (1); Mothers in Action, Study Pamphlet No. 4, Residential Jobs for Unsupported Mothers – A Survey. London, 1971, London, British Library, J/Z0315/11 (19).
81 Mothers in Action, Mothers Alone, September 1969. London, British Library, J/X0315/11 (6).
82 Mothers in Action, Shirley Frost, Sharing Responsibility for the Child, November 1970. London, British Library, J/X0315/11 (7).
83 WAM, 'Relief from Nappies and Baby Talk', n/s, n/d. London, LSE Women's Library Archives, 5WAM/4. Lynn Abrams also discusses WAM. See *Feminist Lives*, 217–218.
84 WAM, Diana Priestley Letter to Grahame Leman, 14 May 1969. London, LSE Women's Library Archives, 5WAM/7.
85 'Mothers Launch Scheme to Get Back to Work', *The Times*, 21 July 1969, 10.
86 'It's Just a Thought', *Liverpool Echo*, 25 July 1969.
87 'How Mrs Priestley Copes with a Co-Op for the Cooped Up', *Birmingham Daily Post*, 13 May 1970.
88 'Housebound Mums Gain Their Freedom', *Aberdeen Press and Journal*, 3 December 1969.
89 WAM, 'WAM Off to a Good Start', *Richmond Times*, September 1969. London, LSE Women's Library Archives, 5WAM/8.
90 no title, n/d. London, LSE Women's Library Archives, 5WAM/8.
91 WAM, Diana Priestley, Guidelines for Starting a WAM Group, 1971. London, LSE Women's Library Archives, 5WAM/3.
92 'They All Came Out to Play', Source Unknown, n/d. London, LSE Women's Library Archives, 5WAM/8.

93 Grahame Leman Letter to Diana Priestley, 11 August 1970. LSE Women's Library Archives, 5WAM/7.
94 Grahame Leman Letter to Pat Brangwyn, 22 July 1969. Emphasis in original. London, LSE Women's Library Archives, 5WAM/7.
95 Grahame Leman Letter to Diana Priestley, 3 August 1970. London, LSE Women's Library Archives, 5WAM/7.
96 'Help Yourselves, Mums of Harrow', *Harrow Observer*, 10 November 1970. London, LSE Women's Library Archives, 5WAM/8.
97 *WAM News*, Summer 1970, 5. London, LSE Women's Library Archives, 5WAM/1.
98 'Let's Dispense with the GUILT', *WAM News*, Winter 1970–1971, 1. Capitalisation in original. London, LSE Women's Library Archives, 5WAM/1.
99 Playspace in Richmond: A Study Initiated by WAM (Working Association of Mothers) and the Richmond Branch of AASE (Association for the Advancement of State Education), Middlesex, July 1972. London, LSE Women's Library Archives, 5WAM/2. 'Where the Action is on Swings and Things', *The Times*, 22 November 1972, 15.
100 Report on the First Meeting of WAM Branches, 23 October 1971. London, LSE Women's Library Archives, 5WAM/3.
101 Helen McCarthy, 'Career, Family and Emotional Work: Graduate Mothers in 1960s Britain', *Past & Present*, 246, Suppl. 15, 2020, 295–317, 300, see also Helen McCarthy, 'Feminism, Selfhood and Social Research: Professional Women's Organizations in 1960s Britain', in *Precarious Professionals: Gender, Identities and Social Change in Modern Britain*, eds Heidi Egginton and Zoë Thomas (London, 2021), 287–304.
102 McCarthy, 'Career, Family and Emotional Work', 303.
103 McCarthy, 'Feminism, Selfhood and Social Research', 287–288.
104 Fred Cooper, 'Loneliness as Crisis in Britain after 1950: Temporality, Modernity, and the Historical Gaze', in *The Routledge History of Loneliness*, eds Katie Barclay, Elaine Chalus, and Deborah Simonton (London, 2023), chapter 11.
105 Ann Oakley, *The Sociology of Housework* (Bristol, 2019 [1974]), 82; Gavron, *The Captive Wife*, 135.
106 Tavistock Institute of Human Relations, Working Association of Mothers, Wellcome Archives, SA/TIH/B/2/79 (file 1 of 2), n/d.
107 Laura Paterson, "I Didn't Feel Like My Own Person': Paid Work in Women's Narratives of Self and Working Motherhood, 1950–1980', *Contemporary British History*, 33:3, 2019, 405–426.
108 Tavistock Institute of Human Relations, Working Association of Mothers, Wellcome Archives, SA/TIH/B/2/79 (file 1 of 2), n/d.

109 *Ibid.*
110 *Ibid.*
111 Diana Priestley Letter to Grahame Leman, 8 October 1969. London, LSE Women's Library Archives, 5WAM/7.
112 Carol Dyhouse, *Students: A Gendered History* (Abingdon, 2006), 99.
113 Caitríona Beaumont, *Housewives and Citizens: Domesticity and the Women's Movement in England, 1928–64* (Manchester, 2013).
114 Tavistock Institute of Human Relations, Working Association of Mothers (file 1 of 2).
115 '350,000 Plead for the Toddlers', *Teddington and Hampton Times*, 5 May 1972. London, LSE Women's Library Archives, 5WAM/4.
116 Diana Priestley, National Campaign for Nursery Education: Reflections on an Outing, 2 May 1972. London, LSE Women's Library Archives, 5WAM/4.
117 'Toddlers Turn Out in Force for Nurseries', *Surrey Comet*, n/d, 1972. London, LSE Women's Library Archives, 5WAM/4.
118 Tavistock Institute of Human Relations, Working Association of Mothers, London, Wellcome Archives, SA/TIH/B/2/79 (file 1 of 2), n/d.
119 Tavistock Institute of Human Relations, Working Association of Mothers, London, Wellcome Archives, SA/TIH/B/2/79 (file 1 of 2), n/d. Capitalisation in original.
120 *Ibid.*
121 Tavistock Institute of Human Relations, Working Association of Mothers, London, Wellcome Archives, SA/TIH/B/2/79 (file 2 of 2), n/d.
122 *Ibid.*
123 Sarah Stoller, 'Forging a Politics of Care: Theorising Household Work in the British Women's Liberation Movement', *History Workshop Journal*, 85, 2018, 95–119, 99.
124 Phone Call with Clare Delpech (April 2015); see also 'Our History'. Retrieved from https://apni.org/history/ [Accessed 1 September 2023].
125 Chris Mahony, 'Obituary: Merton Sandler', *British Medical Journal*, 4, 349, 2014, 6609.
126 APNI, 'History'.
127 *The Association for Post-Natal Illness Annual Report*, 30 June 1990. London, APNI Archive.
128 Thames Television, *Time to Care*, ed. P. Gerhardt (Thames Television, 1990), London, APNI Archive.
129 'Public Opinion: The Column You Write', *Daily Mirror*, 4 August 1989.
130 'A Mum's Nuclear Horrors', *Sunday Mirror*, 13 January 1985.
131 'The Hell of Baby Blues', *Sunday Mirror*, 13 July 1986.

132 'News Round Up', *Aberdeen Press and Journal*, 5 June 1985; 'Group to Help Fight Post-natal Depression', *Aberdeen Press and Journal*, 9 April 1985; 'Why Do I Hate the Way I Look?', *Sandwell Evening Mail*, 24 March 1987.
133 'Helping Mothers to Cope with Depression after Childbirth', *West Briton and Cornwall Advertiser*, 25 January 1982.
134 *The Association for Post-Natal Illness Annual Report*, 30 June 1990, London, APNI Archive.
135 Langhamer, 'Who the Hell Are Ordinary People?', 189.
136 'Group to Help Fight Post-natal Depression', *Aberdeen Press and Journal*, 9 April 1985.
137 Tania McIntosh, *A Social History of Maternity and Childbirth: Key Themes in Maternity Care* (Abingdon, 2012), 113–114; 'Local Maternity Survey Spotlights a "Lonely" Need', *Lichfield Mercury*, 13 October 1967; 'Kindness Call for Mums-to-be Wins Local Sympathies', *Lichfield Mercury*, 7 July 1967; 'Brightening the Maternity Ward', *Birmingham Daily Post*, 21 November 1962; 'Easing the Lot of a Lot of Women', *Birmingham Daily Post*, 3 February 1970; 'Assn. Wants to Hear from Mums', *Bury Free Press*, 26 April 1974.
138 'Local Antenatal Classes Drawing Nearer', *Kilmarnock Standard*, 12 February 1982.
139 'Will You Help Fight Depression?' *Solihull News*, 4 September 1987.
140 'Mum Aims to Help Post Natal Depressives', *Northampton Herald & Post*, 8 November 1990.
141 'Help for Depressives', *Lynn Advertiser*, 12 April 1988.
142 'Great Expectations', *Reading Evening Post*, 25 May 1978.
143 'New Mums Helped in Post Natal Groups', *Huddersfield Daily Examiner*, 20 November 1982.
144 'Trust Aim to Help Mums of the Future', *West Lothian Courier*, 25 April 1986.
145 *Postnatal Forever* Newsletters, London, Wellcome Archives, SA/NCT/D/3/4.
146 NCT, *Scottish Newsletter*, Winter 1989, London, Wellcome Archives, SA/NCT/D/3/4; NCT, *Postnatal Support within the NCT*, July 1982, London, Wellcome Archives SA/NCT/D/3/1.
147 NCT, *Postnatal Resource Pack*, 1992. London, Wellcome Archives, SA/NCT/D/3/1.
148 London, Wellcome Archives, SA/NCT/D/3/5, n/d.
149 Barbara Kott and Jackie Carnell, 'Foreword', in *Postnatal Depression: Focus on a Neglected Issue*, Papers from the HVA/NCT National Conference, London, 18 April 1996. London, Wellcome Archives SA/NCT/D/3/3.

4

The women's liberation movement and mothers' discontent

In the 1960s, Mica Nava was caught between two worlds. The mother of three young children – all of whom had been birthed at home and breastfed, choices that placed her at the 'vanguard of the countercultural climate of the time' – Nava was middle class, politically engaged, a writer, and an artist. Although she 'loved the image of myself with child on hip and at the breast and a trail of lively kids with long hair', she wanted to be 'mobile and adventurous', to earn money of her own. The father of her children could access these political, professional, and economic freedoms, and in 1968, he was contributing to some of the most iconic political protests of that tumultuous year. The bulk of childcare fell to Nava, who 'had no language for the unease' she experienced, while her partner 'participated in the exhilarating political dramas of the moment'.[1]

The following decade would be transformational as women carved their own political drama through the feminist movement, and in so doing created a new language around motherhood – a language that articulated mothers' dissatisfaction in newly political terms. The feminist upsurge would explore the very issues that drove Nava into feminism: the apparent irreconcilability of creative, intellectual, and domestic dreams; the onus on women to carry the burden of domestic labour; the tensions arising from the experience and institution of motherhood, as Adrienne Rich would later describe it.[2] All this was to come when, in September 1969, Nava attended her first meeting of the Tufnell Park women's group, carrying her newborn with her. The next year, she attended the first national conference of the movement, again with her child. There, she listened to Rochelle (Sheli) Wortis's critique of Bowlby's theories about uninterrupted maternal care: for Nava, this paper was 'the mobilising event of the early movement'. Mothering was crucial to Nava's feminist development: 'It was mothering that, beyond anything else, had seemed to me to delimit – as well as to expand – my life in such a momentous way'.[3] Nava was far from alone in being thrust into the feminist movement by the conflicting emotions provoked by motherhood.

The commitment to exploring the politics of mothering, to contesting it, and to improving mothers' experiences emerged as an important strand of work within some parts of the women's liberation movement. Feminist groups emerged in Britain towards the close of the 1960s but coalesced into a more organised movement at the start of the 1970s. It developed in resistance to the renewed emphasis on feminine domesticity that developed in the 1950s; was inspired by working-class women's trade union activism, not least at the Ford factory in Dagenham, and around trawler safety in Hull; emerged from the political movements of the late 1960s, not least the student movement, Black Power, and peace movements; was informed by influential feminist texts that flowed across the Atlantic from the United States; had roots in some of the cultural changes and structural shifts of the 1960s, including increased access to education and contraception; and was shaped by the 1960s culture of permissiveness – a culture that had a 'darker side' for women.[4]

The resulting movement had significant divisions along ideological lines, and diverse groups within the movement placed different degrees of emphasis on the role of motherhood in women's oppression. It is notable, though, that of the first four demands formulated by the movement, developed at the first national conference in 1970, two demands related to reproduction and childrearing: 24-hour nurseries ('we need somewhere for the kids, but we have to choose as to whether the kids will be kept out of the way or given their own space, and whether, freed from children, we just manage to survive through working or make the time to discover who stops us from living') and free contraception and abortion on demand ('we want to be free to choose when and how many kids to have, if any. We have to fight for control over our own bodies, or even the magic pill or (in the case of mistakes) abortion on demand only gives us the freedom to get into a real mess without any visible consequences, we still can't talk of sex as anything but a joke or a battle-ground').⁵ Making motherhood a choice – and crucially a choice that when taken did not oppress, immiserate, or diminish women – was fundamental to women's liberation. Such an interest in motherhood made an exploration of mothers' experiences necessary.

The women's liberation movement shared knowledge about unhappy mothering by developing mechanisms through which it could be made visible, including through consciousness-raising groups, conferences, edited collections, pamphlets, magazines, and the creation of feminist publishing houses. It contested male-generated psychoanalytic and medical approaches to maternal distress, creating an alternative locus of expertise drawn from the political analysis of mothers' lived experiences. Feminist activists used this testimony as evidence of the need for women's liberation. While, as Lynn Abrams has argued, the '1960s liberated women's feelings', it was in the organised women's movement of the 1970s that British mothers' feelings became politicised.⁶ As the well-known feminist maxim underlined, 'the personal is political'. As Nava has observed, this was 'its key maxim but also generated a wider radical reframing and expansion of what constituted the political'.⁷ Childcare was political; the home was political; relationships were political; the hospital, clinic, and consulting room were political. It was consistent, then, that the feelings that arose within these political spaces and environments were political artefacts, too.

This chapter sets out not only what some feminist activists *thought* about motherhood but also what was *felt*, in all its richness, contradictions, and ambivalences. It is apposite here, though, to observe what was 'done' by the movement around mothering: campaigns around the rights of lesbian mothers, around single mothers, around the division of parental responsibilities, around work, around childcare, nurseries, and playgroups, and the ways that motherhood might be made an active choice through abortion and contraception. There is not space to establish the histories of these feminist campaigns here, but these activities demonstrate the practical energy within the movement. This work was connected to the recognition of mothers' full emotional personhood. As the Edinburgh Women's Liberation Group wrote in the mid-1970s:

> Women claim the right, as people, to fail to meet some ideal standard of motherhood... and to judge for themselves how their skills may best be deployed. The best interests of the children will not be served by confining them with a miserably frustrated mother, but by enabling both mother and child to be fulfilled and happy persons.[8]

Giving voice to the miserable frustrations of motherhood was one of the many enduring interventions of the movement.

Mothers, mothering, and the creation of the movement

This chapter suggests an alternative to a narrative put forward by Ann Dally in her influential text, *Inventing Motherhood*, published in 1982. Dally condemned the women's liberation movement for inattentiveness and a lack of nuance around the experience of mothering while praising the movement's overall contribution. 'The attitude of modern feminists towards motherhood and feminist writings about motherhood has on the whole been superficial, lacking in understanding and lacking in awareness of its own deficiencies in this most important area of life', she wrote. This, she explained, stemmed from the influence of texts written by young women who were not yet mothers, and the comparative lack of involvement of older women who, she points out, may have been too involved with the work of mothering to participate. Aside from Betty Friedan's *The Feminine Mystique*, Dally said:

> few of the other important books that led and influenced the movement were written by mothers. It is clear from reading these books that few of the authors had much idea of what motherhood involves and so their attempts to bring it into their theories and suggestions tend to be unsatisfactory and unconvincing. Because the subject has not been fully faced or explored, motherhood is an area in which questioning women's role has had least impact, and the area in which there is the greatest inequality. Meanwhile millions of mothers, conscious of the importance of both what the women's liberation movement is saying to them and of motherhood itself, are confused and nervous... to many it seems impossible to be a good mother in the context of feminism.[9]

Dally was right that motherhood posed some challenging questions for feminists. Certainly, strands of feminist thought emphasised the oppressive and burdensome nature of mothering. But many women in the women's liberation movement were in fact propelled into feminist activism at least in part by their experiences as mothers (rather than, as Dally suggests, turning to the theorisation of motherhood having become a mother within the movement). Michèle Roberts has recalled the key role of young mothers in the movement, writing that a 'current myth about the seventies is that feminists despised mothers and motherhood. Wrong. Women's liberation was started by young mothers'.[10]

Roberts is right: new mothers were instrumental in founding the movement. For instance, an early group in south London emerged from a 'One O'clock Club' for mothers of small children.[11] Jan Williams, one of its members, underlined the centrality of discussions about motherhood to the group.[12] Others followed similar paths; for example, the first women's group that feminist and historian Catherine Hall participated in also grew out of her experience as a new mother in the late 1960s. Hall was, according to her husband, cultural theorist Stuart Hall, 'ready-made for... feminism'. Catherine Hall recalled that, like other left-wing, educated mothers, she was unsettled by the loss of her 'political life,' questioning 'who am I now, what do I do, how do I create this new kind of life with a baby?' and that from conversations around these questions a feminist group emerged. The first feminist playgroups were, she said, stirred by 'the frustrations of motherhood.' Given this, 'childcare was always at the top of the list because that's where we were'.[13] Others had similar experiences. In 1967, Audrey Battersby was 'on my own with three children, and going quietly crazy'. She 'started fishing around for somewhere to put myself politically... I had thought my condition, my disgruntlement if you like, with life and marriage and everything, was personal'. In the end

> It was as a result of talking to other women – about child-rearing mostly – that we decided to have a series of meetings... Somehow or other, people started connecting. More and more meetings started happening... by that time, I was fired up with the desire to do something, I didn't quite know what, but I knew it was to do with being female and being angry.[14]

Val Charlton had a similar experience:

> before having the baby, I thought I'd just carry on working. I was so naive, I had no idea; it was a tremendous shock. It was all embracing; when he was born, I reacted to it very badly. I really hated it; I loved him, but I hated the way of life. I was very isolated, I was in the place all by myself. I thought I was going insane. So I was very typical, I think, of people who were ripe for the women's movement. I think I'd been shocked by a difficult birth, and I was very shaky after that. I just remember that time as absolutely horrendous, exhausted, confused, feeling absolutely terrible. I remember going up to Yorkshire, meeting a couple of friends of mine who also had children the same age, and saying, 'This is ridiculous, we can't live like this, we've got to do something about it'. That was just weeks before I heard about the women's liberation movement.[15]

Sue O'Sullivan had her first child in 1968 and was 'deeply shocked by the experience of giving birth'. The following year:

> [I] found myself sitting somewhat self-consciously in a living room, talking with other women about isolation, feelings of inadequacy, ambivalences towards motherhood, and hearing sympathetic voices confirming, identifying and expanding. I know, even if I can no longer touch its electricity, that I left with a wonderful feeling, a spinning head and a churning stomach.[16]

Alison Fell wrote in *Red Rag*, the Marxist and then Marxist-socialist feminist magazine, that before encountering the women's movement she was

> a housewife living with a man and child in an isolated family situation in a strange city. I make one trip per day to the supermarket, just for a change of scene. I try for jobs and fail because I can't get the child into a nursery... I blame myself for not being 'strong' enough to make it in the world. I blame myself for not being consumed with interest for the child and the man... The conflict between the various ideas of what I should be, and the real trap I'm living in, makes me constantly depressed and guilty.

A friend introduced Fell to a women's liberation group, and 'in the space of an hour the war that was going on inside me began to show itself as a war in which everyone was involved'. It was, she wrote, 'the beginnings of political consciousness'.[17] She explained elsewhere that 'in 1967 I found myself in Leeds as a faculty wife, mother, and depressive'. Involvement with women's liberation 'saved me from a weight of guilt about how badly I fitted into my womanly role'.[18] In 1968, Michèlene Wandor was married with two children, 'still trying to come to terms with being a housewife and mother, though of the highly educated kind'. By 1971, she was involved in women's liberation and struggling to balance childrearing, art, and politics.[19] 'One after another, voices repeat the same confusion', Lynne Segal has reflected, 'often triggered by the arrival of children, however much desired'.[20] Some of these unhappy mothers, adrift at the end of the 1960s and beginning of the 1970s, would go on to form feminism's 'second wave' and chart new shores for feminism.

It is little surprise, then, that babies attended women's liberation conferences. One of the most famous images of the Ruskin conference is of cultural theorist Stuart Hall holding a sleeping child and Henry Wortis sitting with another baby in the creche – a creche that was, importantly, staffed by men. Filmmaker Sue Crockford, a member of the Tufnell Park Women's Liberation group and maker of a documentary about the conference, recalled thinking the idea of a creche staffed by men was 'mildly radical'.[21] Mica Nava has shared a photograph of herself and Crockford, mid-conversation at the conference, both with babies on their laps.[22] Some babies attended the speeches. Marlene Hobsbawm, mother of two young children, recalled that 'There were a lot of young women with babies'. These babies were 'fed more that day than in any other of their whole lives. This was not every hour, this was every four minutes. You felt kind of naked *without* a baby sucking away'.[23] Thus, far from being absent, frustrated mothers of small children were centrally involved with the movement from its beginnings.

Of course, some women also became mothers while active in the movement: in 1980, Liz Heron wrote of a 'latterday feminist baby boom'. These new feminist mothers were, she worried, 'reversing the process' initiated by the movement's 'founding mothers... striving to challenge the mystique – and the material realities – that made them prisoners'. By contrast, these new mothers were 'moving away from us and melting into motherhood'.[24] For other activists, becoming a mother clarified their feminism. Jo Eliot has recalled that 'I really understood what feminism meant when I became a mother... the real inequalities between men and women didn't really kick in until I had a child'.[25] For yet others, the journey into motherhood posed challenging political questions. As Sara Maitland wrote,

> [her daughter] has forced upon me an unwelcome self-knowledge; she has made demands on me which I resent fiercely... She has forced me to confront dark places within my own soul – my desire to possess, to own; selfishness, or egocentricity; real doubts about the purity of my past loves, past actions. And above all she has compelled me to feel both an anger and a bleeding impotence about the position of women in this society, such as I never truly felt when I was far more 'on-the-street' politically active than I am now. I have been obliged to recognise in myself feelings about biology and gender difference and social relationships, which I was able to evade in the years before she was born, and which I cannot analyse away into the accepted modes of feminist orthodoxy.[26]

The transformations that motherhood brought, and the costs it exacted, were visible within the movement.

I am not the first to object to what Lynne Segal has identified as the 'unyielding dogma... that Women's Liberation ignored the needs of mothers'. Segal has challenged such a characterisation, noting that 'back in the beginning many of the key instigators of Women's Liberation were already mothers' who 'fought tirelessly' for nurseries, equitable parenting, child health, respectful gynaecological and obstetric care, the rights of single mothers, children's play spaces, and housing. Segal offers a useful counterpoint to Dally's observation that the movement encompassed younger rather than older mothers:

> The loss of selfhood accompanying motherhood can be greater for those who have as yet only a shaky grip on their adult identities, who have still to find secure sources of recognition and support that might create and sustain them. As younger mothers, we needed to create our own alternatives.[27]

Such an analysis may, itself, however, skim over the contributions of older women to the movement. Lee Comer, whose critique of the family, and of the isolation and demoralisation of the housewife, *Wedlocked Women*, (1974), pointed to the diverse demographic of her women's group in Leeds in 1969,

> We didn't at all fit the neat sociological explanations of the beginnings of feminism in this country, which would have us all to have been spoon-fed girl children of the 50s and 60s, enjoying the fruits of the 1944 Education Act, educated at University to expect success and equality only to be disappointed in love and work... We were, instead, of all ages and classes, grandmothers and teenagers, with more children between us than degrees, drawn together as women, by our commonality, our energy and our will to share in each other's strengths.

Comer saw the 'myth of motherhood' as a 'patriarchal trick'; her commitment to feminist activism was undimmed by motherhood. Her daughter was born in September 1970, 'just as the women's movement began to take recognisable shape'. Motherhood and feminism were, she says, 'inextricably woven... I felt equally responsible to both'.[28] But for others activism and mothering were less easily reconciled and these dual commitments did exact a toll.[29]

Notably, it was not just women's *own* experiences of motherhood that drew them into feminist politics. It was also experiences of being mothered – or a close observation of their mothers' lives – that drew some women to feminism. It is almost a cliche that the feminist politics of the 1970s was a reaction against the claustrophobic domestic ideology of the 1950s and early 1960s. Segal, raised in Australia, recalls her parents' unhappy marriage and has said that she had

> hoped never, ever, to find myself in any situation that could remind me of the regret, frustration, bitterness and interminable rowing that suffused my childhood, as maternal appeasement tried, only to fail and fail again, to soothe the paternal impatience and aggression in the family in which I grew up.

The 'dissenting children of the professional middle classes, like me, would rather have done anything than end up the way they wanted us to be; would rather have gone anywhere than become like our parents: home-owning, married, and hypocritical about sex'.[30] Susan Ardill told Segal that she was 'very much a daughter of a 1950s housewife, who lived a life of low-key depression and little personal satisfaction'.[31] Lynne Harne reflects that in 1968 'all I knew was that I rejected my mother's values and what she wanted me to be, ie educated but married to an educated man and bringing up his children'.[32] Certainly generational tensions and schisms were explored within the movement. Liz Heron wrote in 1984 of the manifold ways that women's lives differed from their mothers' and reflected that

> for some of us, our mothers are difficult to deal with. They were not, perhaps, the warm, supportive, generous and loving beings that sentimentalists see at the core of all women, of all mothers. Mothers are people and motherhood is a condition not likely to bring out the best in people if it is undergone with reluctance (however unacknowledged), with material hardship or with bitterness. Women today, with more room to choose what they want, and with more room to know there is a choice, also have the possibility of being more fulfilled as mothers. But if we reproach our mothers, or feel that they failed us, it is also because of what motherhood had to be – often a relationship that stifled in its enforced bonding of mother and child and was jealous of its very tyranny over both.[33]

Margaretta Jolly notes the sharp intake of breath when women's liberationist oral history interviewees were asked about their mothers.[34] Sheila Rowbotham has claimed that 'One of the most passionate relationships in modern feminist writing is that between mothers and daughters'.[35] Mothers, then, in both writing and memory, occupied a contested and sometimes painful space for feminist activists.

Despite the core role that young mothers played in its establishment, the movement was not always a welcoming place for those with babies. Rahila Gupta recalled that few of her fellow activists asked about her childcare arrangements, and remembered a sense of failure if she had to leave an event in order to take care of her disabled son. 'Motherhood is almost, by definition, the Achilles heel of feminism', she wrote in 1989.[36] In 1980, Sara Maitland argued that the women's movement was 'getting better at the practical support and articulation of the bad sides of motherhood, but we do not really seem to be coming to grips with the reality of that painful, wonderful, destructive, liberating love that many of us feel for our children'.[37] In some ways, this reflects the ambivalent and contradictory emotions that feminists had about being in conventional relationships with men. Reflecting on this tension, Janet Ree remembered that

> I know people have said that it's wrong to perceive the early women's movement as being against children and mothering, and I'm not saying it was actively against them. But what I did pick up as being really primary for women was to be yourself in your own right. And for mothers that meant not falling for the so-called myth of motherhood. I completely accepted this line... but there was a clash for me, even though at the time I didn't allow it to surface. I loved family life... It was a very conventional aspiration. And really the time was not right for those feelings of the family, not in the women's movement of the early seventies.

She recalled that in her local group, 'the last thing anyone talked about was what it felt like to have a baby or to be a mother'.[38] Ree's experience demonstrates the struggle to grasp the meanings of motherhood from a feminist perspective: how to acknowledge and address the meaningful changes motherhood brought, without re-centring or essentialising it in women's lives? It is little surprise, then, that ideologies and experiences of mothering were discussed within the movement.

The 1960s were a transformative moment for women's feelings – it was then that housewives and mothers began to speak more openly about their experiences – and in many ways the 1970s women's movement was building upon the cultures of disclosure established in this earlier decade.[39] What was distinctive about the feminist politics of the 1970s, though, was the intense and explicitly political significance given to women's feelings, and the network for its dissemination it developed. As Alison Fell wrote in 1979:

> In the last decade the explosion of women's liberation consciousness across the world has, for the first time, given many thousands of women the conviction that their voices are important. Women have written leaflets, tracts, herstories, position papers, comics and newspapers in a sustained attack on sexist laws, attitudes and institutions, tearing off the veils of the old femininity and saying (or shouting): 'We are not the women you tell us we are; this is who we are and this is what we want to become; this is our experience'.[40]

These ideas and experiences were shared through a powerful print infrastructure: the magazine *Spare Rib* ran from 1972 to 1993; *Women's Voice* from 1972 to 1982; *Shrew* from 1969 to 1974.[41] Feminist magazines created a means for the 'conspiracy of silence' around distressed motherhood to be broken. Annette Muir wrote in *Shrew* in January 1970 that

> We are bombarded on all sides with the image of motherhood as a radiant woman who has achieved her ultimate fulfilment by holding a sweet-smelling, sleeping baby in her arms. The reality is more likely to be a harassed dishevelled mum with a foul-smelling, yelling baby. I think the shock effect of this gap between myth and the reality is underestimated and not discussed enough... We seem committed to a conspiracy of silence.[42]

How and why, then, did feminist mothers shatter this conspiracy of silence around distress?

'This is our experience': reclaiming and politicising distress

The feminist interest in mothers' distress should be seen within the broader context of the movement's interest in mental health. While in the 1990s academics were able to comment that 'most histories of the second wave of the women's liberation movement do not mention madness or "mental health" as areas of theoretical, political or practical intervention', this has since developed into an area of scholarly interest.[43] Mathew Thomson has described how the British women's movement positioned itself as an antagonist towards and an alternative to conventional psychiatry, for it 'provided the women's movement with a powerful enemy to identify themselves against'. As he demonstrates, though, the women's movement was also able to appropriate the concept of the emotional and psychological self, with magazines like *Spare Rib* extending the 'consciousness of consciousness to a broader audience'.[44] More recently, Kate Mahoney has explored the ways that feminist mental health activism created new sites of therapeutic care in the 1970s and 1980s, and has argued that in the 1990s it shaped national mental health campaigns via the charity MIND.[45]

The women's movement underlined the ways that postwar gender ideologies generated burdens that provoked or exacerbated women's distress. Wandor wrote in a 1972 edition of *Spare Rib* that domesticity was a driving cause of women's mental ill health. Amid an endless cycle of washing and childrearing, 'No-one can understand that you've simply been driven mad and that it isn't a condition that pills or therapy can cure', she argued. The term 'mad' suggested a 'state of dislocation in which you don't know where or who you are', and women became a 'bewildered prize in the perpetual emotional tug of war between husband and children without time or space to worry about where you yourself fit in'. In this fraught situation, Wandor concluded, 'No woman can emerge undamaged'.[46] Patriarchy, it was argued, 'ignores women's emotional needs and punishes them for not conforming to their social role as caretakers of others'.[47] Mainstream mental health care, it was argued, was inadequate to deal with mothers' distress, as this provision was grounded in patriarchal ideas about women's selfhood. Alternative models needed to be created.[48]

Views about the medicalisation of unhappy motherhood varied within the movement: some feminists argued that postnatal depression was diminished and belittled by the medical profession as part of its indifference to women's suffering, while others argued that mothers' unhappiness arose from structural oppressions and was thus medicalised as a means of dismissing women's distress. More agreement occurred around the inability of patriarchal institutions to ameliorate women's unhappiness. The women's movement was sceptical about the potential for women's distress to be cured by traditional institutions. These, they underlined, were embedded in the very systems that perpetuated women's oppression. Indeed, among the papers given at the first national women's liberation conference was a paper that discussed the role of the 'psy' sciences in shaping the conditions of childrearing. Rochelle Wortis, a member of the London Women's Liberation Workshop, argued that 'modern psychology, with its emphasis on individual development, individual achievement and individual advancement, has encouraged the isolation of the adult woman, particularly the mother, and the domestication and subordination of females in society'. Wortis contested the models of childrearing put forward by psychologists and psychoanalysts, paying particular attention to John Bowlby, whose ideas had been 'sharply criticised'.[49] From its early stages as an organised movement, then, the British women's liberation movement identified psychoanalytical ideas about childrearing and the social conditions of mothering as forces that oppressed women. Wortis was not alone: Piri Marcus also argued that psychiatrists had coercive powers:

> There are lots of ways of discouraging mothers from complaining about the present situation of mothering and about the theories and 'science', 'advice' and general attitudes towards – and against – them. The most powerful one is the institutionalisation of either the children she has given birth to, or the children and the mother, or only the mother herself. The mother might be sent to mental hospital, sometimes even to prison; children night be sent to 'children's homes' if the mother 'can't cope'; that is, if she is not fulfilled and satisfied by mothering itself.[50]

By contrast, the women's movement demonstrated that women's discontent was *political* and could be a stimulus for activism. Discontent, it argued, had been depoliticised by male-dominated mental health institutions, which had claimed expertise over the female experience. In the women's movement 'pride of place' was given to 'the lived experience of mental illness, its connections with female construction of self, and to specific feminist therapies such as women's consciousness raising groups'.[51] In the early years of the women's liberation movement, a plethora of sites were established to extract feminist political meaning from personal feeling, including, among others, consciousness-raising groups, encounter groups, and self-help groups. The focus on revealing the psychologically repressed and the emotionally intimate was critical to the feminist political project.

At the first Women and Mental Health Conference in London, held in October 1977, a new definition of 'mental health' was arrived at: 'mental health as self-determination, being able to choose to fit in or not fit in, to change or not'. This statement asserted autonomy and subjectivity in both the understandings of mental health and its treatment, but it also emphasised the extent to which mental health rested on socially defined ideas of what it was to 'fit in', or to seek to change. The 'main issue' that had emerged from the conference, aside from this definition, was the vexed question of whether therapy could ever be feminist:

> The argument is basically between those who believe that when we can't cope we should take time to go through our problems with people who know what they are doing – that therapy makes us better able to go out and be political – and those that believe that personal one-to-one therapy is counter-revolutionary.[52]

Therapists were criticised for reinforcing rather than challenging the gender norms of the postwar period. Writing in *Shrew*, one female psychiatrist took aim at her profession. She noted that female patients presented with complaints that were usually about 'keeping a man, changing a man or finding a man'; concerns that had been 'reinforced' by therapists.[53]

In April 1978, this was given further voice in *Spare Rib*. Sheila Jeffreys, perhaps the best-known proponent of political lesbianism and a significant voice in radical feminism, argued that there could be no such thing as feminist therapy because the relationship duplicated the dynamic of patriarchy: 'precisely the sort of authoritarian and hierarchical set-up which, as women, we are trying to get away from'.[54] The very tools and techniques of therapy were oppressive, argued Jeffreys, who asserted that therapy had been developed by the male ruling class and as such was not value-free. She urged women to return to consciousness-raising, which was 'the basis of the revolutionary struggle of women', and provided a space for the 'development of revolutionary anger and strength with others with whom we can take political action... its purpose is not to make an individual woman feel that she can cope better with her lot, but to make her feel that she need not cope, but must struggle'.[55] The therapist was considered a conservative force that prevented women from rebelling against their oppression. Furthermore, therapy perpetuated a culture of selfhood that fragmented women's experiences. Jeffreys wrote that therapy was the 'separation of the realm of mental health from the rest of our social and political lives'.[56] Feminist therapy, it was suggested, focused on women's internal lives rather than encouraging women to utilise their anger as a revolutionary political force.

Other women strongly disagreed. Writing in *Spare Rib*, one correspondent argued that it was the individualistic nature of therapy that provided emancipation:

> women have a right to choose something they want and maybe they are choosing therapy because it's the *first* thing that's come along which gives them something for themselves – and *why not?* I get sick to the stomach of hearing how I shouldn't be so 'introspective' – why the fuck *not, for once*?[57]

This suggested that feminist therapy, in placing women's experience at the heart of its techniques, subverted cultural ideologies of feminine self-effacement. Other members of the women's liberation movement argued that feminist therapy could be complementary to feminist political activism. Stef Pixner, writing 'For Therapy' in *Spare Rib*, suggested that her experience in therapy had encouraged her to become 'less depressed, more angry, more able to know what I need and act on it'.[58] In another article in *Spare Rib*, Frances Seton 'found that the therapeutic process has given me a greater appreciation of political issues and motivation'. Although she initially viewed entering therapy as an admission of weakness, Seton found that 'Having begun to trust the process, to understand the workings of the psyche and how to use the tools of therapy, I can... apply it to the larger social sphere'. Through therapy, she was able to 'inform my political views with a new understanding of the political importance of psychology'. Here, then, the therapeutic process was positioned as being one that facilitated personal transformation for political ends.[59]

Whereas in the early days of the movement women denounced psychological theories as constructing false dichotomies between male and female personalities – suggesting that all difference was culturally rather than biologically reproduced – by the later years of the movement there was a greater willingness to revisit and redeem some psychological theory.[60] Two psychotherapists from the Women's Therapy Centre in London, founded in April 1976, explained the shift as arising from the new types of knowledge developed in feminist spaces.[61] In feminist organisations, women 'began to acknowledge that this distress might have a logic and life of its own even though its roots lay in the violence and oppression women experience within society'. Feminist therapy revealed the extent to which 'nothing short of a restructuring of social arrangements is required if the conditions that give rise to women's present psychological position are to change fundamentally'.[62] Access to fee-paying feminist therapy precluded economically precarious and working-class women, so alternative mechanisms for disseminating ideas about psychology were taken up.

Feminist groups and publications allowed new ideas to circulate and develop about how to disrupt and change conventional mental health care.[63] The Psychology Group of the Women's Liberation Workshop published an edition of *Shrew* dedicated to psychology in April 1972, explaining that it was initially established to 'examine the liberating possibilities of psychotherapeutic techniques' and to demonstrate the ways that 'therapy is often used to trap women more tightly in their roles', while setting out their aim to explain and explore the various models of psychotherapy that might be useful to the movement.[64] They also encouraged those interested in establishing alternative forms of mental care provision to come to a self-help meeting in North London, where two groups emerged: the Women's Re-evaluation Counselling Group and the Women's Self-Help Therapy Group.[65] The desire to locate the feelings and effects of oppression underpinned these modes of activism.

Consciousness-raising diverged from, challenged, and coalesced with conventional therapeutic approaches to women's mental health. It played a role in nurturing a feminist language that brought the self to the fore as well as acknowledging the oppressive effects of the social and political contexts in which women lived their lives. Consciousness-raising developed at the very inception of the women's movement as a mechanism for grassroots activism and recruitment.[66] In November 1968, Kathie Sarachild of the New York-based Redstockings group read a paper ('Consciousness-Raising: a Radical Weapon') in Chicago that outlined the strategy for consciousness-raising, a paper was later published, gained traction, and then circulated in Britain.[67] Conceived of as a conduit between large-scale social reform and individuals, women organised themselves into small groups and held 'a form of structured discussion in which women connected their personal experiences to larger structures of gender'.[68] This sought to ascribe political meaning to the situation of the individual and to lay the ground for radical change. The practice sought to explore the relationship between personal experiences and structural oppression. 'Consciousness-raising groups are a means whereby women share their often very personal experiences of discrimination and oppression, as a first step towards political understanding of it and resistance to it', one feminist pamphlet published in 1976 explained.[69] The 'very personal' stories shared were collectively validated and this nurtured political understanding.

This route to activism was not clear-cut, however, as consciousness-raising aimed to give voice to women's experience. Groups were founded on the premise that 'sharing private suffering' could be healing and emphasised personal experience as a path to political struggle.[70] 'In consciousness-raising', the Psychology Group of the Women's Liberation Workshop observed, 'women discover the common nature of their problems and this understanding is channelled into a political perspective; the groups have a semi-therapeutic function in that they deal with the emotions aroused by the process of changing'.[71] '"Consciousness raising" was, after all, about consciousness and change: about collective exploration of personal experiences and emotions, in turn leading to the necessity of struggle for personal and social change', Sue O'Sullivan wrote in 1982.[72] The political purpose of consciousness-raising distinguished it from therapy, although both were thought to have potential to make social structures visible through an interrogation of the individual psyche.[73] Consciousness-raising quickly expanded beyond the small group, and editors of feminist magazines such as *Spare Rib* saw themselves as performing a consciousness-raising activity.[74] In 1974, one reader wrote: 'I read your magazine and I find I am right – life is hard, bloody hard. But the knowledge I am not alone and not crazy, makes me feel so much better and stronger'.[75] This feeling of shared experience was reiterated in groups: one member of the Tufnell Park group recalled in *Spare Rib*, that the group served to assure her that 'I need no longer consider myself a candidate for the '"funny farm", since so many of the women arrayed in that small sitting room, despite their surface differences, seemed to share what for so long I had believed to be my own idiosyncratic suffering'.[76]

The need for liberation was not only *felt* by women but was also needed by families. Mica Nava wrote that the social conditioning around motherhood damaged women's mental health, leading them to perform it with 'a kind of manic zeal', and observed that 'there now exist the recognized syndromes of over-mothering and over-control, when children are not allowed to experience themselves as autonomous persons'.[77] Sue Sharpe, a member of the London Women's Liberation Workshop, wrote of the ways women embodied their distress:

> developing minor illnesses, nervous complaints and so on, which are remedied with tranquilizers, sleeping pills, or a quick drink to keep going. 'Mother's little helpers' have performed their silent functions only too long. Living conditions also often aggravate the situation and for example tower-block life, day in day out, has been shown to have a deteriorating effect on mental health.[78]

As Rowbotham noted, while there was 'release' in voicing 'struggles, dependence, exhaustion and rage' of mothering, women also began to expose the 'depression, derangement, violence' they felt.[79]

Mothers, postnatal depression, distress, and liberation

Aged 22, in the early years of the women's movement, Sara Maitland conceived her daughter, Mildred. The pregnancy was easy, Maitland felt well, and she joined women's groups in Oxford that connected her to other pregnant women. Her community was middle-class, white, and intellectual, and she anticipated the pleasure of being both a feminist and a mother. Mildred was born in 1973, and Maitland loved her daughter immediately, deeply, and fiercely. Soon, though, the 'long Oxford summer' was over. Mildred's sleep veered off course, and as her husband went to college, Maitland found herself alone for protracted stretches. Lonely and stressed, Maitland ran the gamut of maternal emotions:

> Sometimes I would go to pick her up feeling furious and resentful and at the touch or sight of her, I would collapse, melted by physical love and tenderness. Sometimes I would be playing with her quite happily when a complete and profound anger would come over me and I would want to kill her.

Afraid, Maitland went to see her doctor and worried that she was experiencing postnatal depression. Her doctor, however, did not agree. 'Rubbish', he responded. Instead, her doctor said it was 'perfectly sane to have strong difficulties in adjusting to being a mother… that small babies were indeed demanding, annoying and boring'. The conversation opened a new understanding of not just her experiences but also the role of the diagnosis of postnatal depression. There was now a trend that ran counter to the proper recognition of postnatal depression, Maitland said, in which 'even sensible worries about concrete realities like housing or money are dismissed as "Baby Blues"; a definition which can and does prevent women themselves coming to face the realities of motherhood'. Society still had a stake in the idea that mothers should unequivocally enjoy life within the nuclear family. If they fell short of this pleasure, 'it is easier to say that we are poor sick things and some nice drugs will make us feel better, than face up to the fact that mothering is an impossible and treacherous job in our society'. The labour of mothering was arduous, the cultural conditions punitive, and the assignation of blame inescapable:

> Mothering is a job which not only demands a unique combination of management responsibilities, manual labour and skilled work, but also goes on seven days a week, twenty-four hours a day and is completely unpaid, unrewarded, and undervalued. Moreover it is a no-win arrangement nowadays: if you devote yourself entirely to your child, you are failing yourself in your duties to self-development, damaging your husband's frail ego and probably 'over-mothering' or 'spoiling' your child. If you do not so devote yourself you are depriving your child of his/her emotional needs. Either way you are isolated and either way, whatever happens, it is *all your fault*.[80]

The accommodations that Maitland and her husband subsequently made were informed by their class, their economic position, and the dynamics of their partnership: adjusting ideas about ideal family size; an emphasis on the administration of family life; and a search for childcare. Not all mothers were, of course, in a position to make effective changes after the contradictions between expectation and experience came to light. Nor, of course, did all distressed mothers encounter doctors who enabled them to interpret their feelings as emerging from particular social and political structures. But the recognition that there was a disjuncture between the representation of motherhood and the lived labour of childcare in 1970s Britain – and that this could play a role in provoking distress and discontent – was an important strand of feminist thought.

Others, too, found that motherhood provoked painful and tumultuous emotions. Sue Cowley – later O'Sullivan – wrote in *Red Rag* that the reality of mothers' lives ran counter to the idealised representations of the affluent and time-rich nuclear family nurtured by psychologists. 'Happy' mothers, left alone with children, could readily transform into 'a screaming witch' or descend into 'a depression'. The solution was community, and having other adults on hand during childcare: 'You can talk with an adult about the children while being with them and it changes so much. You talk about why you lose control, why you can't cope, what funny thing happened yesterday. And, importantly, you can talk about other things besides children. You aren't alone and isolated', she argued.[81] Introducing *Dutiful Daughters*, Sheila Rowbotham and Jean McCrindle observed that 'It is in fact the advent of children into their marriages which causes by far the greatest tensions in these women's lives and forces them into states of nervous irritation and sometimes near breakdown'.[82] The pressures put on mothers of small children were untenable, it was argued. John Bowlby and those who espoused the importance of continuous mothering were accused of creating 'a free-floating guilt some say is well nigh impossible to escape'.[83] Lee Comer – who left school at 16 – wrote *Wedlocked Women* while living with her daughter in the north of England. Comer roundly criticised Bowlby and argued that the contemporary conditions of motherhood were a cornerstone in women's oppression. 'What mothers have to do – and they do it astonishingly well – is to present their families and to the outside world, a smiling face, a face which colludes with the public's hypocrisy and maintains that motherhood is one long succession of fulfilling moments', she argued. Mothers were 'forced to maintain this collusion with each other' through the 'taboo on their experience as mothers'.

> They may be able to share the odd grumble between each other about being tired and overworked, but they cannot speak of their desperation. They cannot talk about what being cooped up all day with their children does to them… nor can they speak of the precarious ambivalence of their situation – of the sometimes overwhelming love they feel for their children which has to vie with their feelings of violence.

Such a context was, Comer argued, 'tailor-made to breed resentment'.[84] Mothers received little recognition or pity for their work or their challenges; in lone fathers, however, loneliness and depression were subjects of handwringing concern.[85] Comer and others argued that misery was provoked by the private and isolated nature of mothers' work, the construction of myths that enforced feelings of inadequacy and shame, and the structuring of society that meant that children were raised in a society riven by racial, sexual, economic, and gendered inequalities.

Sue O'Sullivan attended the Ruskin conference in 1970 while heavily pregnant with her second child. She had not much enjoyed her first experience of mothering, recalling that, at home with her small baby:

> I was floundering badly but I think I must have looked alright… there was pleasure and contentment, but through it all I felt displaced emotionally. I wasn't sure what anything meant. I'd joined the grown-up world of mothers and yet I felt more unsure and lonely than ever before. I could perform all the techniques of motherhood competently, I was riveted by the baby, but I had an awful feeling that being a mother didn't fit me well. I was a failure in what I assumed would come most naturally… this was something different and much more fundamentally fearful and guilt-inspiring.[86]

Her experience with her second son – born shortly after the Ruskin conference – was worse.

> I thought I was never going to surface. I felt unable to express it to anyone. I couldn't call up my women's group and say, 'Get over

here'. Maybe people brought flowers round, but I was back in the nuclear family, and I couldn't get out. I was just a mess; for three months seriously, and then less and less. I was aware of it but I think I blamed myself.

I couldn't tell my doctor about it. I'd go in to see the doctor and I'd end up smiling cheerfully... my husband knew just how desperate I was. He told me afterwards that he was afraid to leave me on my own. Then I started going again to women's groups, to the meetings... for about two or three years I was very constrained and very weighed down with these two little kids. If I look at myself physically in pictures of that time, well, I remember feeling bedraggled, unwashed hair, drudge. Tired.[87]

O'Sullivan was not alone. The women's liberation movement allowed motherhood to be talked about in political terms.[88] It argued that men's control of women's reproductive role was crucial to their oppression and was deeply connected to capitalism and patriarchy. The nuclear family, the movement suggested, maintained women's exploitation. As *Spare Rib* explained in 1983, 'What the nuclear family depends on, of course, is women's unpaid work: bearing and raising children, doing housework, providing sex and emotional support for men... in general, "families" are designed to exploit women'.[89] Postnatal depression signified the medicalisation of women's discontent – the depoliticisation of their frustration – but it was also a product of oppression. In 1972, women's liberation activists argued that women talked about domesticity in 'the tones of a private neurosis to express a social fact – the imposed isolation of her work'.[90] In 1982, Michèle Barrett and Mary McIntosh wrote about the 'tyranny of motherhood', observing that 'it is clear that being a housewife can drive women mad'.[91] O'Sullivan re-emphasised this in the same year. 'We know... that kids and isolated housing drive women mad; that combining shitty capitalist waged work, with unwaged work in the home, with caring for and being responsible for raising children, with all the assumptions of heterosexuality drives many women crazy. Even as they try harder to cope!'[92]

The feminist movement developed a rich literary culture through which women's experiences of mothering and depression could be shared. In *Dutiful Daughters* (1979), Sheila Rowbotham and Jean McCrindle included oral testimony from working-class mother

Linda Peffer, who recalled having her children as 'like a bomb'. The arrival of her daughter did not adhere to the cultural script around maternity:

> You see the thing was that I didn't feel any feeling for Karen [her daughter] whatsoever... I just couldn't cope with the housework, and I just felt that all I done with Karen was just fed and bathed her and kept her, and I just sort of used to burst into tears. And of course I wouldn't tell anybody, because if I tried to tell anyone, you know, they'd think how terrible, you know, she's got this lovely baby, and what a horrible woman she is. So I just went into this absolute deep depression. Really – I mean, I was almost suicidal. Because I felt trapped. There was this little thing lying there, and I had to do everything for her, and nobody told me. You see, you're not really all keyed up with all these instincts.

Gradually, she

> started voicing opinions. It's surprising after you've said it a couple of times how many people say, ooh yes, you know, really – and they start opening up, and you find a hell of a lot of women have felt exactly the same as you, only they've just been so scared to say it.[93]

By giving space to these experiences and stories, the women's movement created richer narratives around motherhood.

These understandings of distressed motherhood were also spread through magazines. As Laurel Forster has argued, the print culture established by the movement was considered a 'potential portal to power'.[94] In the 1970s and 1980s, the magazine *Spare Rib*, for example, published several articles and poems that focused on postnatal depression.[95] In June 1976, Catherine Ballard and Hilary Hackett wrote an article in *Spare Rib* asking

> What then is post-partum depression? According to a consultant gynaecologist:
> It's all bunkum and baloney...
> But a consultant psychiatrist said:
> Bloody gynaecologists and midwives fill my wards with desperate women.[96]

Hormonal explanations obscured the extent to which motherhood engendered a 'dislocation of self', they argued. This redefined women's psychological relationship with motherhood, which psychoanalytic experts had posited as a process of feminine fulfilment. Ballard and Hackett argued that postnatal depression encompassed a range of feelings, including

> shock, insecurity, inadequacy, confusion and resentment; fears about their ability to love or look after the child; inexplicable states of tension and difficulty in relaxing or sleeping; sensations of having lost their 'real selves'; new and unpleasant feelings about their bodies and sexuality; guilt feelings sometimes associated with disappointment about the child's sex or looks; loss of concentration and appetite; an obsession with the baby and its routine.[97]

This is indicative of how the experience of postnatal depression encompassed both emotional responses and sets of behaviours. Ballard and Hackett proposed a model that highlighted the psycho- and social dislocation triggered by childbirth, accounting for its incidence in both working- and middle-class women. For middle-class women, the psychological impact of motherhood was exacerbated by the individualistic emphasis of their social conditioning. They suggested that an environment that cultivated strong links between women would be less prone to provoking distress.

Spare Rib also responded to wider cultural discussions about postnatal depression. For example, in December 1973, the BBC broadcasted a play entitled 'Baby Blues' written by Nemone Lethbridge as part of its 'Play for Today' series on BBC1. The autofictional play followed a new mother in her late thirties, who, depressed after the birth of her much-longed-for first child, discovers her husband is having an affair and experiences psychosis. Spiralling, the protagonist attempts to kill herself and her child. The play caused a splash and was discussed in political magazines and on the radio, as well as in *Spare Rib* in 1974.[98] Lethbridge was on the front cover, and inside the magazine, she discussed her own experiences of mental illness, noting that five days after the birth of her son via caesarean, she 'went out of my mind'. Initially, this took the form of visions and hearing voices, but her experience was protracted: 'I couldn't stop crying for eighteen months'. Her gynaecologist assured her that the 'baby blues' were par for the course, and her 'sensitive and sensible' GP prescribed her a variety of drugs: tryptizol; largactyl; Librium; valium; Tofranil; concordin; Anafranil. Realising that her experience was far from unique, Lethbridge called for a network of support groups to be established.[99] The organisation Depressives Anonymous formed, holding its first national conference in 1974. By the winter of that year, groups spanned the nation.[100] Like MAMA, which spread following a BBC programme about postnatal depression, Depressives Anonymous was given impetus by television, though it retained a more general focus on depression rather than mothers. In 1980, the organisation changed its name to Depressives Associated, reflecting the perception that anonymity exacerbated the stigma of depression; like other self-help groups, the organisation emphasised the comfort that shared experience could bring.[101]

Feminism, childbirth, and midwifery

But feminist interest extended beyond the early phase of mothering and into the experience of becoming a mother itself. Childbirth was, perhaps naturally, often where women's conversations about their experiences of mothering began. While the range of experiences became quickly apparent – some labours were fast, others slow; some labours less painful, some horribly so; some labours enjoyable, some miserable – consciousness-raising conversations drew common experiences to the fore. The conviction that the medical profession handled childbirth with 'indifference and arrogance' emerged, with women feeling they were treated more like livestock than people. The medicalisation and technologisation of childbirth had, feminists argued, rendered labouring women powerless and passive at best, and resulted in traumatic births at worst. No doubt some of these consciousness-raising conversations included women who had hoped to have a 'natural childbirth', inspired by the NCT and prominent advocate Sheila Kitzinger. The feminist anthropologist, prolific author, and antenatal teacher was perhaps the best-known individual postwar proponent of natural childbirth and argued that for most women, childbirth was not a medical event. It could be empowering and even enjoyable, she suggested.

Like Grantly Dick-Read in the 1930s, Kitzinger argued for women's education about and participation in childbirth. She discussed home births, birthing pools, encouraged fathers to be present, if desired, and encouraged women to move around during labour, to squat, be upright, or to use a birthing stool; all measures considered to be empowering. Kitzinger was an advocate for the importance of mothering and mothers. She argued that preparing women for motherhood and childbirth was a complement to liberation from the 'shackles of domesticity' rather than an anathema to it. Women should have knowledge, choices, and power when it came to their fertility and reproduction, Kitzinger argued, and be able to give birth without fear and unnecessary interference.[102] Like women in consciousness-raising groups, Kitzinger argued that hospitals treated women in labour like cattle and framed birth as a political experience that reflected and embodied power relations.[103] Her ideas were widely disseminated; her book *The Experience of Childbirth*, first published in 1962, was republished multiple times and sold over a million copies worldwide.[104] But hospitals, by far the most common site of childbirth following the Cranbrook Report of 1959 and the Peel Report of 1970, proved resistant to ideas about natural childbirth, and rates of induction and interference – epidurals, c-sections, and the use of forceps – were high.

Given this, it is surprising that it was not until 1975 that the prominent feminist magazine *Spare Rib* published a significant feature on childbirth, and when it did so, it emphasised pain above all other issues.[105] The piece came out in favour of hospitals as the right site for childbirth and argued for women's right to medical intervention to relieve pain.[106] Kitzinger was shocked to find herself in conflict with *Spare Rib* when she read the article. The article's authors, she thought, 'unselfconsciously lent their support to the system that I believed was abusing them' and overlooked the acute imbalance of power within the medical system.[107] Kitzinger was not the only reader to respond with concern. Among those who disagreed with the article's conclusions were a trainee NCT teacher and a trainee midwife, who wrote in to argue that women should be able to have babies where they felt safest and most comfortable, to defend natural childbirth, and to encourage the magazine to support beleaguered midwives.[108]

Midwives were also organising, and in 1976, the Association of Radical Midwives (ARM) was established. Set up by student nurses – although its membership soon extended beyond this – ARM sought to resist the trend towards technologised births, to promote midwifery's prestige, skills, and expertise, and to reinforce the agency of birthing women.[109] It set out a vision for maternity services that positioned the relationship between mothers and midwives at the core of good maternity care and stressed the importance of improving education in midwifery.[110] Some of these ideas were set out in leaflets that were illustrated by Polly Kitzinger, Sheila Kitzinger's daughter.[111] Feminism was a key influence. Midwife Mary Cronk remembered

> how much we were an organization rooted in feminism... the influence of the feminist movement was so much a part of our early thinking and work, for women and for midwives, as we tried to raise our own awareness and the awareness of women, that their bodies were theirs, and that they had a say in what happened to them.[112]

Another founding member, Jenny Spinks, also stressed the 'feminist viewpoint' that informed the group's development.[113] Newspapers described the group as a 'small but militant pressure group'.[114] But others distanced themselves from feminism and radicalism. 'Radical' meant getting back to roots, explained the *Birmingham Daily Post* in 1993, which contrasted the image evoked by the organisation's name ('an army of cropped-haired viragos dressed in combat gear and Doctor Marten boots storming delivery rooms, pushing aside fathers and doctors and pulling the plug on the oxygen pump before making off with the mother in labour to give birth, au naturel, in the nearest field') with a more moderate reality. The local spokesperson did not jump to the defence of the characterisation, laughing off the stereotype of the bra-burning feminist. Instead, she played into the discourse of choice, emphasising the organisation's more modest aim to support women to make empowered decisions about and during childbirth.[115]

Disempowering birth experiences could have long-term implications, ARM argued. Community midwife Rachel Celia wrote in 1982 that for most women, birth would be 'frightening, traumatic and lonely', the result of which 'usually presents as a lack of confidence, self denigration and depression', and under which there was 'anger, hurt, tears, anxiety and confusion'. Women were frequently belittled on labour wards, Celia warned, and the denial of the validity of their experience could lead to 'boredom, anxiety or depression which, unrecognised, quickly becomes chronic or moves onto another less direct and easily relieved state'. By contrast, acknowledging mothers' anger about their birth experiences could be transformative: 'I have often seen quite long-term depressions lift after just one discussion where anger and criticism were encouraged; women are remarkably resilient', Celia wrote. Enabling mothers to express their emotions ran counter to women's socialisation, she argued. Dismissing or minimising mothers' rage and sadness did little when mothers felt it was the 'end of the world'. Beyond this retrospective work, midwives could help to diminish the risk of postnatal depression by emphasising to expectant mothers that such a response was a 'reasonable reaction to any new situation'.[116] ARM, therefore, mirrored the women's movement's articulation of the ways that women's emotions were socially circumscribed.

ARM sought to build links with those in related professions and organisations that organised around childbirth, including the NCT and AIMS.[117] It reached out to health visitors to stress their shared goals and complementary concerns.[118] This emphasis on shared concerns was reiterated at its annual conferences.[119] It is notable, though, that at ARM's fourth annual conference, held in May 1984 and attended by 480 people, one non-midwife reminded the audience that ordinary mothers had played a key role in birth activism.[120] She was perhaps thinking of the landmark protest in the active birth movement held on Hampstead Heath in north London just two years before. This protest, triggered by a clash between a mother and the Royal Free Hospital, saw nearly 6,000 women demand the right to have an active birth, and to be allowed to give birth in their chosen position, rather than on their backs as hospitals preferred.[121] The links between mothers, organisations, and professional associations – even those with a feminist lens – needed to be periodically reaffirmed.

Women of colour, Black women, activism, and mothers' distress

Women of colour made critical contributions to the women's liberation movement. However, their experiences within the movement were often marred by silencing.[122] As Marilyn Gayle found, the women's liberation movement was 'almost exclusively white and almost exclusively middle-class'. It 'tended to ignore its own racism and classism'.[123] In the late 1970s, women of colour increasingly formed their own organisations which acted as important and expansive sites of theorisation, solidarity, and resistance. This flourishing would expand further in the 1980s in response to the social and economic policies promoted by the Thatcher government.[124] This autonomous organising highlighted the ways that Black women and women of colour's lives were shaped by residual colonialism and imperialism in the British state.

The intersecting oppressions that Black mothers experienced along the lines of class, race, and gender meant that some of the analyses developed by the women's liberation movement, of which white women comprised the majority of members, were extraneous or unhelpful. In the 1980s, Black mothers and women of colour were engaged in activist work around the family and reproduction in ways that resisted anti-black racism.[125] This necessitated a focus on survival and resistance; women of colour were battling 'sustained fascist and racist onslaughts'.[126] Challenging stereotypes of Black families, defending lone mothers, resisting health inequities, and critiquing white feminist universalising claims about contraception and abortion emerged as critical threads of Black feminist activism. Hazel V. Carby argued that the feminist concepts of 'the family' the 'patriarchy' and 'reproduction' 'become problematic in their application to black women's lives'. Carby observed that 'the black family has functioned as a prime source of resistance to oppression'. The idea of 'dependence' was also flawed: the devaluing of Black men's paid labour and suppression of their place in the labour market had positioned some Black women as heads of households and meant that they were not financially dependent on men, said Carby.[127] For feminists and activists of colour, then, the white feminist characterisation of the family as a site of women's disempowerment neglected the experiences of Black women.

Interactions with healthcare and health professionals could be particularly alienating. One 1979 study, which itself made sweeping generalisations about Asian communities, observed that some pregnant British Asian women were referred to clinics for immigrant populations despite being raised in Britain and speaking perfect English.[128] Amrit Wilson's 1978 study *Finding a Voice* observed that

> Post-natal depression is said to be common among immigrant women generally. Among Asians it affects particularly those who are separated from their families… Often these women, sometimes as young as seventeen or eighteen, suffer alone, no one except their husbands knows about them, or cares. Occasionally they are referred to hospitals, but the treatment they receive sometimes serves only to underline their isolation.[129]

In 1978, women of colour formed a national network, the Organisation of Women of Asian and African Descent (OWAAD). It was a formative influence on Black women's political organising in Britain, with influence extending well beyond its 1983 demise.[130] The effects of racism on women's mental health were amplified by the organisation, which argued that 'you are more prone to a mental breakdown if you live under intolerable conditions… it would seem that we are predisposed to mental health problems, just by being here'. Race, class, and sex shaped access to mental health care. 'So, basically we are not mad', OWAAD wrote

> we are reacting to the shit we face daily, but it is easier for the authorities to label us as being 'mad' as yet another form of social control! We can be locked up in hospitals, drugged or shocked out of our minds or deported – all in the name of treatment.

The social conditions that harmed Black women also prevented their healing through community. OWAAD concluded that 'Stuck up on the seventeenth floor of a tower block with young children and weakened by language difficulties, our sisters are forced to live in isolation and loneliness in the midst of a strange uncaring society'.[131] While Black women's movements did not emphasise the oppressions engendered by normative domesticity, women of colour articulated the emotional and psychological consequences of compounding gendered, class, and racialised oppressions.

Conclusion

This chapter has explored the space occupied by mothers' frustrations, unhappiness, and postnatal depression in the women's liberation movement between the late 1960s and the 1980s. Unhappy motherhood was both a pull to and a topic of discussion within the feminist movement. This is far away from the accusation made by Maureen Freely in the 1990s that feminism had abandoned mothers: mothers and unhappy mothering were important themes, even while the institution of motherhood and the nuclear family were subjects of furious critique.[132] However, its critique of the family garnered more attention than its attentiveness to the emotional lives of mothers. Even Betty Friedan, whose publication of *The Feminine Mystique* in the 1960s did so much to place the spotlight on women's distress, worried in the 1980s that feminists in the United States had ceded the topic of the family to their antagonists.[133] This chapter has argued that feminists in Britain were not blind to mothers' struggles, even while passionate debates about men, the family, and liberation emerged between different ideological strands of the movement. The family was nonetheless a fraught topic. As the first book-length history of the movement – written by movement members – noted,

> Of course, it would be easier to develop a clear political analysis of family life if it were altogether a bad thing… there are ways in which the family can be a source of care, affection, strength and security, as much as it can be a source of physical violence, psychic oppression and social control.[134]

Despite – and in some ways because of – these painful conversations about the family, the movement played an important role in enabling a wider conversation about mothers' struggles. But those within the women's movement engaged with motherhood and with women's wider distress in different ways, shaped by their ideological perspective, political positioning, and personal experiences.

Importantly, the movement enabled mothers to give less sanitised accounts of their experiences. Indeed, by the late 1980s, mothers were able to proclaim their imperfections proudly. Journalist Libby Purves opened her aptly titled book *How Not to Be a Perfect Mother* with the encouraging declaration that 'Under the mantle of every mother lies an ordinary, disgruntled human being'.[135] The movement should be credited with supporting a culture of disclosure around the messy, ambivalent, and contradictory emotions of mothering.[136] However, the movement did not, and could not, successfully overturn some of the practical challenges that would face mothers in the late twentieth century: reconciling full-time work with parenting and the insufficient provision and excruciating cost of early years childcare, for example. Nonetheless, the process of making mothers' discontent visible created new arguments for social reform. One of the movement's most important legacies was to reframe women's discontent as a product of their oppression and to imply the possibility of political solutions to emotional, intimate, and psychological problems.

Women's problems would soon be placed on the academic agenda. Mica Nava, with whom this chapter opened, wrote her first publication *The Family: A Critique of Certain Features* (1972) at the end of her first year as a mature student of sociology at the London School of Economics.[137] Nava was not alone as a feminist looking to sociological training in the 1970s. Indeed, the entrance of feminists and mothers to the sociological discipline would help to carve a new space for discussion about mothers' experiences – and would challenge the discipline to change.

Notes

1 Mica Nava, 'Looking Back: '1968', Women's Liberation and the Family', *Free Associations* 78, 2020, 53–71, 55–62, 55.
2 Adrienne Rich, *Of Woman Born: Motherhood as Experience and Institution* (New York, 1986 [1976]).
3 Nava, 'Looking Back', 55–62.
4 Sue Bruley, '"It Didn't Just Come out of Nowhere Did It?": The Origins of the Women's Liberation Movement in 1960s Britain', *Oral History*, 45, 1, 2017, 67–78.
5 'The Four Demands', in *Once a Feminist: Stories of a Generation*, ed. Michelene Wandor (London, 1990), 242–243. Originally published in *Women's Newspaper*, 1, 6 March 1971.
6 Lynn Abrams, *Feminist Lives: Women, Feelings, & The Self in Post-War Britain* (Oxford, 2023), 185.
7 Mica Nava, "1968' and the Women's Liberation Movement in Britain', *Moving the Social*, 64, 2020, 37.
8 Edinburgh Women's Liberation Group, Nursery Report, c.1974, xi, quoted in Sarah Browne, *The Women's Liberation Movement in Scotland* (Manchester, 2014), 73.
9 Ann Dally, *Inventing Motherhood: The Consequences of an Ideal* (London, 1982), 165–168.

10 Michèle Roberts, *Paper Houses: A Memoir of the '70s and Beyond* (London, 2008), 50.
11 Anna Coote and Beatrix Campbell, *Sweet Freedom: The Struggle for Women's Liberation* (London, 1982), 16.
12 Quoted in 'Nine Years Together: A History of a Women's Liberation Group', *Spare Rib*, 9 (April 1978), quoted in Coote and Campbell, *Sweet Freedom*, 16.
13 Catherine Hall and Stuart Hall, quoted in Margaretta Jolly, *Sisterhood and After: An Oral History of the UK Women's Liberation Movement, 1968–Present* (Oxford, 2019), 195–197.
14 Audrey Battersby, *Once a Feminist: Stories of a Generation* (London, 1990), 113–120, 113–114.
15 Val Charlton, *Once a Feminist: Stories of a Generation* (London, 1990), 160–170, 161–162.
16 Sue O'Sullivan, 'From 1968', in *'68, '78, '88: From Women's Liberation to Feminism*, ed. Amanda Sebestyen (Dorset, 1988), 51–62, 52.
17 Alison Fell, 'Everyday Offensives: Notes on Ideology', *Red Rag*, 6, 1973, 18.
18 Alison Fell, 'Rebel with a Cause', in *Truth, Dare or Promise: Girls Growing Up in the 50s*, ed. Liz Heron (London, 1985), 11–25, 24–25.
19 Michelene Wandor, 'A Diary in Keeping', in *'68, '78, '88: From Women's Liberation to Feminism*, ed. Amanda Sebestyen (Dorset, 1988), 1–4, 1–2.
20 Lynne Segal, *Making Trouble: Life and Politics* (London, 2007), 62.
21 Sue Crockford, 'In the Beginning We Demanded'. Retrieved from https://www.bl.uk/collection-items/in-the-beginning-we-demanded#:~:text=Sue%20Crockford%20was%20a%20member,the%20film%20A%20Woman's%20Place [Accessed 1 July 2023].
22 Nava, 'Looking Back', 59.
23 Marlene Hobsbawm, *Once a Feminist: Stories of a Generation* (London, 1990), 121–125, 123.
24 Liz Heron, 'The Mystique of Motherhood', in *No Turning Back: Writings from the Women's Liberation Movement 1975–80*, ed. Feminist Anthology Collective (London, 1981), 138–140, 139. First published in *Time Out*, 553, 7–21 November 1980.
25 Jo Eliot, in *Personal Histories of the Second Wave of Feminism*, summarised from interviews by Viv Honeybourne and Ilona Singer, Volumes One and Two, Feminist Archive South, 91. Retrieved from http://feministarchivesouth.org.uk/wp-content/uploads/2013/02/Personal-Histories-of-the-Second-Wave-of-Feminism.pdf [Accessed 1 October 2024].

26 Sara Maitland, *Why Children?* Eds Stephanie Dowrick and Sibyl Grundberg (London, 1980), 78–91, 79.
27 Segal, *Making Trouble*, 84–88.
28 Lee Comer, 'From 1969', in *'68, '78, '88: From Women's Liberation to Feminism*, ed. Amanda Sebestyen (Dorset, 1988), 84–89.
29 Segal, *Making Trouble*, 135.
30 Lynne Segal, *Straight Sex: The Politics of Pleasure* (London, 1994), 2.
31 Segal, *Making Trouble*, 66.
32 Lynne Harne, 'From 1971: Reinventing the Wheel', in *'68, '78, '88: From Women's Liberation to Feminism*, ed. Amanda Sebestyen (Dorset, 1988), 63–71, 63.
33 Liz Heron (Ed.), 'Introduction', in *Truth, Dare or Promise: Girls Growing Up in the 50s* (London, 1985), 1–9, 8–9.
34 Margaretta Jolly, *Sisterhood and After: An Oral History of the UK Women's Liberation Movement, 1968–Present* (Oxford, 2019), 5.
35 Sheila Rowbotham, *The Past is Before Us* (Boston, MA, 1989), 11.
36 Rahila Gupta, 'Giving Birth Again', in *Balancing Acts: On Being a Mother*, ed. Katherine Gieve (London, 1989), 94–106, 105–106.
37 Maitland, *Why Children?*, 79.
38 Janet Ree, *Once a Feminist: Stories of a Generation* (London, 1990), 93–106.
39 Abrams, *Feminist Lives*.
40 Alison Fell (ed.), 'Introduction', in *Hard Feelings: Fiction and Poetry From Spare Rib* (London, 1979), 1–6, 1.
41 Laurel Forster, 'Spreading the Word: Feminist Print Cultures and the Women's Liberation Movement', *Women's History Review*, 25, 5, 2016, 812–831. For more on mothering and feminist print cultures, see Sarah Crook, 'Writing about Mothering and Childcare in the British Women's Liberation Movement, 1970–85', in *Women's Periodicals and Print Culture in Britain, 1940s–2000s*, eds Laurel Forster and Joanne Hollows (Edinburgh, 2020), 351–365.
42 Annette Muir, 'On Having Children', *Shrew*, January 1970.
43 Tamsin Wilton, 'Madness and Feminism: Bristol Crisis Service for Women', in *Feminist Activism in the 1990s*, ed. Gabriele Griffin (London, 1995), 28–40, 32. See, for example, Nancy Tomes, 'Feminist Histories of Psychiatry', in *Discovering the History of Psychiatry*, eds Mark Micale and Roy Porter (Oxford, 1994), 348–383.
44 Mathew Thomson, *Psychological Subjects: Identity, Culture, and Health in Twentieth-Century Britain* (Oxford, 2006), 279–281.
45 Kate Mahoney, *Feminist Mental Health Activism in England, c.1968–95* (Manchester, 2023).
46 Michelene Wandor, 'Family Everafter', *Spare Rib*, 5, 1972, 10–13, 12.

47 Bristol Women's Therapy Centre, 'Talking with Women in Bristol', *Spare Rib*, 102, 1981, 6–8, 8.
48 For a discussion of this, see Sarah Crook, 'The Women's Liberation Movement, Activism and Therapy at the Grassroots, 1968–1985', *Women's History Review*, 27, 7, 2018, 1152–1168, from which some of this chapter is drawn. The author extends her thanks to the journal for its permission to reprint parts of it here.
49 Rochelle P. Wortis, 'Child-Rearing and Women's Liberation', in *The Body Politic: Women's Liberation in Britain 1969–1972*, ed. M. Wandor (London, 1972), 124–130, 124.
50 Piri Marcus, 'Motherhood: A Letter', in *Sweeping Statements: Writings from the Women's Liberation Movement 1981–83*, eds H. Kanter et al. (London, 1984), 296–298, 297.
51 L.J. Jordanova, 'Mental Illness, Mental Health: Changing Norms and Expectations', in *Women in Society: Interdisciplinary Essays*, ed. Cambridge Women's Studies Group (London, 1981), 95–114, 97.
52 Ruth Wallsgrove, 'Choosing to Fit In…Or Not Fit In', *Spare Rib*, 65, 1977, 13.
53 'A Psychiatrist's View', *Shrew*, 4, 2, 1972, 3.
54 Sheila Jeffreys, 'Against Therapy', in *Women's Health: A Spare Rib Reader*, ed. Sue O'Sullivan (London, 1987), 142–145, 143.
55 *Ibid.*, 143–144.
56 *Ibid.*
57 Claire Betti, 'Letters Forum', *Spare Rib*, 71, 1978, 36.
58 Stef Pixner, 'For Therapy', *Spare Rib*, 69, 1978, 20–21.
59 Frances Seton, 'Opening Myself to Change', *Spare Rib*, 44, 1976, 30–32, 32.
60 Lynne Segal, *Is the Future Female? Troubled Thoughts on Contemporary Feminism* (London, 1987), 117–122. See Juliet Mitchell, *Psychoanalysis and Feminism* (Harmondsworth, 1974).
61 Sheila Ernst and Marie Maguire (Eds), 'Introduction', in *Living with the Sphinx: Papers From the Women's Therapy Centre* (London, 1987), 1–29, 8.
62 Luise Eichenbaum and Susie Orbach, 'Separation and Intimacy: Crucial Practice Issues in Working with Women in Therapy', in *Living with the Sphinx: Papers from the Women's Therapy Centre*, eds Sheila Ernst and Marie Maguire (London, 1987), 49–67, 49–50.
63 Thomson, *Psychological Subjects*, 280.
64 Editorial, *Shrew*, 1972, 4, 2, 1–2.
65 Carol Morrell, 'On Not Being the Hostess with the Mostest', *Spare Rib*, 16, 1973, 37–38.

66 Sue Bruley, 'Consciousness-Raising in Clapham: Women's Liberation as 'Lived Experience' in South London in the 1970s', *Women's History Review*, 22, 5, 2013, 717–738.
67 Kathie Sarachild, 'Consciousness-Raising: A Radical Weapon', in *Feminist Revolution*, ed. Kathie Sarachild (New York, 1978),A144–150. See also Kathie Sarachild, 'A Program for Feminist 'Consciousness Raising', *Notes from the Second Year: Women's Liberation, 1970*, ed. Shulamith Firestone, 78–80, available at http:// library .duke .edu/ digitalcollections/ wlmpc _wlmms01039/.
68 Baxandall & Gordon, *Dear Sisters*, 13.
69 Bodleian Library, M91B638 'Women's Liberation, an Introduction', 1976, 7.
70 Jordanova, 'Mental Illness', 97.
71 Editorial, *Shrew*, 4, 2, 1972, 1–2, 1.
72 Sue O'Sullivan, 'Passionate Beginnings: Ideological Politics 1969-72,' *Feminist Review*, 11, 1, 1982, 70–86, 71.
73 Luise Eichenbaum and Susie Orbach, *Understanding Women* (Middlesex, 1985), 26.
74 Marsha Rowe, ed. 'Introduction', in *Spare Rib Reader: 100 Issues of Women's Liberation* (Middlesex, 1982), 13–22, 19.
75 Ann Scott, 'Why Is Your Magazine So Depressing?', *Spare Rib*, 34, 1974, 8.
76 Belsize Lane Women's Group, 'Nine Years Together', in *Spare Rib Reader: 100 Issues of Women's Liberation*, ed. Marsha Rowe (Middlesex, 1982), 561–575, 566.
77 Mica Nava, 'The Family: A Critique of Certain Features', in *The Body Politic: Women's Liberation in Britain 1969–1972*, ed. M. Wandor (London, 1972), 36–44, 39.
78 Sue Sharpe, 'The Role of the Nuclear Family in the Oppression of Women', in *Body Politic: Women's Liberation in Britain 1969–1972*, ed. M. Wandor (London, 1972), 138–145, 141.
79 Sheila Rowbotham, 'To Be or Not to Be: The Dilemmas of Mothering', *Feminist Review*, 31, 1989, 82–93, 82.
80 Maitland, *Why Children?*, 78–88.
81 Sue Cowley, 'Thatcher's Nurseries: Expansion or Containment?', *Red Rag*, 4, July 1973, 3–5, 4–5.
82 Sheila Rowbotham and Jean McCrindle (eds), *Dutiful Daughters: Women Talk About Their Lives* (Middlesex, 1989), 4.
83 Heron, 'The Mystique of Motherhood', 139.
84 Comer, *Wedlocked Women*, 181.
85 *Ibid.*, 183–184.
86 Sue O'Sullivan, *I Used to be Nice* (London, 1996), 40–41.

87 O'Sullivan, *Once a Feminist: Stories of a Generation* (London, 1990), 214–226, 220–222.
88 Rowbotham, 'To Be or Not to Be'.
89 'A to Z of Feminism', *Spare Rib*, 136, 1983, 29–30.
90 Jan Williams, Hazel Twort, and Ann Bachelli, 'Women and the Family', in *The Body Politic: Women's Liberation in Britain 1969–1972*, ed. M. Wandor (London, 1972), 31–36, 31–32.
91 Michele Barrett and Mary McIntosh, *The Anti-Social Family*. 2nd ed. (London, 1991), 61.
92 O'Sullivan, 'Passionate Beginnings', 85.
93 Linda Peffer, *Dutiful Daughters: Women Talk about Their Lives*, eds Jean McCrindle and Sheila Rowbotham (Middlesex, 1979), 378–389.
94 Forster, 'Spreading the Word', 812.
95 See, for example, Rebecca Smith, 'Postnatal Depression', *Spare Rib*, 98, 1980, 46; Diane Walters, 'Who's Birthing the Baby – Postnatal Depression and Maternity Hospitals', *Spare Rib*, 118, 1982, 22–23.
96 Catherine Ballard and Hilary Hackett, 'My World Became the Size of the Baby', in *Spare Rib Reader: 100 Issues of Women's Liberation*, ed. Marsha Rowe (Middlesex, 1982 [first printed *Spare Rib*, June 1976]), 384–393, 384.
97 Ibid., 384.
98 *Spare Rib*, 21, 1974, front matter.
99 Nemone Lethbridge, 'News: Postscript to Baby Blues', *Spare Rib*, 21, 1974, 17.
100 For more on Lethbridge and Depressives Anonymous, see Fabiola Creed, 'Nemone Lethbridge's Play *Baby Blues* on BBC Television: Maternal Mental Illness Narratives, Stigma and Support in 1970s Britain', *Women's History Review*, 34, March 2024, 1–25.
101 'Getting Rid of Depression with Talk and Sympathy', *The Times*, 5 January 1982.
102 Sheila Kitzinger, *The Experience of Childbirth*. 4th ed. (London, 1978), 22–25, 15.
103 Kitzinger, *Passion for Birth*, 224.
104 Lesley Page, 'Kitzinger (née Webster), Sheila Helena Elizabeth (1929-2015), Anthropologist and Childbirth Activist', in *Oxford Dictionary of National Biography* (Oxford, 2019). Retrieved from https://www.oxforddnb.com/view/10.1093/odnb/9780198614128.001.0001/odnb-9780198614128-e-110338 [Accessed 28 August 2024].
105 Sue O'Sullivan (ed.), 'Discussing Childbirth', in *Women's Health: A Spare Rib Reader*, ed. Sue O'Sullivan (London, 1987), 303.

106 *Ibid.*; Valerie Charlton and Annette Muir, 'Birthpangs', in *Women's Health: A Spare Rib Reader*, ed. Sue O'Sullivan (London, 1987), 304–315 [first published in *Spare Rib* 36, June 1975].
107 Sheila Kitzinger, *A Passion for Birth* (London, 2015), 156.
108 Cindy Harris and Marianne Scruggs, 'Castor Oil, Epidurals and Home Births', in *Women's Health: A Spare Rib Reader*, ed. Sue O'Sullivan (London, 1987), 316–317 [first published in *Spare Rib* 38, August 1975].
109 Barb Tanner and Jo Rob, 'What Do ARM Midwives Want?', in *Radical Midwifery: Celebrating 21 Years of A.R.M.*, eds Margaret Jowitt and Ishbel Kargar (Lancashire, 1997), 18–19.
110 Wellcome Archives, WQ100 1986A84v, The Association of Radical Midwives, *The Vision: Proposals for the Future of Maternity Services* (Lancaster, 1986).
111 Kitzinger, *Passion for Birth*, 191.
112 Mary Cronk, 'Foreword', in *Radical Midwifery: Celebrating 21 Years of A.R.M.*, eds Margaret Jowitt and Ishbel Kargar (Lancashire, 1997), 8–11, 8.
113 Jenny Spinks, 'A Personal View of the ARM', in *Radical Midwifery: Celebrating 21 Years of A.R.M.*, eds Margaret Jowitt and Ishbel Kargar (Lancashire, 1997), 15–16.
114 'The Battle over Who Delivers Your Baby', *Express and Star*, 14 April 1981.
115 'Radical Approach to Birth', *The Birmingham Post*, 5 May 1993.
116 Rachel Celia, 'Valuing and Validating Feelings', in *Radical Midwifery: Celebrating 21 Years of A.R.M.*, eds Margaret Jowitt and Ishbel Kargar (Lancashire, 1997 [first published Summer 1982]), 120–124, 120–122.
117 Notices, *Staines & Ashford News*, 5 February 1987; 'It's Better for Baby', *Edinburgh Evening News*, 20 April 1989.
118 Pippa MacKeith, 'Annotation: The Association of Radical Midwives', *Health Visitor*, 52, 5, 1979, 174.
119 Wellcome Archives, P12134, Association of Radical Midwives, The Practising Midwife, Report of the 1982 National Conference (London, 1982).
120 Wellcome Archives, P12136, Association of Radical Midwives, Working for Change, Report of the 1984 National Conference, Oxford, May 1984 (London, 1984), 40.
121 Claire Bowes, 'Janet Balaskas: Campaigner for Active Birth Movement'. Retrieved from https://www.bbc.co.uk/news/health-17589544 [Accessed 29 August 2024].

122 Natalie Thomlinson, *Race and Ethnicity in the Women's Movement in England, 1968–1993* (Basingstoke, 2016).
123 Marilyn Gayle, 'Sex Doesn't Fit, Race Doesn't Fit', in *'68, '78, '88: From Women's Liberation to Feminism*, ed. Amanda Sebestyen (Dorset, 1988), 116–125, 124.
124 Jade Bentil, '"We Were Fire-Fighting Against Thatcher and the System She was Putting Forward": The Black Women's Movement and the Boundaries of Nationhood in Thatcher's Britain', in *Resist Organize Build: Feminist and Queer Activism in Britain and the United States during the Long 1980s*, eds Sarah Crook and Charlie Jeffries (New York, 2022), 75–116.
125 *Ibid.*
126 Heidi Safia Mirza, *Black British Feminism: A Reader* (London and New York, 1997), 8.
127 Hazel V. Carby, 'White Women Listen! Black Feminism and the Boundaries of Sisterhood', in *The Empire Strikes Back: Race and Racism in 70s Britain*, Centre for Contemporary Cultural Studies (London, 1986 [1982]), 212–235, 214–215.
128 Alix Henley, *Asian Patients in Hospital and at Home* (Kent, 1979), 73.
129 Amrit Wilson, *Finding a Voice* (London, 1978), 21–22.
130 Beverley Bryan, Stella Dadzie, and Suzanne Scafe, 'The Heart of the Race: Black Women's Lives in Britain', in *Black British Feminism, a Reader*, ed. Heidi Safia Mirza (London and New York, 1997), 42–44, 42.
131 OWAAD, 'Black Women and Health', in *No Turning Back: Writings From the Women's Liberation Movement 1975–80*, ed. Feminist Anthology Collective (London, 1981), 145–149.
132 Maureen Freely, 'Keeping Mum', *Everywoman*, November 1995, 10–12.
133 Betty Friedan, *The Second Stage* (Boston, MA, 1998 [1981]), 70.
134 Anna Coote and Beatrix Campbell, *Sweet Freedom: The Struggle for Women's Liberation* (London, 1982), 100–101.
135 Libby Purves, *How Not to Be a Perfect Mother* (London, 1988), 11.
136 Paula Nicholson, 'Motherhood and Women's Lives', in *Introducing Women's Studies: Feminist Theory and Practice*, eds Diane Richardson and Victoria Robinson (Basingstoke, 1993), 201–223.
137 Nava, '1968 and the Women's Movement', 37; see Mica Nava, 'The Family: A Critique of Certain Features', in *The Body Politic: Women's Liberation in Britain 1969–1972*, ed. Michelene Wandor (London, 1972), 36–44.

5

Feminist sociology, research, and visibility

> depression, *see* motherhood, full-time
> Index, Sue Sharpe, *Double Identity: The Lives of Working Mothers* (Middlesex, 1984), 245.

From the 1970s onwards, mothers' accounts of postnatal distress were increasingly explored, analysed, and interpreted through a sociological lens. This was, I suggest, facilitated by the expansion of social science research during the 1960s and, most importantly, driven by the entrance of feminists into the academy in the 1970s and 1980s. As Ann Oakley has said, the women's liberation movement 'swept into the world of academia a whole new set of debates and terminologies and demands'.[1] This chapter contributes to the body of scholarship that sees social scientists as instigators as well as interpreters of social change.[2] Feminist social scientists were conscious of being agents for changing attitudes, approaches, and cultures around childbirth and the social conditions of mothering. They developed new concepts, approaches, and methods to make sense of women's and mothers' lives. Research methodologies have their own histories. The intensive interview was in its 'golden age' during the 1960s; by the 1980s, it was in its 'mature middle age', and by the following decades, it had 'become increasingly choreographed'.[3] Feminist sociologists established formative work on mothers' distress during and following this 'golden age' of the interview. Their interviews created new evidence of mothers' experiences and feelings, giving priority to mothers' self-reported and self-narrated experiences. The infrastructure of the social sciences – scholarly organisations, journals, conferences – allowed ideas about disordered motherhood to be communicated and circulated within the academy, while popular non-fiction presses gave 'lay' audiences access to some of these emergent academic discourses about distressed mothering.

This chapter circles back to the sociologist Ann Oakley. Oakley's early life mapped onto some of the most significant trends for women in postwar Britain. She was raised within a 'nuclear' family – that which was held up as the ideal in postwar Britain; she was university educated but graduated into domesticity and maternity in the 1960s; discontented, her life was transformed by the emergence of a feminist consciousness in the 1970s; in the ensuing decades, she combined motherhood and paid work. Oakley's academic career, however, was less typical, and here she should be seen as a pioneer within a field that historians are increasingly turning to as offering distinctive insights into postwar life. Oakley's contributions to sociology were, in part, a product of her own experiences: 'I am a feminist, an academic sociologist, and a woman with children. I was not a feminist until I had children, and I became a sociologist as an escape from the problems of having children', she has written.[4] Feminist sociologists, of whom Oakley was one, made the emotional and psychological struggles of mothering young children legible in the 1970s and the 1980s. This work challenged the 'sociological unimagination'[5] around childbirth ('the first form of mothering labour') and the intimate terrain of women's lives.[6] It deepened academic understandings of motherhood and shone a light on what Betty Friedan had, in the early 1960s, called 'the problem that has no name': married housewives' misery.[7]

Here I am treating the sociological imagination as a productive, reflective, and reflexive force: productive, as by fixing research value onto subjects, they come to assume wider social meaning; reflective, because the connections that are made between topics – postnatal depression and life events, or postnatal depression and precarious housing, or postnatal depression and inexperience with babycare, or postnatal depression and medicalisation, or postnatal depression and poor support networks – reflect wider preoccupations; and reflexive, because it pioneered new connections between the personal and the research-focused.[8]

While this chapter homes in on female feminist researchers and their work during the 1970s and 1980s, vectors other than gender were important in the creation of these new sociological lenses. Crucially, not all feminist sociologists or sociology students in this period were middle class. Access to post-secondary education after a period of paid work or motherhood was a driver of women's social mobility during the 1970s.[9] The social sciences – which included sociology, economics, and psychology – witnessed an expansion in student numbers, particularly within polytechnics, which sought to widen participation.[10] Interviews with working-class mothers returning to post-secondary education underlined that their take up of these learning and training opportunities was driven in part by a sense that they opened up new and improved future possibilities, but also by a sense that this was something that they could do for themselves, rather than as part of their caring roles. In the late 1970s, Sue Sharpe's study of working mothers, for example – the damning index of which opened this chapter – noted that many mothers were taking up opportunities for further education and training despite the additional challenges this commitment engendered.[11] Some of these working-class social sciences students stayed within academia and shaped the new research agendas that emerged in the 1970s. These backgrounds informed their sociological work and were proudly worn alongside other identities: sociologist Liz Stanley, for example, has described herself as 'Working class by birth, a Northerner in England by choice, and a lesbian by luck'.[12]

As Mike Savage has shown, the creation of the postwar welfare state saw a 'remarkable new role for social scientific expertise' develop in the 1950s and 1960s. The new techniques, approaches and methodologies of these social sciences 'mined down to reveal mundane, ordinary life', and were 'implicated in a broader process of building a modern, rational, post-imperial nation'.[13] It was in these years that the initial rumblings of sociological interest in women's experiences of domestic life could be discerned, and that the ground was laid for its ensuing expansion. But while Savage looks to a wider field of social research and investigation, my interest here is primarily in the development of feminist sociology within the academy. As I show, the vissitudes of the academy shaped the kinds of sociological work that was produced within it and determined who was able to undertake this work. Within this chapter, the chronological arc follows periods in sociology that have been demarked as 'expansion' (1950–67), 'revolt' (1968–75), and, following 1976, the 'years of uncertainty'.[14]

Of course, feminist sociologists who joined the discipline in the 1970s and 1980s built on wider trends in the field. There was, for example, preexisting work on women's lives that sought to stimulate policy reform and to change public discourses.[15] They were not the first cohort of researchers to have explicitly political sympathies: Michael Young and Peter Willmott's postwar investigations, which included *Family and Kinship in East London* (1957) and *The Symmetrical Family* (1973), reflected their affinity with the Labour Party (indeed, Young wrote the Labour Party's 1945 manifesto, and both authors worked within the party's research department from 1945 to 1951).[16] Nor did feminist sociologists initiate sociological interest in the family – Young and Willmott's landmark 1957 study of life in urban Bethnal Green and suburban Debden (which they called 'Greenleigh'), for example, played a foundational role in embedding ideas about 'traditional' models of working-class social and familial life in the public imagination.[17] Indeed, as Jon Lawrence has recently observed, in the decades that followed, this particular study was identified by feminist scholars as bearing outsize responsibility for circulating romanticised notions about relationships between working-class mothers and their kin.[18] Neither Ann Oakley nor, earlier, her father Richard Titmuss – who supervised Michael Young's doctorate – held much truck with the methodological rigour of *Family and Kinship,* and Oakley's own doctorate, published as *The Sociology of Housework* one year after the publication of Young and Willmott's *The Symmetrical Family,* came to very different conclusions about the division of labour within the home. As she has recently explained, her work showed 'there was nothing remotely symmetrical' about *The Symmetrical Family.*[19] Furthermore, female sociologists pioneered new strands and research methodologies well before the conceptual frameworks and organising ideas of the 1970's feminist movement came into being, laying the groundwork for the women who would come after them. In the 1950s, for example, researcher Elizabeth Bott (who saw herself as an anthropologist rather than a sociologist, despite making fundamental contributions to sociology) made the in-depth interview a 'part of the repertoire of sociology', enabling sociology to frame itself as an empirical subject, with interests and approaches that were distinct from psychology.[20] Despite these pre-existing fields of research and scholarly approaches, the feminist sociology of the 1970s and 1980s was distinct from the work that preceded it. As Helen McCarthy has said, 'it was only from the 1970s that feminist researchers explicitly connected the articulation of women's experience to the development of collective strategies of resistance'.[21] Unlike earlier works, feminist social science was in conversation with ideas about women's liberation, a broader political project. These researchers were emboldened by the intellectual and social networks fostered by feminism. Women's liberation provided encouragement that went beyond intellectual stimulus. Oakley reflects that 'the ideology, politics and practice of organised feminism provided a playground away from the university, a sounding board, and, above all, a comfort blanket'.[22]

The feminist sociological work that developed in the 1970s reshaped social science. New areas of research were developed, and as Oakley wrote, 'Sociologies "of" were reframed as sociologies "for" – specifically for women, with the construction and communication of knowledge about their lives and experiences treated as an emancipatory act'.[23] Feminist sociology contributed to the expansion of knowledge about, and offered alternative understandings of, mothers' distress. This chapter argues that the academic interest in maternal distress was facilitated by the postwar expansion of sociology and was transformed by the entrance to the social sciences of an interconnected network of feminist researchers.

Hannah Gavron and the 'captive wife'

One of the forerunners to this interconnected network – whose pioneering work laid the ground for later studies – was Hannah Gavron (née Fyvel). In 1964, Gavron submitted a doctoral thesis to Bedford College, London. The thesis, 'The Position and Opportunities of Young Mothers – Progress or Retrogression (A study of the difficulties confronting young mothers in the contemporary family based on a comparative study of working class and middle class families)' aimed to examine 'the problems confronting a young mother with small children today'.[24] Her work identified the loneliness, lack of confidence, and boredom of middle- and working-class young mothers. The subject was one with which she had a personal affinity; she had two young sons. The research had not been easy; she had faced resistance and scepticism within her department, and had encountered delays in surmounting some of the key hurdles of doctoral progression. The monograph that emerged from the thesis – *The Captive Wife: Conflicts of Housebound Mothers* – was published for a wider, non-academic readership in 1966, and has subsequently become much cited. By its publication, though, Hannah Gavron had taken her own life.

Hannah Gavron was born in 1936, the daughter of the Jewish intellectual T.R. Fyvel and Mary Fyvel. She read sociology at Bedford College, starting her degree at age twenty when she was already married. Aged twenty-one, she became pregnant, and, with the support of her head of department, Gertrude Williams, she extended her degree and gave birth to her first son, Simon, in April 1958, and to another son, Jeremy, in 1961. Having achieved the rare feat of a first-class degree, she began work on her doctorate in 1960, for which she interviewed young 'housebound mothers', both middle- and working-class, based in Kentish Town, London, about their experiences and aspirations.[25] Gavron's work contributed to a cluster of studies of the family that emerged around the same time, forming a part of a wider sociological and medical explorations of the home and its changing structures, but was distinctive in its foregrounding of women's experiences. Here there was no romanticisation of the home, and no mystification of the labours of mothering. In their stead there was a clear-eyed view of the ways that the expectations and conditions of childrearing converged to make mothering an arduous and isolated undertaking. Working-class women were particularly tied to their children, she found, with opportunities to assert themselves as individuals paling in comparison to better resourced middle-class women.[26]

At this point in the 1960s there were few senior women in British academia, and so few to whom Gavron could look as a role model. Little surprise, then, that the environment in which she worked was somewhat inhospitable to her topic and her ambition. In his recent book about his mother's life, Jeremy Gavron has argued that her work encountered resistance from her supervisors. Although her thesis was finished in 1964, she was made to wait until 1965 to hear if it had been approved, a delay that her father attributed to the 'masculine sloth' of her supervisor, Ronald Fletcher, author of the well-known *The Family and Marriage in Britain* (1962). Her applications for two jobs at the LSE were rejected, rebuffs that Jeremy Gavron suggests may have owed something to sexism: a lecturer at the LSE recalled Ann Oakley's father, Richard Titmuss, chair of Hannah Gavron's interview board, commenting not on Gavron's interview performance but on her makeup.[27] The culture of the LSE and Bedford were not, contemporaries affirmed, supportive of women's careers, and numerous contacts of Hannah Gavron's suggested that it was possible that her prospects were actively limited by senior male academics, to whom she represented the discomforting stirrings of a nascent feminist consciousness.[28] There was hope, though, for by 1964 Gavron had two books under contract with Routledge – one an introduction to sociology, the other a contract for what would become *The Captive Wife*.[29] She edged closer to gaining a stronger foothold within the academy, too, for in 1965 Gavron was offered a job at the Institute of Education with the sociologist Basil Bernstein.[30] She took her own life on December 1965, before she could take it up, and would not see the impact that *The Captive Wife* quickly achieved upon its publication the following year.

Despite its scholarly tone and somewhat austere style (it was, the first page explained, intended to 'throw some more light on patterns of family life' and to 'test further' the results of related sociological studies – hardly sensationally framed aspirations) upon publication *The Captive Wife* was picked up by national newspapers, tapping as it did into a wider set of social anxieties about women and the family.[31] The *Sunday Mirror*, for example, used the book to discuss the difficulty of defining social class; the *Daily Telegraph* urged readers not to 'scoff' at Gavron's suggestions about how the lives of young mothers could be improved, on the basis that happy mothers raised happier children; the *Evening Standard* noted that the study was part of a wider research picture, explaining that 'we've no excuse for not knowing what's wrong with us these days. We've got the surveys to tell us. Asking, answering, analysing. Looking us over, listening, documenting'.[32] It also permeated the local press, and in this setting the humdrum framed the diffusion of Gavron's social analysis of mothers' experiences, making acknowledgement of mothering's challenges – as an earlier chapter explored in more depth – *ordinary*. The *Coventry Standard*, for example, published an article about *The Captive Wife* alongside an article about the 'newest, zaniest craze' for 'see-through shoes and boots'.[33] The *Birmingham Post* focused on potential solutions.[34]

Other national newspapers encouraged empathy and action. The *Scotsman* directly addressed its readers, drawing attention to the way that mothers' struggles with loneliness and isolation undermined marital balance and harmony, as well as destabilising women's identities:

> How can you develop as a person if your career is suddenly cut from under your feet and you are snatched from a full and stimulating life and set down in a bright little kitchen whose very brightness you quickly grow to hate? In the evening you listen to your husband's account of his day. He may have found his work taxing, his workmates infuriating, but at least he has been OUT. And when he says 'And how did your day go?' and you reply, 'oh, all right, Susie wet her pants eight times' – well, he'll soon stop asking.

In the 1960s these bright little kitchens were increasingly crowded with the aspirant technology of domestic appliances, but for the wives within them their sheen was a mirage. The *Scotsman* used the piece to explain the issues that had stirred the creation of the National Housewives Register (founded in 1960), and encouraged its readers to be proactive. 'If there is no group and no single members in your area, why not start one?', it asked.[35] Lynn Abrams has explored the National Housewives Register as an example of how women responded at the grassroots to the changed landscapes of postwar Britain and widened their own social networks. For educated women, 'active involvement could be a springboard to a new career and a new identity', she has argued.[36] The idea of the 'captive wife' was enduring and adaptable. In 1982, the Welsh *Daily Post* worried that Gavron's 'captive wife' still existed. 'Today's female prisoner is the working wife who dutifully performs a boring and unrewarding job so her husband and children may enjoy the benefits of a two-income family', it explained. This working mother faced a 'dull day's work sandwiched between a frenetic early morning organising her family before she goes to work and a weary evening trying to do in a few hours what today's pampered full-time housewife takes all day over'. The 'Valium-gulping housewife living from coffee morning to coffee morning' may have receded, but 'the working mum, forever dreading Monday morning' might 'replace her as the victim-of-the-decade'.[37] The *Post* captured what feminist researchers found in the 1970s and 1980s – employed mothers of young children were obliged to undertake a 'second shift' at home.[38] In many ways the book was, feminist Lynne Segal wrote, 'an early messenger of what was to come'.[39]

Women and feminists in sociology

Change within sociology occurred quickly in postwar Britain. In 1950, the sociology department at the LSE was the only one of its kind; the expansion of higher education at the end of the decade, and the acceleration of growth after the Robbins Report of 1963, benefited both the sciences and the social sciences. Sociology departments 'popped up like mushrooms after a spring rain' at the expanding 'Redbrick' institutions as well as the new 'plateglass' universities.[40] These new departments created new teaching posts for sociologists and enrolled increasing numbers of students.[41] Between the 1940s and the early 1970s, the number of undergraduates studying sociology increased from around 200 to nearly 4,000 – not including those at the Open University or at polytechnics.[42] These students became increasingly vocal towards the end of the 1960s. Indeed, sociology found itself at the crux of the decade's student revolts.[43] Julius Gould, professor of sociology at Nottingham University, wrote in 1968 that sociology 'appeals, not least in Britain, to a generation that seems, both puzzlingly and enviably, free from the shackles of the past'.[44] Sociology was a field seen to have political potential.

The expansion – at least until the cuts and retreats of the 1980s began – of the social sciences did not, however, mean that female researchers had an easy path. Women sociologists were in the minority.[45] Feminist sociologists were liable to occupy precarious positions within the academy, sometimes holding multiple short-term posts at a time and struggling to secure funding.[46] Moreover, there was a 'pipeline' problem. In 1975, a study of women in sociology conducted by a working group within the British Sociological Association (BSA, founded in 1951), found that childcare arrangements posed considerably greater challenges to female than male survey respondents.[47] As sociologists Helen Roberts and Diana Woodward observed in the early 1980s, 'it is not marriage and *parenthood* which disadvantages an academic career, but marriage and *motherhood*'.[48] Women also found academic institutions bureaucratic, slow, and frustratingly divorced from external organisations (birth activist and anthropologist Sheila Kitzinger recalled her brief employment at a university in the early 1980s as an uneasy time, and concluded that she could not create change through any such 'authoritarian organisation').[49]

Nonetheless, feminist researchers were confident in the importance of their work. In her 1982 presidential address to the BSA, Margaret Stacey commented that:

> What is true of women workers may also be true of women academics. We have fought hard for the places we have got; some of us have had to deny ourselves children for them; many carry the double burden, but we want our paid work. Women's jobs may be more at risk even than those of the men, but women know what we have to fight for and why it is worth it.[50]

Like Oakley, Stacey's journey to the fore of sociology was both ordinary and extraordinary: ordinary, in the way she encountered resistance based upon her status as a wife and mother; extraordinary, in the influence that she went on to exert in the field. Born in 1922 to feminist parents, Stacey read sociology and social work at the LSE, graduating in 1943. A member of the Labour Party, she married in 1945 and, after teaching in Oxford, she moved with her husband to Swansea in Wales, where her husband took up a position in political studies. The couple adopted and fostered children, and had biological children. As for many women in her generation, during this period of childrearing, Stacey was not in paid employment. She found that Swansea resisted giving her a job 'because I was married with children'. After a decade, it relented, appointing her to an academic post in 1961, and in the 1970s, Stacey took up a Chair at Warwick. In 1970, she published work on children in hospital, marking a shift towards research on gender and health. This study emerged from her own experience ('I got into that because I was the mother of young children who hadn't always been treated very kindly in hospital'). She described feminism as a significant influence, 'in the sense that words for concepts became available, which one couldn't appropriately articulate before, because the words weren't there'.[51]

Stacey was part of a generation of feminist social scientists able to use a growing publishing infrastructure, including but not limited to academic journals, to share their expertise. Leading mainstream sociological journals were established or revitalised between 1950 and 1967, and feminists also established their own academic journals, which provided important spaces to explore motherhood.[52] Mica Nava, who had been drawn into women's liberation by an interest in the family, was a member of the *Feminist Review* editorial collective.[53] Michèle Barrett (born 1949), who studied sociology at Durham and Sussex universities before joining City University London as a sociology lecturer in 1977, and Mary McIntosh (born 1936), who taught sociology at Leicester University and the Polytechnic of the South Bank, London, before accepting a position at the University of Essex, were both members of this editorial collective and co-authors of *The Anti-Social Family* (1982). In this they observed that 'it is clear that being a housewife can drive women mad, though why they tend so often to experience depression and "nerves" rather than, say, anger or revolt is perhaps less clear'.[54] This challenge was published by Verso/New Left Books, a publishing house founded in 1970.

Crucially, then, feminist sociologists published outside scholarly journals. Their writing about motherhood and the family was made available in paperback form, enabling a wider diffusion of their ideas. Pelican Books, published by Penguin, had a key role as a distributor of non-fiction to a wide audience.[55] It also had an important role, along with other publishers, in making knowledge about mothers' lives and experiences available outside the academy. For example, Gavron's *The Captive Wife* was initially published by Routledge in 1966, but was then published by Pelican in 1968 before entering reprint several times across the 1970s. Of course, publishers were also gatekeepers. Helen Roberts set out the challenge of securing a publisher for her edited collection, *Doing Feminist Research*. Initially rejected by an editor who advised that it would only find a 'rather small and specifically feminist market', the book was picked up by Routledge. Rather than having a 'rather small' market, *Doing Feminist Research* entered reprint multiple times.[56] Looking to these paperbacks, then, helps us to understand the ways that feminist sociological research slipped outside campus walls and into libraries, bookshops, and homes.[57]

Given the circulation of feminist sociology through non-academic publishing and its dialogue with the women's liberation movement, it is little surprise that conversations developed within feminist sociology extended beyond the boundaries of the academy. Inspiration, however, flowed both ways, and feminist sociologists were informed by feminist thinking outside universities. Sociologists Sheila Allen and Diana Leonard Barker observed that 'much of the current exchange of information, research, and interest in sexual divisions and society has occurred outside and thus without the supports and advantages of the formal academic structure'.[58] Feminist sociology was therefore informed by conversations occurring across academic disciplines and outside university settings.[59] Of course, the relationship between academic feminism and groups outside the academy was not always easy. In 1979, the Leeds Revolutionary Feminist Group published a pamphlet that was highly critical of academic feminists.[60] Sociologist Liz Stanley and sociologist and social worker Sue Wise took issue with some of this criticism. An explicitly feminist stance was more likely to impede than promote their careers, they argued.[61] The relationship between social science and women's liberation was contested, then, but the flows of influence were indubitable.

Feminist sociology

For some feminists, early iterations of the social sciences were part of the apparatus that had justified women's oppression.[62] The task for feminist sociology, then, was significant: to challenge, reorient, and reshape a discipline that had played a role in oppressing women. Others pointed to the ways that traditional sociological analyses had marginalised women, singling out class analysis as particularly prone to erroneously deriving women's experiences from men's positions. Such arguments were transformative for the field. Beverley Skeggs has argued that 'second wave feminist pioneers in sociology... presented incontrovertible evidence that could not be ignored, evidence that also made its way into the media and eventually government policy'.[63] Major impetus to this project arrived in 1974 when the BSA held its first gender-themed conference on the topic of 'Sexual Divisions'.[64] Two volumes emerged from the event: *Dependence and Exploitation in Work and Marriage*, and *Sexual Divisions and Society*, both published in 1976. Introducing *Sexual Divisions and Society*, editors Sheila Allen and Diana Leonard Barker commented on the revitalisation of the feminist movement and the movement's relationship with scholars:

> some sociologists have become personally involved or sympathetic to these movements and used their professional skills to analyse and relate sociological material on relevant problems. They have recognised that there were serious lacumae [sic] and biases in current sociological accounts and looked to the movements for impetus and reanalysis; and the movements have given encouragement and an audience to those who have long been interested in the area.

'The result of this', they wrote, was a 'significant, creative spurt'.[65] The conference exposed the power of feminist sociological approaches. Alongside other papers, Christine Delphy critiqued the economic role of marriage, centring the importance of childcare; Sally Macintyre problematised the idea of 'normal' reproduction, pointing out the different ways that medical professionals responded to married and unmarried pregnant women's reports of depression and ambivalence; Hilary Rose and Jalna Hanmer considered the patriarchal context of reproductive technologies.[66]

Sociology maintained a fruitful relationship with the emergent subject of women's studies. In Britain, women's studies emerged in adult education and community-based education, driven by women who were active in the women's movement.[67] In the 1970s, courses on women proliferated at the undergraduate level, and programmes on Women's Studies were initiated at the MA level.[68] Women's studies was, as Oakley said, necessarily interdisciplinary, so 'work done in the fields of social policy, social psychology, and social anthropology has fed into the concerns of women's studies in sociology'.[69] Within cultural studies, too, feminist groups formed. As the women's studies group within the Centre for Contemporary Cultural Studies (CCCS) at the University of Birmingham observed, 'it is through the questions that feminism poses, and the absences that it locates, that feminist research and women's studies are constituted as one part of the struggle for the transformation of society'.[70] Anthropology, which had a longer history, was another field that feminists entered in the 1970s. Pat Caplan, for example, was a founding member of the Anthropology Department at Goldsmiths. Born in 1944, she graduated from the School of Oriental and African Studies, University of London with a BA in African Studies (Swahili branch) in 1963, gaining a PhD in social anthropology in 1968. She read Betty Friedan's *The Feminine Mystique* shortly before she found out she was pregnant. In an oral history interview, she explained that becoming a mother, taking on caring responsibilities, and being introduced to feminism were linked:

> once I had a baby, I realised – well, I mean, I'd realised it, to some extent, becoming a wife, but even more so becoming a mother, that it did put a lot of constraints on what you could do, but more importantly, how people saw you… I think I was probably very receptive to the message of feminism, as I could feel myself getting pushed into a sort of wife/mother/housewife role – these were the sort of pressures that were coming, and I didn't like them. I recognised that all those things needed to be done, and I didn't resent doing them one iota… But the kind of messages that feminism gave, I think, resonated very strongly with women like me, who'd been very highly educated and who thought that there were no barriers to whatever we wanted to do, and suddenly we discovered with the rude shock of, 'It's not quite like that, actually!' So I got involved in feminism.[71]

This involvement connected her to broader feminist intellectual networks and groups. These subjects – women's studies, anthropology, and cultural studies, to name just a few – and academic groups created additional and overlapping academic spaces for research into mothers' lives (and women's lives more broadly) and sites for the development of new methodological and theoretical approaches to knowledge production.

Feminist sociology encouraged reflexivity about the research process and researchers' positionality. The process of knowledge production was attentive to the politics of such an endeavour. As Dale Spender argued in the early 1980s, the ethos of the 'personal is political' was fundamental to feminist research. 'Feminists have focused on "research on research"', she wrote:

> and have been extremely critical of the way in which knowledge has for so long been presented as a *fait accompli* with little or no acknowledgement of the part played by the personal in the process of producing such knowledge. Instead of trying to be 'detached', feminists are blatantly 'involved' in the knowledge which they are producing and unlike the traditional model in which the researcher is presumed to be 'outside' the subject matter being researched, feminist contributions frequently testify to the way in which women are changed by the research process.[72]

Particular institutions took up this mantle. At the University of Manchester, the sociology department established 'Studies in Sexual Politics' to '"give voice" to feminist sociological work produced in the tradition of the Manchester department'. This tradition was one of close concern with research processes and a tilt towards ethnographic approaches.[73] Sociologist Liz Stanley started teaching in the department in 1977 and was the series' main editor. The series, she set out, drew attention to the processes of knowledge production and aimed to avoid the production of 'alienated knowledge'.[74] In the 1980s, she and Sue Wise explained that the 'guiding principle' for feminist research ought to be 'using feeling and experience as the basis for explicating the personal and the everyday': this meant abandoning the pretence of impartiality and omnipotence.[75] The emphasis on processes and position, then, was both a part of, and distinct from, longer disciplinary trends.

Feminist sociologists examined how materials used by sociology, such as the records kept in antenatal clinics, could result in the 'the self-perpetuation of lay, sociological and clinical assumptions about the social world', allowing them to 'take on a quality of legitimacy and solidity'.[76] It was not just the collection of data that feminist sociologists examined, of course. Vital work was done around developing new concepts to understand women's lives. In her presidential address to the BSA in 1982, Stacey argued that:

> Sociological concepts and terms... were devised by men about the male world of the public domain and about the family as it was seen by those men. Those concepts and terms have a crippling effect on any attempt to understand the world of women... These concepts and terms are quite inappropriate to deal adequately with the private world of the family.[77]

One of the tasks of feminist sociology, then, was to develop new concepts for examining the 'world of women'. As Oakley pointed out, for feminism 'the task is not merely one of adding women in to the discourse, but of reconstituting the discipline itself'.[78]

In the 'early days of feminist sociology... the main focus of writing on methods was intensely *practical*'.[79] Feminist sociologists argued that research processes needed to make women visible and not to generalise from the experience of men. Helen Roberts argued that sexism was an ideology that 'generalises from the experience of one section of society, men, to create an explanation of the experience of both men and women'. The ideology of sexism 'is expressed in sociology by methodologies that ignore sexual divisions and do not "see" the experience or situation of women'. By contrast, feminism was 'a feature of ideological conflict, and does not of itself attempt an "unbiased" or "value-free" methodology'. Instead, it forged a 'dialectic at the ideological level' which 'creates the conditions in which a non-sexist methodology might be approached'.[80] Survey research came in for particular critique, with feminists arguing that it commodified women's oppression and obscured important aspects of their lives. 'Large scale and questionnaire surveys have an inbuilt conservatism', Oakley wrote in 1985. 'They do not allow people to range freely in the realm of their more utopian visions of prenatal clinics, delivery rooms, and obstetrical or midwifery bedside manners'. Such approaches were also insufficiently sensitive, she claimed, and it was 'unlikely that the statistically common and personally disabling "soft" outcome of postpartum depression, for example, will be tapped satisfactorily in a large questionnaire survey, and certainly its antecedent social and medical care factors are unlikely to be found using this approach'.[81]

Hilary Graham argued for a technique of sociological interviewing that was more akin to 'storytelling'; the narrative tradition 'presumes only that the speaker has a story which she is prepared to share with others'.[82] Oakley argued that conventional prescriptions around the sociological interview reinscribed masculine power relations. In her work on the transition to motherhood, she had defied methods textbooks, working to flatten the conventional hierarchy. She explained that

> I regarded sociological research as an essential way of giving the subjective situation of women greater visibility not only in sociology, but, more importantly in society... Interviewing women was, then, a strategy for documenting women's own accounts of their lives...The interviewer [w]as an instrument for promoting a sociology for women – that is, a tool for making possible the articulated and recorded commentary of women on the very personal business of being female in a patriarchal capitalist society.[83]

The emphasis placed on 'sisterhood' in early feminist thinking about methodologies has been criticised for emphasising gender at the expense of other axes of differences, including race and social class.[84] Class, education, and race were important power vectors within the interview relationship. Indeed, other female social scientists found that while it was easier to establish a rapport with female interviewees, social class and educational background played a central role in shaping contributors' responses.[85]

Nonetheless, a common theme that emerged in sociological reports was interviewees' appreciation of the opportunity to discuss their lives. Janet Finch, chair of the BSA from 1983 to 1984, found that her female interviewees frequently told her, 'I've really enjoyed having someone to talk to'.[86] Oakley was so struck by this as a theme that it contributed to her development of a subsequent research project.[87] It was a finding shared with research conducted outside the academy: in the 1980s an NCT study of disabled mothers' experiences reported that the interviews had 'opened a floodgate'.[88] As other historians have explored, participation in social research offered contributors opportunities to perform and demonstrate the desirable skills of self-management and personal agency.[89] That is not to say, however, that asymmetries of power, class, and position in the knowledge-production process did not remain.

It was against this asymmetrical context that feminist researchers considered the ways that women's experiences were presented within academic research. For example, in *Becoming a Mother*, Oakley's interviewees are quoted extensively. This, she explained, was due to 'the fact that the women said it all much better, and much more clearly or directly, than a sociologist could ever do'.[90] Oakley inverted typesetting norms by placing her comments in italics. Later, Oakley reflected on this choice, arguing that:

> In those early stages what was desperately needed was publicly accessible information from women about their own experiences... I found it difficult to jump in there as another kind of expert and reduce all these vivid descriptions and intelligent reflections to the status of figures that could be statistically manipulated.[91]

From Here to Maternity was important for reasons well beyond this inversion of typesetting norms, of course: together with *Women Confined*, its academic counterpart, it initiated new conversations around motherhood. Feminist work opened up new areas of life to sociological inquiry, not least the structuring and experience of childbirth, the family, marriage, and mothering. Writing in 1989, historian Jane Lewis celebrated the work that feminists had done to invigorate the study of the family.[92]

Medicalisation and childbirth

In the late 1970s Sally Macintyre called for greater sociological interrogation of childbirth.[93] By the mid-1980s, this call had been taken up, if not answered, and Oakley wrote that medical sociology had developed a defined interest in how pregnant women felt about their care. As a result, social scientists – particularly female social scientists, who led this research – had become recognised for their work on obstetric patients.[94] Feminist sociologists were working against a background of growing public and academic interest in women's experiences of childbirth: that 'incredibly labour-intensive, tiring, sweaty, bloody and personal form of women's work', as Joanna Bourke has framed it.[95] Oakley says that the sociology of childbirth was informed by movements outside the academy: feminism, healthcare activism, medicalisation, and changed attitudes to healthcare.[96] It is notable, though, that researchers' own experiences of labour sometimes played a crucial role in encouraging an academic interest in birth, and stirred the creation of methodologies that centred women. As Oakley has written, looking back on her first labour, 'I remember myself as a passive patient, bewildered, afraid and alone, controlled rather than controlling, his birth more their achievement than mine'. She 'did not understand that I was delivered of my identity at the same time, prevented from being the central figure in the central drama of my life'. Her second baby was born at home, a 'non-event' in comparison. Her third child was born in a hospital but without drugs; it was the only birth that she felt she was 'directing the course of events'.[97] Childbirth, she felt, was a moment of transition and transformation, but it was also a moment at which mothers were deprived of control. Within this context, medicalisation – a concept that entered the sociological literature in the 1970s, and that is rather more critical than the literal meaning of 'to make medical' – was taken up by feminist researchers as a means of understanding how ostensibly normal, healthy expectant mothers were cast as patients and childbirth transformed into a medical procedure.[98] Researchers argued that the medicalisation of labour and rigidity of the hospital setting exacerbated mothers' distress. Feminism 'helped to nourish the sociological study of childbirth by querying particularly that division between the public and the private which had served so well to hide reproductive labour from the sociological gaze', says Oakley.[99]

The impact of these rapid changes to childbirth was also being contested outside the disciplinary boundaries of sociology. Statistician Marjorie Tew, whose book *Safer Childbirth: A Critical History of Maternity Care* (1990) challenged the hypothesis that medicalisation and hospitalisation were responsible for the decline in maternal and infant mortality, was employed as a part-time research statistician in a Department of Orthopaedic Surgery while she interrogated the evidence that underpinned claims about the benefits of medical intervention. For fifteen years she conducted her investigations 'alone on a voluntary basis in [her] spare time', during a 'dogged lonely campaign'. It was only when her first article on maternity care was published in 1977 that she 'became aware... that some doctors, some midwives and some women concerned with childbearing and with women's rights actually welcomed statistical confirmation of the apprehensions their experiences raised about the benefits of the new medicalized maternity care'.[100] Tew suggested that some steps that were ostensibly taken in the name of safety were actually taken to avoid inconvenience. The induction rate, for example, was 13 per cent in 1958, rising to 13.4 per cent in 1964, then to 26 per cent in 1970, and to 39.4 per cent in 1974. Such figures suggested that inductions were being used to address the 'irritating uncertainty' around delivery.[101] Public attention was brought to the issue in October 1974 when the *Sunday Times* reported on the rising rates of induction, asking if such a 'revolution' was what women wanted.[102] In December 1974, the issue of inductions for convenience was raised in parliament, and Barbara Castle, Secretary of State for Social Services, noted that she had received concerned letters from the public.[103] Public unease grew in January 1975 when the BBC show *Horizon* discussed the topic.[104] An investigation into induction was launched by the Department of Health and Social Security soon after.[105] The following year, a group of student midwives interested in the status of midwifery and in the experiences of labouring women came together; the Association of Radical Midwives came out of this 1976 meeting.[106]

It was against this medical, cultural, and intellectual background that Ann Oakley's sociological studies of motherhood emerged. Her 'Transition to Motherhood' project was closely attentive to women's experiences of childbirth. Women in her study recounted their experiences of medicalised births and inhumane postnatal care: of being frightened by health professionals into fear of their looming labour; of being given medication without full consent; of being given extensive episiotomies; and of the distress caused by the noise and disruption of the hospital ward while 'lying in'.[107] One interviewee reflected: 'that was sort of the atmosphere of the hospital, in the hospital everyone was depressed. It was much more like leaving a mental hospital than this happy maternity hospital'.[108] Another said she felt 'more exhausted. But it was labelled postnatal depression. The sister, and everyone else picked it up, and said yes: that's postnatal depression. I said to the sister, Piccadilly Circus is more restful than this place'.[109] Drawing from the same research,

Women Confined argued that childbirth was a 'natural act shaped by cultural rhetoric'.[110] This cultural rhetoric was informed by 'scientific' beliefs about optimal birth and women's natural character: '"Science" has a hidden curricula of moral evaluations that masquerade as fact', Oakley wrote.[111] Drawing on this, Oakley connected postnatal depression to a technologised birth. Her findings were 'unequivocal', she said,

> The demonstration of a connection between depression and technology constitutes a major condemnation of the feminine paradigm. Instead of implicating women as the causes of their own postpartum mental disorder (either through personality weakness or hormone imbalance), the medical management of childbirth is characterized as a process that controls not only childbirth but women as well. Women's situation as mothers can thus be seen as partially at least located in their subjection to a system of medical monopoly.[112]

Her conclusions reflected her interviewees' comments on their treatment in hospital. One mother had nightmares about forceps; another said, 'I do blame the hospital' for a birth that left her feeling unwell and tired.[113] However, in some cases, mothers were upset not by the medical interventions in and of themselves, but rather by a more general lack of respect and information. In a Scottish study, a working-class first-time mother summarised this in 1982:

> I had everything. I was induced, then they kept speeding up and slowing down the contractions and I had an epidural and forceps and an episiotomy. And through it all they didnae tell ye anything. It wis terrible. I felt like a lump of mince.[114]

Another working-class mother recommended that,

> They should tell you a lot more aboot what's going on. You're kept in the dark all the time and ye just worry and imagine things. Yer imagination runs away wi' you and ye think o' the worst.[115]

The importance of the experience of childbirth was picked up in literature aimed at informing lay audiences about postnatal depression. 'To deny the impact of birth itself is to ignore the experience and opinions of mothers', wrote advice columnist Maggie Comport in 1987. She worried that within medicine 'obstetric procedures have become magic rituals, above question and with a frightful momentum of their own'.[116] This emphasis on the consequences of withholding information and power from labouring women is reflected in oral histories of maternity care, which have found that the technologisation of birth and the imposition of medicalised procedures prompted less discontent among mothers than the perception that they had not been heard, respected, or informed.[117]

How did Oakley's interviewees articulate the experience of postnatal depression, and how did she interpret it? One mother explained that:

> I sometimes think [her daughter] is a cow. I *hated* her at first... I just wished she'd never been born, couldn't bear her... I was just miserable, tearful, crying at everything, at the slightest thing... I just wanted to die... What have I done? Why have I got this baby? What am I going to do?

Another mother said: 'I kept thinking I'd never be able to cope with him and do anything else at all... to feel that bad with it, I don't think I've ever cried so much in all me life'.[118] In *Women Confined*, Oakley addressed postnatal support groups as part of her proposed changes to the social processes around childbirth and motherhood. While the 'content and ideological charter' of postnatal support groups run by social workers and health visitors 'may not accord with the diagnosis of this book, their existence promotes the idea that lack of "adjustment" following childbirth is a normal occurrence', she conceded. Moreover, 'it also recognizes the important clinical observation that the repeating and reliving of a "bad" experience in a therapeutic context can aid the development of "mastery": the passivity of the self as victim in the original experience may in this way be surmounted'.[119]

Oakley was critical of the medical and psychological framing of postnatal depression. Writing in *Women Confined*, she argued that

> the term itself is of primary ideological importance, since it is the main psychological construct expressing an assessment of 'poor' outcome, a failure on the part of women to achieve reproductive and feminine normality. It is, of course, essential that postnatal depression should

appear to be a technical concept – a clinical term evolved by experts to describe a clinical syndrome: the covert ideological function of 'science' is exactly expressed in the hidden character of such 'technical' evaluations.

The explanations for postnatal depression – as stemming from a hormonal imbalance or a 'disturbance of, or in, femininity' were poorly evidenced and flawed, Oakley suggested.[120] She instead focused on the ways that becoming a mother entailed loss, changed identity, and low self-esteem, as well as the role of medicalised childbirth. This shifted attention to the 'induced self-negation' of mothering. 'Science', she wrote, 'responding to an agenda of basically social concerns, has provided the label "post-natal depression" as a pseudo-scientific tag for the description and ideological transformation of maternal discontent'.[121] Reflecting on the research, Oakley underlined that her interviewees'

> accounts of postnatal depression were not accounts of depression, they were accounts of exhaustion, sleep deprivation, the shock of being precipitated into a new occupation, a mother without – often any kind of previous training – exposure to surgery, to institutionalization in hospital, and all these things we know are stressful to human beings, so you didn't need to have any special explanations of women as women, you just needed to understand that childbirth is a human life event and it can have these kinds of consequences.[122]

Growing the field

The mid-1970s were therefore a fertile time for the consideration of motherhood. Oakley's 'Transition to Motherhood' project began in 1974, and a research project by Hilary Graham and Lorna McKee began the following year. Graham and McKee's project, conducted between 1975 and 1978, was based on 200 women in a northern town, 100 of whom were expecting their first child and 100 of whom were expecting their second. This research was influential: before it had even been completed it was referenced in a House of Lords debate to evidence the inadequacies of antenatal care.[123] The need for the study arose from an awareness of the challenges – including postnatal depression and child abuse – faced by mothers and children and the dissatisfactions with maternity care uncovered in epidemiological studies and surveys of patient experiences. The research revealed that 34 per cent of mothers experienced poor physical health in the first month after birth, dropping to 27 per cent between one and five months. Worse levels of emotional health were revealed: 49 per cent of respondents said they had experienced postnatal depression. These findings led the researchers to conclude that there was an enhanced need for an understanding of the 'emotional stresses of early motherhood', and how these related to poor physical health. The authors noted that their interviews had revealed mothers' feelings about the various losses early motherhood brought about: income, friendship, and confidence.[124]

Oakley's work on mothers was picked up in a study collaboratively conducted by sociologist Bie Nio Ong on a deprived Oldham estate. Ong noted the ambivalence articulated by the pregnant women, even while they adhered to social scripts that emphasised the positive aspects of mothering. Some interviewees did mention postnatal depression, she notes, but this was used to indicate that any anticipated negative emotional experiences would be only temporary. Following the birth, these ambivalences became more marked and contradictory, Ong observed, with one mother saying, 'I feel great, I'm on top of the world. Sometimes I feel a bit depressed and tied in. I then get annoyed with my husband'. Another mother said, 'I get a bit ratty sometimes. Motherhood? I enjoy *all* of it'. Ong suggested that apparent contradictions implied that mothers constructed motherhood as having discrete experiences, a paradigm that meant 'They can thus conform simultaneously to the public expression of the joy of motherhood and have private feelings of depression'.[125]

Ong noted the ways that class shaped the women's experiences of maternity care ('Antenatal care is based on certain assumptions, derived from middle class culture, which are not necessarily consonant with women's own preoccupations'), and emphasised the power inequalities imposed by the medical framework around antenatal care and childbirth. This medicalisation, Ong said, 'reduces women to maternity cases'; the report argued that 'in order to close the gap between women and professionals we have to understand the wider cultural, social and political context in which pregnancy and childbirth are located'.[126] Like other researchers, Ong reflected positively on the interview experience for the women she engaged with, arguing that it was a 'therapeutic tool' that 'enables respondents to talk openly about the pressures, anxieties, hopes and fears of this stage of their lives'.[127] This sociological research, then, aspired to have a more direct and personal social impact than raising the visibility of complaint.

Women's experiences were shaped by racism. In 1986, researcher Caroline Currer highlighted how the racism experienced by Asian mothers resulted in their exclusion from the public realm, in effect sequestering them with their children.[128] Currer noted

> one woman could not let her children out to play at all due to the attacks on them – and seven children at home in the holidays confined to two living rooms was nearly driving her mad. (I use the term colloquially but literally too, if depression can be termed as 'madness').[129]

Sociological research, then, was one of the mechanisms by which the realities of mothering in an unequal society – structured by race, class, and gender – could be made visible.

Feminist sociological studies brought attention to mothers' anger and argued that it was a normal response to the toll of unsupported childcare. Graham and McKee's study demonstrated the prevalence of anger in new mothers. Indeed, 60 per cent of the mothers admitted that there had been times when they felt anger directed towards the baby (the authors note this was more often experienced by the mothers of girls, those breastfeeding, and first-time mothers); indeed, 81 per cent of the mothers studied reported that their experiences of early motherhood had made them 'more sympathetic' to baby batterers. Graham and McKee concluded that 'anger, far from being an abnormal or pathological response' was in fact an 'endemic feature of the early weeks of motherhood'. Given this, they argued health education programmes should acknowledge that 'anger is a common, reasonable and understandable response to the stresses of twenty-four hour babycare'. Further, the policy recommendations proposed that strategies for 'dealing with the problem of anger' should be focused on mothers' social context, including physical, emotional, and material conditions.[130] This transformed anger from an individualised failing to an indication of the need for support.

Graham argued for a 'sociological perspective on child abuse which takes account of the context, and particularly the constraints, of contemporary motherhood' as 'child abuse can not be seen simply as a reflection of individual pathology, but rather as a response to social and psychological pressures which are woven into the fabric of mothers' lives'. Graham asked not why some parents succumbed, but why the majority, suffering acute tiredness and stress, did not.[131]

Other feminist sociologists also explored the social and economic contexts of mothers who abused their children. Bie Nio Ong researched abusing mothers in the 1980s, arguing that 'how motherhood is portrayed in the literature – and this of course reflects the dominant ideas in our society – abuses women as people'. Child abuse should not be individualised, she argued, explaining that it stemmed from the 'violence of the institution of motherhood'. 'Women as mothers are violated in their personal growth because they are expected to cope, no matter what the circumstances', she argued. She stressed the lack of options available to low-income young women that rendered early motherhood an appealing option. Her interviews, conducted in accordance with feminist methods, revealed the stark gendered divisions of labour, even when husbands were out of paid work. The mothers' caring work took place in a background of poverty and financial struggle.

Like Hannah Gavron's earlier work, Ong found that her interviewees did not exist within the kinship networks set forth in (idealised) representations of working-class life. This isolation came through in her interviewees' comments, with one mother saying that

> He [husband] was drinking – no support at all. And in the night it was me up, up, and the kids were up at five in the morning. So, I reached out for help. I was asking the welfare for help for a long time. I didn't get any help. Nobody came... So, I coped for another three months. Then I hit Eddy. I just snapped... I just smacked him across the face and then somebody reported me, that I was beating him up.

Ong also observed the comparative acceptability of illness rather than being a 'non-coper'. A mother told her that being on my own with the two kids, that's what got me depressed. I had no one to help me or cope with the kids... my friend went to see the psychiatrist you know, to sort my problems out and why I was getting depressed and how she could help me. And he said 'she needs a lot of friends, she needs people to come down and see her...' And she put her foot down (confronted the husband) and took me out.

Such testimonies allowed Ong to explore the legitimising role that illness could play. However, as she observed, illness also individualised women's problems and focused professionals' efforts to 'restore women to a position in which they can cope again with the demands of motherhood'. Ong proposed that professionals should consider

> how the notion of coping itself is oppressive and pathological. In view of the structural and material circumstances in which many women have to carry out their mothering role, it is no wonder that they break under the strain: how can we expect someone to cope, living in a one-bedroomed house with two children, with no support from her partner and little money to spend?

Such a focus shifted attention from the individual to the social, material, and structural environment in which women mothered.[132]

Given these shared findings around maternal isolation and desperation it is little surprise that feminist researchers collaborated. In 1986, Graham and Oakley drew together their research to consider the differences between the ways that mothers and doctors viewed pregnancy. The piece considered the ways that the physical landscape of antenatal clinics and a perceived hierarchy of expertise facilitated brusque interactions and encouraged patient passivity, as well as the treatment of pregnancy as a potentially abnormal event. The researchers proposed two routes to change. One adhered to the existing organisational model (they suggested redesigning antenatal clinics, for example), and a second proposed 'alternative patterns of care'. This second route involved more 'fundamental changes... to ameliorate the conflicts between doctors and mothers'. Oakley and Graham argued that it might be necessary to transform the system itself and proposed changes that shifted power back into the hands of mothers and midwives.[133] Feminist sociological research examined the world as it was, but also suggested ways that areas affecting women's and mothers' lives could be remapped along more equal and radical lines.

By the close of the 1980s, women had not only disputed existing paradigms but had also created new ways of conceptualising serious unhappy motherhood. At the LSE, for example, psychologist Paula Nicholson undertook doctoral research that argued that while postnatal depression was not an 'objective reality', it did 'exist "culturally" and enables women to make sense retrospectively of their experience and attach a meaning via this label'. Nicholson was critical of both clinical and non-feminist social science explicatory paradigms around postnatal depression: the 'life events' model put forward within non-feminist social science recognised the stress of mothering but continued to see women as 'individually vulnerable' and proposed solutions that emphasised support for these mothers rather than transformation of ideas about women's psychology; the medical model also saw postnatal depression as an individualised problem, albeit one that was grounded in illness. By contrast, Nicholson put forward a mother-centred approach that looked at the meanings attached to events by mothers themselves.[134] In 1990, Nicholson noted the normality of mothers' feelings of loss, sadness, and grief after childbirth. Midwives and health visitors, she suggested, could help mothers 'develop a new understanding of her place in the world after such a dramatic upheaval'.[135] As this book has shown, health visitors and midwives also played an important role in women's transition into motherhood.

Conclusion

In the early 1980s, Hilary Graham explained the appearance of successful motherhood as the work of *coping*:

> the more successful a mother is, the less apparent her presence becomes as she moves unobtrusively through the home, contending quietly with the demands of housework, husband and children. In other words, to cope successfully is to deny yourself a voice: the best mother is one who is seen but not heard.[136]

In 1970s and 1980s Britain, feminist sociology was one of the mechanisms that gave some mothers back their voice – both as researchers and as participants in research. Feminist sociology brought to the fore mothers who did not adhere to the expectation of *coping*. Studies that centred mothers' voices exposed mothering as both pleasurable and oppressive; the home as claustrophobic; and women's relationship with their children as often fraught. This chapter has argued that feminist sociology, informed by the political analyses developed within the women's liberation movement, helped to make mothers' distress visible. This had implications for medicine as well as the wider culture. As psychologist Judy Dunn wrote in a piece titled 'Unhappy Mothers' for the *London Review of Books* in 1980,

> There is every reason to suppose that what is now making it impossible for doctors to continue to ignore the difficulties of mothers is not only the articulate and insistent voice of the women's movement, but the scale on which scientific research has documented the cost of the stress under which many mothers live.[137]

Feminist sociology in the area of motherhood helped to inscribe new understandings that held space for stress, emotional ambiguity, ambivalence, and anger. The energy and analysis that feminist sociologists brought to the study of motherhood were vital, even in the face of structural challenges within the academy, which made use of their precarious labour, was sometimes hostile to their arguments, and sometimes marginalised their ideas. Of course, feminist sociology should not be seen in isolation. Feminist interventions into the academy shaped conversations across subjects. In 1981, feminist and academic Dale Spender wrote that feminist 'discoveries' soon crossed disciplinary boundaries when the illusion of particularity was destroyed, and it became apparent that the 'problem of male dominance in the construction of knowledge... manifested itself across disciplines'.[138] It is telling that issues identified by the feminist movement, not least childbirth, motherhood, work, and childcare, have endured as areas of scholarly and activist interest. This is both a marker of the movement's success in centring these concerns within academia and a marker of public policy's failure to grasp them.

But one of feminism's most profound impacts on the academy was to force a reckoning with women's full humanity. As Skeggs says, feminist sociologists worked with ideas in different ways: as diagnosis, as description, as evidence for policy, as critique, as a call to political action, to legislate, always an attempt to 'speak truth to power'. All these techniques can both inscribe and undo.[139]

The impact of feminism in sociology was to develop new approaches, new analyses, and new fields, and to centre women's voices. The ultimate aim of her sociology, Oakley said, was 'to actually improve people's lives… it's about having some kind of practical impact, and sometimes you have that by opening a debate, by making people argue, and by highlighting an issue'.[140] Oakley is right: lives can be improved by opening new conversations and shifting the locus of expertise within them. Just as Sheila Kitzinger sought to develop a language and body of knowledge about childbirth that belonged to women themselves, feminist sociology played a role in disseminating narratives of mothering rooted in women's own experiences.[141] It is this that helped to change the unhappy mother from being a 'stock figure' of popular culture to an active agent: she was an expert about herself.

Notes

1 Ann Oakley, *Father and Daughter: Patriarchy, Gender and Social Science* (Bristol, 2014), 225.
2 Lise Butler, 'The Social Scientific Turn in Modern British History', *Twentieth Century British History*, 2022, hwac015, https://doi.org/10.1093/tcbh/hwac015
3 Mike Savage, 'History and Sociology: A Twenty-First Century Rapprochement?', *Twentieth Century British History*, 33, 3, 2022, 416–431, 429.
4 Ann Oakley, *Becoming a Mother* (Oxford, 1979), 2.
5 Ann Oakley, *Women Confined: Towards a Sociology of Childbirth* (Oxford, 1980), chapter three.
6 Joanna Bourke, 'Becoming the 'Natural' Mother in Britain and North America: Power, Emotions and the Labour of Childbirth Between 1947 and 1967', *Past & Present*, 246, Suppl. 15, 2020, 92–114, 93.
7 Adrienne Rich, *Of Woman Born: Motherhood as an Experience and Institution* (London and New York, 1986 [1976]); Betty Friedan, *The Feminine Mystique* (New York, 1963), 15–16.

8 Jennifer Leachman, 'A Longitudinal Study of Preparation for Childbirth, Pain in Labour and Postnatal Depression', Unpublished PhD Thesis, University of Bath, Bath, 1988, 88.
9 Eve Worth, 'Women, Education and Social Mobility in Britain during the Long 1970s', *Cultural and Social History*, 16:1, 2019, 67–83.
10 Worth, 'Women, Education and Social Mobility', 74; Peter Mandler, 'Educating the Nation IV: Subject Choice', *Transactions of the Royal Historical Society*, 27, 2017, 17.
11 Sue Sharpe, *Double Identity: The Lives of Working Mothers* (Middlesex, 1984), 237–238.
12 Liz Stanley (ed.), *Feminist Praxis: Research, Theory and Epistemology in Feminist Sociology* (London and New York: Routledge, 1990), Bio.
13 Mike Savage, *Identities and Social Change in Britain Since 1940: The Politics of Method* (Oxford, 2010), vii.
14 A.H. Halsey, *A History of Sociology in Britain: Science, Literature and Society* (Oxford, 2004).
15 Helen McCarthy, 'Social Science and Married Women's Employment in Post-War Britain', *Past & Present*, 233, 1, 2016, 269–305. See, for example, Margery Spring Rice, *Working-Class Wives*. 2nd ed. (London, 1981 [1939]), 18–20; Alva Myrdal and Viola Klein, *Women's Two Roles* (London, 1956); Judith Hubback, *Wives Who Went to College* (London, 1957); Pearl Jephcott, *Married Women Working* (London, 1962).
16 For more on Michael Young, see Lise Butler, *Michael Young, Social Science, and the British Left, 1945–1970* (Oxford, 2020).
17 Michael Young and Peter Willmott, *Family and Kinship in East London* (London, 1957); For more see Halsey, *A History of Sociology in Britain*, 127–128; see, for example, John Newson and Elizabeth Newson, *Infant Care in an Urban Community* (London, 1964), as well as the other texts that came out of this Nottingham project.
18 Jon Lawrence, '"Inventing The 'Traditional Working Class': A Re-Analysis of Interview Notes from Young and Willmott's *Family and Kinship in East London*', *The Historical Journal*, 59, 2, 2016, 567–593, 569.
19 Ann Oakley, *Father and Daughter: Patriarchy, Gender, and Social Science* (Bristol, 2014), 58–59.
20 Mike Savage, 'Elizabeth Bott and the Formulation of Modern British Sociology, *The Sociological Review*, 56, 4, 2008, 57–605, 600.
21 Helen McCarthy, 'Feminism, Selfhood and Social Research: Professional Women's Organizations in 1960s Britain', in *Precarious Professionals: Gender, Identities and Social Change in Modern Britain*, eds H. Egginton and Z. Thomas (London, 2021), 287–304, 302–303.

22 Oakley, *Father and Daughter*, 225.
23 Ann Oakley, 'Interviewing Women Again: Power, Time and the Gift', *Sociology*, 50, 1, 2016, 195–213, 196.
24 Hannah Gavron, 'The Position and Opportunities of Young Mothers – Progress or Retrogression (A Study of the Difficulties Confronting Young Mothers in the Contemporary Family Based on a Comparative Study of Working Class and Middle Class Families)', Unpublished PhD Thesis, Bedford College, University of London, London, 1964, 1.
25 P. Thompson, 'University of Essex, Department of Sociology: "Interview with Ann Oakley" in "Pioneers of Social Research, 1996–2018" 4th Edition', UK Data Service [Distributor], 2019-04-08, SN:6226, Para. 57. http://doi.org/10.5255/UKDA-SN-6226-6, https://discover.ukdataservice.ac.uk//QualiBank/Document/?cid=q-52d8e1d2-72ae-446c-a2d6-4ddde8771299.
26 Hannah Gavron, *The Captive Wife: Conflicts of Housebound Mothers* (London, 1968 [1966]), 89.
27 Jeremy Gavron, *A Woman on the Edge of Time* (London, 2016 [2015]), 146 and 223.
28 *Ibid.*, 226–227.
29 *Ibid.*, 129–134.
30 *Ibid.*, 152.
31 Gavron, *The Captive Wife*, 9.
32 'When Does a Woman Know She is Middle Class?', *Sunday Mirror*, 15 May 1966; 'The Housebound Housewife', *The Daily Telegraph*, 5 May 1966; 'The Loneliness of the Stay-at-Home-Mother', *Evening Standard*, 5 May 1966.
33 'Tragedy of Captive Wives', *Coventry Standard*, 16 June 1966.
34 'How to Free "the Captive Wife"', *Birmingham Post*, 5 May 1966.
35 'Loophole for the Captive Wife', *The Scotsman*, 15 July 1968.
36 Abrams, 'The Self and Self-Help', 203–204.
37 'What's in it for the Working Wife?', *Daily Post: The Paper for Wales*, 7 April 1982.
38 Ellen Malos, *The Politics of Housework* (Cheltenham, [1980], 1995).
39 Lynne Segal, 'The Politics of the Family: Laing and Esterson in Context', *Journal of Psychosocial Studies*, 11, 1, 2018, 104–125, 119.
40 Peter Mandler, 'The Rise of the Social Sciences in British Education, 1960–2016', in *The History of Sociology in Britain*, ed. Plamena Panayotova (Cham, 2019), 218–299, 283.
41 Jennifer Platt, 'The History of the British Sociological Association', *International Sociology*, 17, 2, 2002, 179–198.
42 Halsey, *A History of Sociology in Britain*, 89.

43 *Ibid.*, 117–118.
44 Julius Gould (ed.), 'The Power of Politics', in *Penguin Social Sciences Survey 1968* (Middlesex, 1968), 9–10.
45 Jennifer Platt, 'The Women's Movement and British Journal Articles, 1950–2004', *Sociology* 41, 5, 2007, 961–975; Sara Delamont, *Feminist Sociology* (London, 2003), 29.
46 Beverley Skeggs, 'The Dirty History of Feminism and Sociology: Or the War of Conceptual Attrition', *Sociological Review*, 56, 4, 2008, 670–690, 674; Ann Oakley, *Social Support and Motherhood* (Oxford, 1992), 76–92.
47 Helen Roberts, 'Some of the Boys Won't Play Any More: The Impact of Feminism on Sociology', in *Men's Studies Modified: The Impact of Feminism on the Academic Disciplines,* Ed. Dale Spender (Oxford, 1981), 73–81, 74.
48 Helen Roberts and Diana Woodward, 'Changing Patterns of Women's Employment in Sociology: 1950–80', *The British Journal of Sociology*, 32, 4, 1981, 531–546, 540.
49 Sheila Kitzinger, *A Passion for Birth* (London, 2015), 186–189.
50 Margaret Stacey, 'B.S.A. Presidential Address: Social Sciences and the State: Fighting Like a Woman', *Sociology*, 16, 3, 1982, 406–421, 419.
51 P. Thompson, 'University of Essex, Department of Sociology, 'Interview with Margaret Stacey', in "Pioneers of Social Research, 1996–2018" 4th Edition', UK Data Service [Distributor], 2019-04-08, SN:6226, Para. 1–336. http://doi.org/10.5255/UKDA-SN-6226-6, https://discover.ukdataservice.ac.uk//QualiBank/Document/?id=q-4d7d478a-802b-4242-b8b6-8fe8050a8b98
52 'Toward a Feminist Theory of Motherhood', *Feminist Studies*, 4, 2, 1978.
53 Nava, 'Looking Back', 65.
54 Michèle Barrett and Mary McIntosh, *The Anti-Social Family* (London, 1982), 59.
55 Peter Mandler, 'Good Reading for the Million: The 'Paperback Revolution' and the Co-Production of Academic Knowledge in Mid Twentieth-Century Britain and America', *Past & Present*, 244, 1, 2019, 235–269.
56 Helen Roberts (ed.), 'Ten Years On', in *Doing Feminist Research* (London, 1990 [1981]), xiii–xxi, xiv.
57 Lucy Delap, 'Feminist Bookshops, Reading Cultures and the Women's Liberation Movement in Great Britain, c. 1974–2000', *History Workshop Journal*, 81, 2016, 171–196, 172.

58 Sheila Allen and Diana Leonard Barker (Eds), 'Sexual Divisions and Society', in *Sexual Divisions and Society: Process and Change* (London, 1976), 1–24, 1.
59 Margaret Stacey, 'The Division of Labour Revisited or Overcoming the Two Adams', in *Practice and Progress: British Sociology 1950–1980*, eds Philip Abrams, Rosemary Deem, Janet Finch, and Paul Rock (London and New York, 1981), 172–190, 190.
60 Leeds Revolutionary Feminist Group, 'Every Single Academic Feminist Owes Her Livelihood to the WLM', Unpublished Paper, WRRC Summer School, Bradford, 1979.
61 Liz Stanley and Sue Wise, *Breaking Out: Feminist Consciousness and Feminist Research* (London, 1983), 26–27.
62 Kate Millett, *Sexual Politics* (London, 1985 [1971]), 177–178.
63 Skeggs, 'The Dirty History', 676–677.
64 Allen and Leonard Barker, 'Sexual Divisions and Society', 20.
65 *Ibid.*, 1.
66 Christine Delphy, 'Continuities and Discontinuities in Marriage and Divorce', 76–89; Hilary Rose and Jalna Hanmer, 'Women's Liberation, Reproduction, and the Technological Fix', 199–223; Sally Macintyre, '"Who Wants Babies?": The Social Construction of "Instincts"', 150–173 (quote from 171); all in Allen and Leonard Barker, *Sexual Divisions and Society*.
67 Sue Jackson, 'Networking Women: A History of Ideas, Issues and Developments in Women's Studies in Britain', *Women's Studies International Forum*, 23, 2000, 1–11.
68 Kelly Coate, 'The History of Women's Studies as an Academic Subject Area in Higher Education in the UK: 1970–1995', Unpublished PhD Thesis, Institute of Education, University of London, London, 1999, 10.
69 Ann Oakley, 'Women's Studies in British Sociology: To End at Our Beginning?', *The British Journal of Sociology*, 40, 3, 1989, 442–470, 443.
70 Women's Studies Group (Ed.), 'Women's Studies Group: Trying to Do Feminist Intellectual Work', in *Women Take Issue: Aspects of Women's Subordination*, Centre for Contemporary Cultural Studies Editorial Group, (London, 1978), 7–17, 7.
71 P. Thompson, 'University of Essex, Department of Sociology: "Interview with Pat Caplan" in "Pioneers of Social Research, 1996–2018" 4th Edition, UK Data Service' [Distributor], 2019-04-08, SN:6226, Para. 1–296. http://doi.org/10.5255/UKDA-SN-6226-6, https://discover.ukdataservice.ac.uk//QualiBank/Document/?id=q-51c8f358-2ce1-4012-b00f-87ce4bbe5a50

72 Dale Spender (ed.), 'Introduction', in *Men's Studies Modified: The Impact of Feminism on the Academic Disciplines* (Oxford, 1981), 1–10, 2.
73 Liz Stanley (ed.), 'Feminist Praxis and the Academic Mode of Production: An Editorial Introduction', in *Feminist Praxis: Research, Theory and Epistemology in Feminist Sociology* (London and New York, 1990), 3–15, 3.
74 Stanley, 'Feminist Praxis', x, 12.
75 Stanley and Wise, *Breaking Out*, 178.
76 Sally Macintyre, 'Some Notes on Record Taking and Making in an Antenatal Clinic', *The Sociological Review*, 26, 3, 1978, 595–612, 608.
77 Margaret Stacey, 'Social Sciences and the State: Fighting Like a Woman', *Sociology*, 16, 3, 1982, 406–442, 407.
78 Oakley, 'Women's Studies in British Sociology', 444.
79 *Ibid.*, 61.
80 Roberts, 'Women and their Doctors', 7–29, 15.
81 Ann Oakley, 'Doctors, Maternity Patients and Social Scientists', *Birth*, 12, 1985, 161–166.
82 Hilary Graham, 'Surveying Through Stories', in *Social Researching: Politics, Problems, Practice*, eds C. Bell and H. Roberts (London, Boston, MA, Melbourne and Henley, 1984), 104–124, 107–120.
83 Ann Oakley, 'Interviewing Women: A Contradiction in Terms?', in *Doing Feminist Research*, ed. Helen Roberts (London, 1981), 30–61.
84 Ann Phoenix, 'Practicing Feminist Research: The Intersections of Gender and "Race" in the Research Process', in *Researching Women's Lives from a Feminist Perspective*, eds Mary Maynard and June Purvis (London, 1994), 49–71.
85 Jocelyn Cornwall, *Hard-Earned Lives: Accounts of Health and Illness from East London* (London, 1984), 13.
86 Janet Finch, 'It's Great Having Someone to Talk to': The Ethics and Politics of Interviewing Women', in *Social Researching: Politics, Problems, Practice*, eds Colin Bell and Helen Roberts (London, 1984), 70–87, 74.
87 Oakley, *Social Support and Motherhood*, 14.
88 National Childbirth Trust, *The Emotions and Experiences of Some Disabled Mothers* (London, 1985), 8.
89 Helen McCarthy, 'Feminism, Selfhood and Social Research: Professional Women's Organizations in 1960s Britain', in *Precarious Professionals: Gender, Identities and Social Change in Modern Britain*, eds Heidi Egginton and Zoë Thomas (London, 2021), 287–304.
90 Oakley, *Becoming a Mother*, 5.

91 Ann Oakley, *From Here to Maternity* (London, 1986), 2–3.
92 Jane Lewis, 'Introduction', in *The Goals of Social Policy: Conference Papers*, eds Martin Bulmer, Jane Lewis, and David Piachaud (London, 1989), 131–140, 131.
93 Sally Macintyre, 'The Management of Childbirth: A Review of Sociological Research Issues', *Social Science and Medicine*, 11: 8, 1977, 477–484.
94 Oakley, 'Doctors, Maternity Patients and Social Scientists', 165.
95 Joanna Bourke, 'Becoming the 'Natural' Mother in Britain and North America: Power, Emotions and the Labour of Childbirth Between 1947 and 1967', *Past & Present*, 246, suppl. 15, 2020, 92–114, 93.
96 Ann Oakley, 'The Sociology of Childbirth: An Autobiographical Journey Through Four Decades of Research', *Sociology of Health and Illness* 38, 5, 2016, 689–705, 689.
97 Oakley, *Becoming a Mother*, 2–3.
98 Peter Conrad, 'Medicalization and Social Control', *Annual Review of Sociology*, 18, 1992, 209–232.
99 Oakley, 'The Sociology of Childbirth', 692.
100 Marjorie Tew, *Safer Childbirth? A Critical History of Maternity Care* (London, 1998 [1990]), viii–ix.
101 *Ibid.*, 156.
102 'Childbirth Revolution', *The Times*, 12 October 1974.
103 'Surveys Arranged on Induction of Childbirth', *The Times*, 20 December 1974.
104 'A Time to be Born', *Horizon*, BBC, January 1975.
105 'Survey Begun on Attitudes to Induced Births', *The Times*, 15 March 1975.
106 Caroline Flint, 'On the Brink: Midwifery in Britain', in *The Midwife Challenge*, ed. Sheila Kitzinger (London, 1988), 22–41, 35. For more on ARM see Chapter 4.
107 Oakley, *Becoming a Mother*, 127–142.
108 *Ibid.*, 130.
109 *Ibid.*, 127.
110 Oakley, *Women Confined*, 293.
111 *Ibid.*, 5.
112 *Ibid.*, 150–151.
113 *Ibid.*, 148–149.
114 James McIntosh, 'Models of Childbirth and Social Class: A Study of 80 Working Class Primigravidae', in *Midwives, Research and Childbirth*, vol. 1, eds Sarah Robinson and Ann M. Thomson (London, 1995 [1989]), 189–214, 197–198.
115 *Ibid.*, 205.

116 Maggie Comport, *Towards Happy Motherhood: Understanding Postnatal Depression* (London, 1987), 27.
117 Angela Davis, 'Women's Experiences of the Maternity Services in Berkshire and Oxfordshire, c. 1970–1990', in *Western Maternity and Medicine, 1880–1990*, eds Janet Greenlees and Linda Bryder (London, 2013), 129–146, 129.
118 Oakley, *Becoming a Mother*, 143–146.
119 Oakley, *Women Confined*, 297.
120 *Ibid.*, 53.
121 *Ibid.*, 277.
122 Ann Oakley interview with Social Science Space, 4 February 2013. Retrieved from https://www.socialsciencespace.com/2013/04/podcast-ann-oakley-on-womens-experience-of-childbirth/ [accessed February 2023].
123 Perinatal Mortality and Morbidity, HL Deb 02 May 1978 vol 391 cc122–67, 141.
124 Hilary Graham and Lorna McKee, *The First Months of Motherhood: Summary Report of a Survey of Women's Experiences of Pregnancy, Childbirth, and the First Six Months After Birth* (London, 1980), 1.
125 Bie Nio Ong, *Our Motherhood: Women's Accounts of Pregnancy, Childbirth and Health Encounters*. A Family Service Units Discussion Paper (London, 1983), 14. Emphasis in original.
126 *Ibid.*, 9–10.
127 *Ibid.*, 7.
128 Caroline Currer, 'Health Concepts and Illness Behaviour: The Case of Some Pathan Mothers in Britain', Unpublished Doctoral Thesis, University of Warwick, Warwick, 1986, 146–147.
129 *Ibid.*, 147.
130 Graham and McKee, *The First Months*, 24–33.
131 Hilary Graham, 'Mothers' Accounts of Anger and Aggression Towards their Babies', in *Psychological Approaches to Child Abuse*, ed. N. Frude (London, 1980), 39–51.
132 Bic Nio Ong, 'Child Abuse: Are Abusing Women Abused Women?', in *Feminist Practice in Women's Health Care*, ed. Christine Webb (Chichester, 1986), 163–182.
133 Hilary Graham and Ann Oakley, 'Competing Ideologies of Reproduction: Medical and Maternal Perspectives on Pregnancy', in *Concepts of Health, Illness and Disease: A Comparative Perspective*, eds Caroline Currer and Meg Stacey (London, 1986), 99–115, 115.

134 Paula Nicholson, 'The Social Psychology of "Post Natal Depression"', Unpublished Doctoral Thesis, London School of Economics, London, 3, 78, 424.
135 Paula Nicholson, 'Understanding Post-Natal Depression: A Mother-Centred Approach', *Journal of Advanced Nursing*, 12, 1990, 689–695, 694.
136 Hilary Graham, 'Coping: Or How Mothers Are Seen and Not Heard', in *On the Problem of Men*, eds Scarlet Friedman and Elizabeth Sarah (London, 1982), 101–116, 105.
137 Judy Dunn, 'Unhappy Mothers', *London Review of Books*, 2, 14, 17 July 1980. Retrieved from https://www.lrb.co.uk/the-paper/v02/n14/judy-dunn/unhappy-mothers [Accessed 25 September 2024].
138 Spender, 'Introduction', 2.
139 Skeggs, 'The Dirty History', 683.
140 Oakley interview with Social Science Space.
141 Kitzinger, *Passion for Birth*, 9.

Conclusion

In December 1983, the author Angela Carter wrote about her recent experience of antenatal and maternity care at the hands of the NHS: the stern female doctor, taking her joke as literal; the hospital set for closure; the compulsion to bond immediately with her baby. This duty to bond, she wrote,

> Constrained affection; what resentment it will breed, in time. It's all part of the mystification in which the process of childbirth is so richly shrouded. For he is doomed to love us, at least for a significant initial period, because we are his parents. The same goes for us. That is life. That's the hell of it.[1]

Carter was in her forties – an 'older mother' in society's eyes. And this, of course, is the other background to mothering in British society: always too much of something. Too old; too young; too devoted; too independent; too strict; too lenient; too present; too absent; too bonded; not bonded enough. Mothering, within these social confines – the invisible guard rails of culturally sanctioned maternity – is condemned, too often, to mystification and constrained affection.

This book began its life when I had no children, and it ends when I have three (aged six, four, and one, at the time of writing). They are phenomenal, hilarious, life-affirming, and deeply, *deeply* loved. When I step back from the daily minutiae of care (the hunt for matching socks, the locating of snacks, the running of baths, the wiping of sticky hands) I am able to see that nurturing them is, for me, a multilayered ritual of hope. But the minutiae is massive, and the writing of this book has been a reminder that women have long been talking about mothering as *hard work*. Across the postwar period, women have claimed the emotional lives of mothers as a bellwether for injustices, inequalities, and structural problems. Poor housing, poor social support, and inadequate access to power, rest, and respite; mothers' emotional worlds are depleted by political and social choices not to address these problems. Mothers have long been organising in ways that seek to address these challenges, too: by forming self-help groups, writing to local newspapers, demanding better maternity care, and campaigning for childcare. Some organisations explored in this book were explicitly political, while the politics of other groups have been implicit or implied. Some groups were avowedly feminist; others wore their feminism lightly, while still laying claim to the value of mothers' happiness and health as important *in itself*, not just as a vehicle for the improvement of the family unit. The book made three interconnected arguments around visibility, experience, and meanings, suggesting that invested communities made mothers' unhappiness visible using a variety of mechanisms; that distressed mothers had agency in this process in a way that laid claim to experiential expertise; and that mothers' unhappiness attained political meanings via the work of feminist writers, sociologists, and health visitors.

Still, in some ways, it is remarkable that the challenges of mothering – the elements of the act itself that are 'too much' – have endured. Jacqueline Rose's argument that motherhood is where, in the West, 'we lodge, or rather bury, the reality of our own conflicts, of what it means to be fully human' rings true.[2] Other problems are products of economics and poor planning. Put another way, they are the products of political and social choices. For too many women the experience of childbirth is scary, disempowering, and impersonal. Childcare remains under-resourced, under-funded, and out of reach for many. Employers individualise parents' struggles (the fact that school finishes at 3.10, work finishes at 6, and small children need to be fed and bathed and read to and put to bed by 7 is *our problem;* requests that we work at weekends or at night when there is no childcare is *our problem*). Housing remains precarious for a great number of families. Public spaces treat infants, and mothers, as a messy inconvenience. Have you tried to get on a bus with a double buggy? Have you changed a nappy on a squalid public toilet floor? Have you tried to cross a busy road with restless toddlers and multiple shopping bags? These hostilities do not trigger postnatal depression, but they do make mothering, sometimes, *too much*. Urban design is, in both form and function, hostile to people with small children.[3] As Sheila Kitzinger observed in 1978, it is not a matter of making minor concessions to mothers ('a pram park here and a baby changing room there') but of 'working out the conditions which have to be met for mothers to be able to put their best into mothering and for families to have the kinds of environment in which they can flourish'.[4] But so far, we have tinkered – made only the smallest concessions – and not reckoned with this environmental or cultural overhaul. Mothers are held at a distance. And underpinning mothers' – and indeed fathers' – tolerance of these cumulative indignities is the banal, routine, exhausting, and extraordinary impulse of overriding parental love. That, to borrow from Carter, is the hell of it.

What accounts for the stubborn endurance of these adversities? It is convenient and, within neoliberalism, politically expedient to look away from the plight of struggling parents – particularly parents who do not fall within the white, middle-class, heteronormative family ideal. And it is, no doubt, these parents who care for their infants in the most challenging of circumstances. The [nuclear] family continues to be an acclaimed unit. But recent political discourse has attached 'hard-working' as an epithet to this already loaded category. The appellation 'hard-working', here, implies *paid* work. The hardest working families, though, are those with the fewest resources; in these, parents have nowhere to fall back on when they need a rest, and their worry-work is sprawling and elemental. Those families we look away from: those mothers are on their own. But the endurance of structural challenges is also, perhaps, because caring for small infants is axiomatically transitory, tiring, and time-consuming. It is perhaps only at its borders, when one reaches the shoreline of parenting an older child, with the freedom created by relative self-sufficiency and independence, that one can take stock and look askance at how hard some of that early care work really was. But by then, for most, the outrage has passed.

Modern mothers have more outlets than ever before to discuss the underbelly of parenting. Internet forums, podcasts, and social media provide new outlets for maternal complaint. There is a burgeoning field of autobiography and autofiction that explores some of the ambivalences and ambiguities mothers navigate. This book has considered some of the forerunners to these contemporary conversations, spaces, and organisers, looking at how mothers' unhappiness was brought to light by five communities between the late 1940s and the late 1980s. Some of the mechanisms towards visibility have stemmed from the medical domain – the particular professional pressures brought to bear upon general practitioners during the early years of the NHS, for example. Other mechanisms have been activist, academic, professional, or social, or a combination of these. The focus on the mechanisms of visibility has rested on the idea that mothers' work, worry, and unhappiness were not created in the postwar period but rather that it saw an expansion of opportunities for their exploration. This expansion was driven by interested and invested communities, among whom numbered general practitioners, health visitors, unhappy mothers in self-help and mutual care groups, feminist activists, and feminist sociologists. Many of these categories overlapped, and all contained mothers. They were driven by a range of professional, personal, and political (and personal *as* political) motivations. This book, then, looked towards diverse efforts to give unhappy motherhood voice across the postwar period.

Some might argue that the particular vehicles for visibility set out here have had their day. The tensions between the structures of modern life and the leap into maternity are best explored 'not [in] the political tract or sociological potboiler but mass-market fiction', wrote a poet and novelist in the *London Review of Books* in 2003. It was in fiction that 'feminist and retro impulses can be resolved, or blurred, through a judicious combination of truth-telling (it's a man's world, and the man is a swine) and fantasy'.[5] But the communities explored here established some of the discourses of permissible truth-telling about mothering.

The speakability of maternal discontent remains uneven. The voices of white, middle-class mothers are heard more readily than those from marginalised, oppressed, disadvantaged, and disempowered communities. But even the most privileged mothers might hear that malign social hiss: *you chose this*. One of the *leitmotifs* of this book has been that while women might choose to become mothers, they do not choose the social, cultural, and economic conditions within which mothering is performed. Discontent with these has been a site of women's organising. But 'mother' is still an emotionally loaded noun, 'to mother' a verb without margins.[6] There remains a disconnect between the expectations placed on mothers and the support available to them.

This book looked at efforts to render unhappy mothers ordinary and to create community around them. This is perhaps best exemplified by the articles about mothers' self-help groups placed in local newspapers by local mothers. These articles firmly framed unhappiness as something experienced by ordinary women with young children: 'we are your neighbours' it implied. In some ways, the very ordinariness of distress has worked against mothers. As Vivienne Welburn observed in the 1970s,

> There is nothing so very unusual about the difficulties which women encounter when they arrive home with a new baby. We are not moved to anger or pity by the image of a tired mother alone with a screaming baby. It is too domestic and familiar, too common and undramatic to excite our interest.[7]

More recently, writer Rachel Cusk expressed a similar sentiment when she suggested in her memoir that she had the 'gloomy suspicion that a book about motherhood is of no real interest to anyone except other mothers... the experience of motherhood loses nearly everything in its translation to the outside world'.[8] Cusk was, reassuringly, mistaken; *A Life's Work* was widely read and reviewed (although its honesty about maternal ambivalence was not always welcomed).[9] Since it was published in the early 2000s Cusk's memoir has been joined by a rich stream of other works on motherhood as a social, political, and historical phenomena.[10] There is, therefore, a thriving field of writing that takes motherhood and mothers seriously. Much of this literature has argued that motherhood is profoundly political and can, with work, have radical potential.[11] Feminist thinking about, through, and around the experience and conditions of motherhood shows no sign of abatement.

The book began in the medical domain – with general practitioners' impetus to research mental health and their practice populations – and took in the activist, academic, and professional landscapes. It began at the beginnings of the NHS, in the upheaval of the immediate postwar years and the new welfare state, and it ends on the cusp of the 1990s, with its promise of free-floating individualistic success. Across these decades, postnatal depression had gained a foothold in the medical domain. Mothers' advocacy had shifted registers, found new outlets, and founded new organisations. From the 1960s onwards, mothers increasingly agitated around unhappiness. Medicine, activism, and sociology had created spaces for the discussion of women's discontent, albeit in very different ways. Mothers' discontent appeared in medical journals, feminist anthologies and magazines, sociological articles, health visitors' case notes, self-help groups' pamphlets, and letters to newspapers. Some mothers wrote furiously in fiction, poetry, and prose. Some were, as author Anne Enright observed pithily of Angela Carter, 'profoundly suspicious of all this mothering malarkey'.[12] Mothers' experiences of everyday discontent are, then, spread across archives. The story these archives tell is one of changing expertise. Expertise about unhappy mothering became increasingly acknowledged to be shared among researchers and mothers themselves. Experience became its own knowledge framework. And, as this book has shown, for some mothers, discontent was a stimulus for political and social work.

Notes

1 Angela Carter, 'Notes from a Maternity Ward', *New Statesman*, 24 September 2015 [December 1983]. Retrieved from https://www.newstatesman.com/long-reads/2005/09/notes-from-a-maternity-ward [Accessed 1 June 2023].
2 Jacqueline Rose, *Mothers: An Essay on Love and Cruelty* (London, 2018), 1.
3 Leslie Kern, *Feminist City: Claiming Space in a Man-Made World* (London, 2020), 28.
4 Sheila Kitzinger, *Women as Mothers* (Glasgow, 1978), 270–271.
5 Katha Pollitt, 'Dream On', *London Review of Books*, 25, 17, 11 September 2003. Retrieved from https://www.lrb.co.uk/the-paper/v25/n17/katha-pollitt/dream-on [Accessed 25 September 2024].
6 With thanks to Sarah Knott for the important and resonant framing of 'mother is a verb'. For this see Sarah Knott, *Mother Is a Verb: An Unconventional History* (New York, 2019).

7 Vivienne Welburn, *Postnatal Depression* (Glasgow, 1980), 112.
8 Rachel Cusk, *A Life's Work: On Becoming a Mother* (London, 2008 [2001], 9.
9 Rachel Cusk, 'I Was Only Being Honest', *The Guardian*, 21 March 2008. Retrieved from https://theguardian.com/books/2008/mar/21/biography.women [accessed 5 March 2025].
10 Helen Charman, *Mother State: A Political History of Motherhood* (London, 2024) and Lucy Jones, *Matrescence: On the Metamorphosis of Pregnancy, Childbirth and Motherhood* (London, 2023)
11 This has been considered within the scholarly field of motherhood studies. See, for example, Andrea O'Reilly (Ed.), *Feminist Mothering* (Albany, NY, 2008) and Andrea O'Reilly, *Maternal Thinking: Philosophy, Politics, Practice* (Toronto, 2009).
12 Anne Enright, 'Diary: Lessons from Angela Carter', *London Review of Books*, 33, 4, 17 February 2011. Retrieved from https://www.lrb.co.uk/the-paper/v33/n04/anne-enright/diary [Accessed 17 September 2024].

Bibliography

Unpublished Primary Sources

Wellcome Collection

Association of Radical Midwives, *The Practising Midwife, Report of the 1982 National Conference* (London: Association of Radical Midwives, 1982). P12134.

Association of Radical Midwives, *The Vision: Proposals for The Future of Maternity Services* (Lancaster: The Association of Radical Midwives, 1986). WQ100 1986a84v.

Association of Radical Midwives, *Working for Change, Report of the 1984 National Conference, Oxford, May 1984* (London: Association of Radical Midwives, 1984). P12136.

Dennis, Margaret, *The First Few Weeks of Motherhood: Some Suggestions for New Mothers*. Oxford Post-Natal Support Group, The National Childbirth Trust, Handbook No. 2, December 1974. SA/NCT/D/3/1.

Health Visitors' Association, *Health Visitors & Mental Health* (London: Health Visitors' Association, 1968). WY115 1968h43h.

Kott, Barbara and Jackie Carnell, 'Foreword', *Postnatal Depression: Focus on A Neglected Issue*, Papers from the HVA/NCT National Conference, London, 18 April 1996. SA/NCT/D/3/3.

Mansfield, Rosaleen, 'An Historical Survey of Postnatal Support', SA/NCT/D/3/1.

Marris, Tyrrell, *The Work of Health Visitors in London: A Survey, 1969*. Greater London Council Research Department of Planning and Transportation, County Hall, London. Research Report No. 12 (London: Greater London Council, 1971). K51004.

Mothers Talking About Postnatal Depression (London: National Childbirth Trust, 1983), SA/NCT/A/7/1.

NCT, Meeting of Postnatal Committee, 7 May 1980. SA/NCT/D/3/1.
NCT, Postnatal Committee Publications – Who Are They For? SA/NCT/A/7/1.
NCT, *Postnatal Depression Support*. 2nd Ed. (London, National Childbirth Trust, 1997). SA/NCT/D/3/5.
NCT, *Postnatal Forever* Newsletters. SA/NCT/D/3/4.
NCT, *Postnatal Resource Pack*, 1992. SA/NCT/D/3/1.
NCT, *Postnatal Support Within The NCT*, July 1982, SA/NCT/D/3/1.
NCT, *Scottish Newsletter*, Winter 1989, SA/NCT/D/3/4.
R. Ann Abel, *Nursing Attachments to General Practice: Staff Implications for Schemes for Attachment of Local Health Authority Staff (Health Visitors and Home Nurses) to General Practice*, Study No. 1. Department of Health and Social Security Social Science Research Unit (London: HMSO, 1969). K50675.
Report of the Medical Officer of Health for Haringey (London, 1972), 43. https://wellcomecollection.org/works/q2n7ay26.
Tavistock Institute of Human Relations, Working Association of Mothers, SA/TIH/B/2/79 (File 1 of 2).
Tavistock Institute of Human Relations, Working Association of Mothers, SA/TIH/B/2/79 (File 2 of 2).
Transcript of an Interview Conducted by Dr. M.J. Bevan with Anthony Ryle, 'an Oral History of General Practice C. 1935–1952' (Oxford, 1995). GP 29.
Waumsley, L. 'Postnatal Support Now', Postnatal Pack: Resources for Co-ordinators and Supporters, NCT Postnatal Committee, 1987. SA/NCT/D/3/3.
Women Public Health Officers' Association, *The Function and Case Load of Health Visitors* (London, 1953). WY115 1953w87f.

British Library

Joint Consultative Committee of Institutions Approved by The Minister of Health for The Training of Health Visitors, and of Organisations of Health Visitors. (1939). Health Visiting as a Career. London. YD.2005a.1665.
Meet-A-Mum Association. (1988). Behind the Painted Smile: An Insight into Postnatal Depression. MAMA. 95/03037.
Meet-A-Mum Association. (1992). Go Forth and Multiply But... What is the Impact of a New Baby on the Family, a MAMA Study Day. YK/1996/A.20.
Meet-A-Mum Association. (1993). Lifting the Veil of Silence: On Emotional Problems after Childbirth. 95/03034.

Meet-A-Mum Association. (1996). Friendship and Support for All Mothers. Surrey. YK1996/A.18338.
Mothers in Action. (1969). Mothers Alone. J/X0315/11 (6).
Mothers in Action. (1970). Shirley Frost, Sharing Responsibility for the Child. J/X0315/11 (7).
Mothers in Action. (1971). Penny Milsom, Unsupported Mothers on Social Security. J/X0315/11.
Mothers in Action. (1971). Study Pamphlet No.4, Residential Jobs for Unsupported Mothers – A Survey. London. J/Z0315/11 (19).
Mothers in Action. (1972). Alternative Care for Children Under Five. J/X0315/11 (11).
Mothers in Action. (1972). Housing Sheet. J/X0315/11 (4).
Mothers in Action. Plan for Day Care. J/X0315/11.
Mothers in Action. Plan for Housing. J/X0315/11.
Mothers in Action. Plan for Pregnancy. J/X0315/11.
Mothers in Action. Working Mothers' Charter: For the Benefit of Working Mothers and Their Children. J/X0315/11 (15).
Mothers in Action. J/X0315/11.

LSE Women's Library

Mothers in Action

Constitution, 12 May 1972, 5MIA/01.
Constitution, 28 September 1968, 5MIA/01.
Correspondence Re. Membership/Mailing List, 'Mothers in Action'. 5MIA/05/01.
Minutes and Supporting Papers, 1971, 5MIA/02/01.
Papers Re. Margaret Deshmane Membership, 'to All London Members'. 5MIA/05/02.
Press Statement, 'The Future of Mothers in Action', 1 March 1972, 5MIA/02/02.

Working Association of Mothers (WAM)

'Help Yourselves, Mums of Harrow', *Harrow Observer*, 10 November 1970, 5WAM/8.
(n.d.). *Relief From Nappies and Baby Talk*, 5WAM/4.
Leman, G. (22 July 1969). Letter to Pat Brangwyn, 5WAM/7.
Leman, G. (3 August 1970). Letter to Diana Priestley, 5WAM/7.
Leman, G. (11 August 1970). Letter to Diana Priestley, 5WAM/7.

Let's Dispense with the GUILT. (Winter 1970–71). *Wam News*, 1, 5WAM/1.
Playspace in Richmond: A Study Initiated by WAM (Working Association of Mothers) and The Richmond Branch of AASE (Association for the Advancement of State Education). (July 1972), 5WAM/2.
Priestley, D. (14 May 1969). Letter to Grahame Leman, 5WAM/7.
Priestley, D. (1971). *Guidelines for Starting a WAM Group*, 5WAM/3.
Priestley, D. (8 October 1969). Letter to Grahame Leman, 5WAM/7.
Priestley, D. (2 May 1972). National Campaign for Nursery Education: Reflections on an Outing, 5WAM/4.
Report on The First Meeting of WAM Branches, 23 October 1971, 5WAM/3.
Source Unknown. (n.d.). *They All Came Out to Play*, 5WAM/8.
Wam News. (Summer 1970). 5WAM/1.
WAM Off to A Good Start. (1969). *Richmond Times*, 5WAM/8.

Association for Post-Natal Illness (APNI)

The Association for Post-Natal Illness Annual Report, 30 June 1990.
Thames Television, 'Time to Care', (ed.) Gerhardt, P. Thames Television, 1990.

Royal College of General Practitioners

Psychiatry and the General Practitioner Working Party, 1956–1958. ACE G12-1.
Research Committee of The Council, 11 June 1957. ACE G4-2.

Bodleian Library

'Women's Liberation, an Introduction' (1976). M91B638.

Theses

Brannen, J. M. (1990). *A Study of New Mothers and Employment: Social Constructions and Constraints* (Unpublished Doctoral Thesis). Institute of Education, University of London, London.
Coate, K. (1999). *The History of Women's Studies as an Academic Subject Area in Higher Education in the UK: 1970–1995* (Unpublished Doctoral Thesis). Institute of Education, University of London, London.
Currer, C. (1986) *Health Concepts and Illness Behaviour: The Case of Some Pathan Mothers in Britain* (Unpublished Doctoral Thesis). University of Warwick, Warwick.

Elston, M.A. (1986) *Women Doctors in the British Health Services: A Sociological Study of Their Careers and Opportunities* (Unpublished Doctoral Thesis). University of Leeds, Leeds.

Gavron, H. (1964). *The Position and Opportunities of Young Mothers – Progress or Retrogression (A Study of the Difficulties Confronting Young Mothers in the Contemporary Family Based on a Comparative Study of Working Class and Middle Class Families)* (Unpublished Doctoral Thesis). Bedford College, University of London, London.

Leachman, J. (1988). *A Longitudinal Study of Preparation for Childbirth, Pain in Labour and Postnatal Depression* (Unpublished Doctoral Thesis). University of Bath, Bath.

Nicholson, N. (1988). *The Social Psychology of "Post Natal Depression"* (Unpublished Doctoral Thesis). LSE, London.

Stewart, M. (1940). *Psychology in General Practice* (Unpublished Doctoral Thesis). University of Edinburgh, Edinburgh.

UK Data Service

Thompson, P. University of Essex, Department of Sociology: 'Interview with Ann Oakley' in 'Pioneers of Social Research, 1996–2018' 4th Edition, UK Data Service [Distributor], 2019-04-08, SN:6226. http://doi.org/10.5255/UKDA-SN-6226-6, https://discover.ukdataservice.ac.uk//Qualibank/Document/?Id=Q-99fb7d87-8c39-44e0-B209-2546d49b338d.

Thompson, P. University of Essex, Department of Sociology: 'Interview with Pat Caplan' in 'Pioneers of Social Research, 1996–2018' 4th Edition, UK Data Service [Distributor], 2019-04-08, SN:6226. http://doi.org/10.5255/UKDA-SN-6226-6, https://discover.ukdataservice.ac.uk//QualiBank/Document/?id=q-51c8f358-2ce1-4012-b00f-87ce4bbe5a50.

Wiggins, M. (2013). *Looking Back on Becoming a Mother: Longitudinal Perspectives on Maternity Care and the Transition to Motherhood* [Data Collection]. Colchester: Economic and Social Research Council. http://doi.org/10.5255/UKDA-SN-850818, Grant Reference ES/J006343/.

Published Sources

Newspapers

Aberdeen Evening Express
Aberdeen Press and Journal
Birmingham Daily Post
Bury Free Press

Coventry Standard
Daily Mirror
Daily Post: The Paper for Wales
Dundee Evening Telegraph
East Kilbride News
Eastbourne Herald Chronicle
Evening Standard
Hayes & Harlington Gazette
Huddersfield Daily Examiner
Kent Messenger
Kilmarnock Standard
Lichfield Mercury
Liverpool Echo
Lynn Advertiser
North Wales Weekly News
Northampton Herald & Post
Nottingham Evening Post and News
Reading Evening Post
Sandwell Evening Mail
Sheffield Independent
Solihull News
Staines & Ashford News
Sunday Mail
Sunday Mirror
Teddington and Hampton Times
The Daily Telegraph
The Glamorgan Gazette
The *Guardian*
The Scotsman
The Times
West Briton and Cornwall Advertiser
West Lothian Courier
Worthing Herald

Books and Articles

'A New Look for a New Decade', *Health Visitor*, December 1989, 62, 12, 357.
'A Psychiatrist's View', *Shrew*, 4, 2, 1972, 3.
'A to Z of Feminism', *Spare Rib*, 136, 1983, 29–30.
'Antenatal Care: Who Needs It?' *Health Visitor*, January 1988, 61, 1, 29.
'Child Benefit Frozen Again', *Health Visitor,* December 1989, 62, 12, 358.

'Childcare', in *Spare Rib Reader: 100 Issues of Women's Liberation*, Ed. Marsha Rowe (Middlesex, 1982), 105–28.
'Clinical Research in General Practice', *British Medical Journal,* 1, 3299, 1924, 550.
'Conference: TUC Women on the Alert', *Health Visitor,* May 1990, 63, 5, 151.
'Depression in General Practice', *British Medical Journal*, 2, 5469, 1965, 1052–53.
'Depression', *Medical Care*, 2, 4, 1964, 195–96.
'Drugs for Depression', *British Medical Journal*, 2, 5408, 1964, 522–23.
'Future Scope of General Practice. Medical Advisory Committee's Report', *British Medical Journal*, 2, 5361, 1963, 861–63.
'HEA Refuses to Publish Report Linking Unhealthy Diet to Poverty', *Health Visitor,* December 1989, 62, 12, 359.
'Health Visitors', *British Medical Journal*, 2, 3070, 1919, 572.
'Housing and Support Needs for Young Single Mothers', *Health Visitor,* November 1989, 62, 11, 326.
'HVA Slams White Paper Proposals', *Health Visitor*, May 1989, 62, 5, 141–42.
'Market Forces the Pace', *Health Visitor,* January 1990, 63, 1, 1.
'Medical Sociology and General Practice', *The Journal of The Royal College of General Practitioners,* 27, 178, 1977, 263.
'No Mothers Need Apply', *Spare Rib*, 95, June 1980, 12.
'Post Natal Depression: Does It Exist?' *Health Visitor*, May 1990, 63, 5, 154–55.
'Psychotherapy and the General Practitioner', *British Medical Journal*, 2, 4986, 1956, 235–36.
'Racism and Health Visiting', *Health Visitor,* October 1984, 57, 10, 291.
'Records in General Practice', *British Medical Journal,* 2, 5352, 1963, 309.
'Research in General Practice', *British Medical Journal*, 2, 4896, 1954, 1100–101.
'Shades of Opinion: Members' Thoughts on Merger Partners', *Health Visitor,* November 1989, 62, 11, 329–30.
'Suburban Neurosis Up to Date', *The Lancet*, 271, 7012, 1958, 146–47.
'Tackling Racism in the NHS', *Health Visitor,* December 1989, 62, 357.
'The Four Demands', in *Once a Feminist: Stories of a Generation,* Ed. Michelene Wandor (London, 1990), 242–43.
'The G.P. At The Crossroads', *British Medical Journal,* 1, 4655, 1950, 709–12.
'The Man Who Loved Children', *TIME Magazine*, 10 March 1998. Retrieved from https://time.com/archive/6732499/the-man-who-loved-children-dr-benjamin-spock-1903-1998/ [Accessed 19 September 2024].

'Towards the Health Centre', *British Medical Journal*, 2, 4732, 1951, 113–14.
'Unity Call in Fight against White Paper', *Health Visitor,* November 1989, 62, 11, 327.
'Use of Medical Records', *British Medical Journal,* 1, 4816, 1953, 941.
'What Mothers Think of You', *Health Visitor*, September 1988, 61, 9, 262.
'Women "Hit Hardest" by NHS Reform', *Health Visitor*, December 1989, 62, 12, 362.
Abel-Smith, Brian, *The National Health Service: The First Thirty Years* (London, 1978).
Abrams, Lynn, *Feminist Lives: Women, Feelings, & The Self in Post-War Britain* (Oxford, 2023).
———, 'Heroes of Their Own Life Stories: Narrating the Female Self in The Feminist Age', *Cultural and Social History*, 16, 2, 2019, 205–24.
———, 'The Self and Self-Help: Women Pursuing Autonomy in Post-War Britain', *Transactions of The Royal Historical Society*, 29, 2019, 201–21.
———, Fleming, Linda, Hazley, Barry, Wright, Valerie, and Kearns, Ade, 'Isolated and Dependent: Women and Children in High-Rise Social Housing in Post-War Glasgow', *Women's History Review,* 28, 5, 2019, 794–813.
Ackner, Brian, 'Imipramine and 'Reactive' Depression', *British Medical Journal*, 1, 5185, 1960, 1570.
Akester, Joyce M., and Macphail A.N., 'Health Visiting and General Practice', *The Lancet,* 284, 7356, 1964, 405–08.
Aldrich, C. Knight, 'Psychiatric Consultation in General Practice', *The Lancet* 285, 7389, 1965, 805–08.
Alibhai, Yasmin, 'Burning in The Cold', in *Balancing Acts: On Being a mother,* Ed. Katherine Gieve (London, 1989), 24–40.
Allen, Ann Taylor, *Feminism and Motherhood in Western Europe, 1890–1970: The Maternal Dilemma* (Basingstoke, 2005).
Allen, Sheila, and Barker, Diana Leonard (Eds), 'Sexual Divisions and Society', in *Sexual Divisions and Society: Process and Change* (London, 1976), 1–24.
Armitage, Phyllis, C., *Health Visiting: The New Profession* (London, 1927).
Arnold-Forster, Agnes, 'Ordinary People and the 1979 Royal Commission on The NHS', *Twentieth Century British History*, 34, 2, 2023, 275–98.
Backett, E.M., Shaw, L.A., and Evans, J.C.G., 'Studies of a General Practice (I) Patients' Needs and Doctors' Services: A Description of Method', *Proceedings of the Royal Society of Medicine*, 46, 9, 1953, 707–12.
Backhouse, Roger E., and Fontaine, Philippe (Eds), 'Introduction', in *A Historiography of the Modern Social Sciences* (Cambridge, 2014), 1–28.

Badinter, Elizabeth, *Mother Love: Myth and Reality: Motherhood in modern history* (New York, 1981).
Balint, Michael, 'Psychotherapy and The General Practitioner: I', *British Medical Journal*, 1, 5011, 1957, 156–58.
Ballard, Catherine, and Hackett, Hilary, 'My World Became the Size of the Baby', in *Spare Rib Reader: 100 Issues of Women's Liberation*, Ed. Marsha Rowe (Middlesex, 1982), 384–93.
Bardon, Desmond, 'Forewords', in Maggie Comport, *Towards Happy Motherhood: Understanding Postnatal Depression* (London, 1987), ix.
Bar-Haim, Shaul, "The Drug Doctor': Michael Balint and the Revival of General Practice in Postwar Britain', *History Workshop Journal*, 86, 2018, 114–32.
———, *The Maternalists: Psychoanalysts, Motherhood, and the British Welfare State* (Philadelphia, 2021).
Barrett, Michele, and Mcintosh, Mary, *The Anti-Social Family* (2nd ed.) (London, 1991 [1982]).
Battersby, Audrey, in *Once A Feminist: Stories of a Generation* (London, 1990), 113–20.
Beaumont, Caitríona, *Housewives and Citizens: Domesticity and the Women's Movement in England, 1928–64* (Manchester, 2013).
———, 'What *Do* Women Want? Housewives' Associations, Activism and Changing Representations of Women in the 1950s', *Women's History Review*, 26, 1, 2016, 147–62.
———, 'The "Housewife as Expert": Re-thinking the Experiential Expertise and Welfare Activism of Housewives' Associations in England, 1960-1980', in *Everyday Welfare in Modern British History: Experience, Expertise and Activism*, ed. Caitríona Beaumont, Eve Colpus and Ruth Davidson (Cham, 2024), 71-93
———, Colpus, Eve, and Davidson, Ruth, 'Introduction', in *Everyday Welfare in Modern British History: Experience, Expertise and Activism*, ed. Caitríona Beaumont, Eve Colpus and Ruth Davidson (Cham, 2024), 1-24.
Bell, Rita, 'Hailsham Mums' Newsline', *Health Visitor*, February 1989, 62, 2, 59–60.
Belsize Lane Women's Group, 'Nine Years Together', in *Spare Rib Reader: 100 Issues of Women's Liberation*, Ed. Marsha Rowe (Middlesex, 1982), 561–75.
Bentil, Jade, 'We Were Fire-Fighting Against Thatcher and The System She Was Putting Forward': The Black Women's Movement and the Boundaries of Nationhood in Thatcher's Britain', in *Resist Organize Build: Feminist and Queer Activism in Britain and The United States*

During The Long 1980s, Ed. Sarah Crook and Charlie Jeffries (New York, 2022), 75–116.
Berridge, V.A., Christie, D.A., and Tansey, E.M. (Eds), 'Public Health in the 1980s and 1990s: Decline and Rise', in *Wellcome Witnesses to Twentieth Century Medicine*, Vol. 26 (London: Wellcome Trust Centre for the History of Medicine at UCL, 2006), 20–21.
Berry, Liz, 'The Republic of Motherhood', *The Republic of Motherhood* (London, 2018), 1–2.
Betti, Claire, 'Letters Forum', *Spare Rib*, 71, 1978, 36.
Beverley Bryan, Dadzie, Stella, and Scafe, Suzanne, 'The Heart of the Race: Black Women's Lives in Britain', in *Black British Feminism, a Reader*, Ed. Heidi Safia Mirza (London and New York, 1997), 42–44.
Billingham, Kate, Jane, Morrell, and Clive, Billingham, 'Reflections on The History of Health Visiting', *British Journal of Community Health Nursing*, 1, 7, 1996, 386–92.
Bivins, Roberta, *Contagious Communities: Medicine, Migration, and The NHS in Post War Britain* (Oxford, 2015).
———, and Thomson, Mathew, 'Anniversary fever? History and the culture of NHS celebration', *Modern British History*, 36, 1, 2025, hwae066, https://doi.org/10.1093/tcbh/hwae066.
Bodkin, N.J., et al. 'The General Practitioner and the Psychiatrist: A Study in Co-operation', *British Medical Journal*, 2, 4838, 1953, 723–25.
Borkman, Thomasina, 'Experiential Knowledge: A New Concept for the Analysis of Self-Help Groups', *Social Service Review*, 50, 3, 1976, 445–56.
Borsay, Anne, and Hunter, Billie (Eds), *Nursing and Midwifery in Britain since 1700* (Basingstoke, 2012).
Bourke, Joanna, 'Becoming the 'Natural' Mother in Britain and North America: Power, Emotions and the Labour of Childbirth Between 1947 and 1967', *Past & Present*, 246, suppl. 15, 2020, 92–114.
Bowlby, John, *Care Child and The Growth of Love*. 2nd ed. (Harmondsworth, 1973 [1953]).
———, *Maternal Care and Mental Health* (Geneva, 1951).
Boyd, Catherine, and Sellers, Lea, *The British Way of Birth* (London, 1982).
Breen, Dana, *The Birth of a First Child: Towards an Understanding of Femininity* (London, 1975).
Brennan, Rose, 'You've Come a Long Way', in *'68, '78, '88: From Women's Liberation to Feminism*, Ed. Amanda Sebestyen (Dorset, 1988), 240–43.
Briscoe, Monica, 'The Detection of Emotional Disorders in the Post Natal Period by Health Visitors', *Health Visitor*, November 1989, 62, 2, 336–37.

Briscoe, Monica, and Lindley, Penny, 'Identification and Management of Psychosocial Problems by Health Visitors', *Health Visitor*, 55, 4, 1982, 165–69.

——, et al. 'Long Term Social Work in A Primary Health Care Setting', *The British Journal of Social Work*, 13, 5, 1983, 559–78.

Bristol Women's Studies Group, *Half the Sky: An Introduction to Women's Studies* (London, 1979).

Bristol Women's Therapy Centre, 'Talking with Women in Bristol', *Spare Rib* 102, 1981, 6–8.

Brockington, Ian, 'Preface', in *Motherhood and Mental Illness*, Eds R. Kumar and I. Brockington (London, 1982).

Brown, George W., and Harris, Tirril, *Social Origins of Depression: A Study of Psychiatric Disorder in Women* (London, 1989 [1978]).

Browne, Sarah, *The Women's Liberation Movement in Scotland* (Manchester, 2014).

Bruley, Sue, 'Consciousness-Raising in Clapham: Women's Liberation as 'Lived Experience' in South London in the 1970s', *Women's History Review*, 22, 5, 2013, 717–38.

——, "It Didn't Just Come Out of Nowhere Did It?': The Origins of the Women's Liberation Movement in 1960s Britain', *Oral History*, 45, 1, 2017, 67–78.

Bryan, Beverley, Dadzie, Stella, and Scafe, Suzanne, *Heart of the Race: Black Women's Lives in Britain* (London, 1985).

Bryder, Linda, 'Mobilising Mothers: The 1917 National Baby Week', *Medical History* 63, 1, 2019, 2–23.

Busfield, Joan, *Men, Women and Madness: Understanding Gender and Mental Disorder* (Basingstoke, 1996).

Butler, Lise, 'The Social Scientific Turn in Modern British History', *Twentieth Century British History*, 33, 3, 2022, 445–50.

Butler, Lise, and Young, Michael, *Social Science, and the British Left, 1945-1970* (Oxford, 2020).

Cain, Ruth, 'A View You Won't Get Anywhere Else'? Depressed Mothers, Public Regulation and 'Private' Narrative', *Feminist Legal Studies* 17, 2009, 123–43.

Carby, Hazel V., 'White Women Listen! Black Feminism and the Boundaries of Sisterhood', in *The Empire Strikes Back: Race and Racism in 70s Britain* (London: Centre for Contemporary Cultural Studies, 1986 [1982]), 212–35.

Carstairs, G.M., 'Incidence of Psychiatric Cases in General Practice', *Edinburgh Medical Journal*, 58, 2, 1951, 72–81.

Celia, Rachel, 'Valuing and Validating Feelings', in *Radical Midwifery: Celebrating 21 Years of A.R.M.*, Ed. Margaret Jowitt and Ishbel Kargar

(Lancashire: Association of Radical Midwives, 1997 [Summer 1982]), 120–24, 120–22.

Charlton, Val, in *Once a Feminist: Stories of a Generation* (London, 1990), 160–70.

Charlton, Valerie, and Muir, Annette, 'Birthpangs', in *Women's Health: A Spare Rib Reader*, Ed. Sue O'Sullivan (London, 1987), 304–15. [Originally published in *Spare Rib* 36, June 1975].

Charman, Helen, *Mother State: A Political History of Motherhood* (London, 2024).

Chettiar, Teri, 'Democratizing Mental Health: Motherhood, Therapeutic Community and the Emergence of the Psychiatric Family at the Cassel Hospital in Post-Second World War Britain', *History of The Human Sciences*, 25, 5, 2012, 107–22.

———, "More than a Contract': The Emergence of a State-Supported Marriage Welfare Service and the Politics of Emotional Life in Post-1945 Britain', *Journal of British Studies*, 55, 3, 2016, 566–91.

———, *The Intimate State: How Emotional Life Became Political in Welfare-State Britain* (New York, 2023).

Clapson, Mark, *Invincible Green Suburbs, Brave New Towns: Social Change and Urban Dispersal in Postwar England* (Manchester, 1998).

Clark, Helen, and Carnegie, Elizabeth, *She Was Aye Workin': Memories of Tenement Women in Edinburgh and Glasgow* (Oxford, 2006).

Clark, June, 'Mothers' Perceptions of Health Visiting', *Health Visitor*, September 1984, 57, 9, 265–68.

Clayton, Thomas, and Gordon, John, 'Psychosis After Childbirth: Ecological Aspects of a Single Impact Stress', *American Journal of The Medical Sciences*, 238, 1959, 363–88.

Collings, J.S., 'General Practice in England Today: A Reconnaissance', *The Lancet*, 255, 6604, 555.

Colpus, Eve, *Female Philanthropy in the Interwar World: Between Self and Other* (London, 2018).

Comer, Lee, *Wedlocked Women* (Leeds, 1974).

———, 'From 1969', in *'68, '78, '88: From Women's Liberation to Feminism*, Ed. Amanda Sebestyen (Dorset, 1988), 84–89.

Comport, Maggie, *Towards Happy Motherhood: Understanding Postnatal Depression* (London, 1987).

Conrad, Peter, 'Medicalization and Social Control', *Annual Review of Sociology*, 18, 1992, 209–32.

Cooper, Fred, 'Loneliness as Crisis in Britain After 1950: Temporality, Modernity, and the Historical Gaze', in *The Routledge History of Loneliness*, Eds Katie Barclay, Elaine Chalus, and Deborah Simonton (London, 2023), Chapter 11.

Coote, Anna, and Campbell, Beatrix, *Sweet Freedom: The Struggle for Women's Liberation* (London, 1982).
Cornwall, Jocelyn, *Hard-Earned Lives: Accounts of Health and Illness from East London* (London, 1984).
Council for the Education and Training of Health Visitors, *An Investigation into the Principles of Health Visiting* (London, [1980], 1982).
Cowan, David, "Modern' Parenting and the Uses of Childcare Advice in Post-War England', *Social History*, 43, 3, 2018, 332–55.
Cowley, Sue, 'Thatcher's Nurseries: Expansion or Containment?', *Red Rag*, 4, 1973, 3–5.
Cox, John, and Holden, J., *A Guide to The Edinburgh Postnatal Depression Scale* (London, 2003).
———, Holden, J., and Sagovsky, Ruth, 'Detection of Post-Natal Depression: Development of the Ten Item Edinburgh Postnatal Depression Scale', *British Journal of Psychiatry,* 150, 1987, 782–86.
———, and Wisner, Katherine, 'Recollections on the Early Days of the Marcé Society for Perinatal Mental Health from Professor John Cox', *Archives of Women's Mental Health,* 19, 1, 2016, 197–200.
———, 'Thirty Years with The Edinburgh Postnatal Depression Scale: Voices from the Past and Recommendations for the Future', *The British Journal of Psychiatry*, 214, 3, 2019, 127–29.
Crane, Jennifer, *Child Protection in England: Expertise, Experience, and Emotion* (Basingstoke, 2018).
———, "Save Our NHS': Activism, Information-Based Expertise and the 'New Times' of the 1980s', *Contemporary British History,* 33, 1, 2019, 52–74.
Creed, Fabiola, 'Nemone Lethbridge's Play Baby Blues on BBC Television: Maternal Mental Illness Narratives, Stigma and Support in 1970s Britain', *Women's History Review*, 34, 2024, 1–25.
Cronk, Mary, 'Foreword', in *Radical Midwifery: Celebrating 21 Years of A.R.M.*, Ed. Margaret Jowitt and Ishbel Kargar (Lancashire, 1997), 8–11.
Crook, Sarah, 'The Women's Liberation Movement, Activism and Therapy at the Grassroots, 1968–1985', *Women's History Review*, 27, 7, 2018, 1152–68.
———, 'Writing About Mothering and Childcare in the British Women's Liberation Movement, 1970–85', in *Women's Periodicals and Print Culture in Britain, 1940s-2000s,* Eds Laurel Forster and Joanne Hollows (Edinburgh, 2020), 351–65.
Cross, Gwenith Siobhan, '"A Midwife at Every Confinement": Midwifery and Medicalized Childbirth in Ontario and Britain, 1920–1950', *Canadian Bulletin of Medical History*, v31, 2, 2014, 139–59.

Curtice, Lisa, 'Talking About How Difficult We Find It', *Health Visitor*, 62, 11, November 1989, 343.

Cusk, Rachel, *A Life's Work: On Becoming a Mother* (London, [2001] 2008).

——, 'I Was Only Being Honest', *The Guardian*, 21 March 2008. Retrieved from https://theguardian.com/books/2008/mar/21/biography.women [accessed 5 March 2025].

D'Cruze, Shani, 'Women and the Family', in *Women's History: Britain, 1850-1945* Ed. June Purvis (London: 1998), 51-83.

Dally, Ann, *Inventing Motherhood: The Consequences of an Ideal* (London, 1982).

Dalton, Katharina, *Depression After Childbirth: How to Recognise and Treat Postnatal Illness* (Oxford, [1980] 1989).

Daniells, N.C., 'Meeting the Challenge of Change', *Royal Society of Health Journal*, 80, 4, 1960, 356–59.

Davidson, Ruth, 'Working-Class Women Activists: Citizenship at the Local Level', in *Alternatives to State-Socialism in Britain: Other Worlds of Labour in the Twentieth Century*, Eds Peter Ackers and Alastair Reid (Basingstoke, 2016), 93–121.

Davies, Celia, 'General Practitioners and the Pull of Prevention', *Sociology of Health & Illness*, 6, 1984, 267–89.

——, 'The Health Visitor as Mother's Friend: A Woman's Place in Public Health, 1900–14', *Social History of Medicine*, 1, 1, 1988, 39–59.

Davies, Margaret Llewelyn, *Maternity: Letters From Working Women* (London, 1978 [1915]).

Davies, Pauline, *Trapped: Unmarried West Indian Mothers in Handsworth*. Papers on Community & Youth Work, No. 2. Department of Community and Youth Work, Westhill College (Selly Oak, Birmingham, 1983).

Davis, Angela, 'Choice, Policy and Practice in Maternity Care since 1948', *History & Policy*, 30 May 2013. Retrieved from https://www.historyandpolicy.org/policy-papers/papers/choice-policy-and-practice-in-maternity-care-since-1948 [Accessed 6 August 2024].

——, *Modern Motherhood: Women and Family in England, 1945–2000* (Manchester, 2012).

——, 'Wartime Women Giving Birth: Narratives of Pregnancy and Childbirth, Britain c. 1939–1960', *Studies in History and Philosophy of Science Part C: Studies in History and Philosophy of Biological and Biomedical Sciences*, 47, B, 2014, 257–66.

——, 'Women's Experiences of the Maternity Services in Berkshire and Oxfordshire, c. 1970–1990', in *Western Maternity and Medicine, 1880-1990*, Eds Janet Greenlees and Linda Bryder (London, 2013), 129–46.

———, 'Childminders and the Limits of Mothering as Experiential Expertise, England c.1948-2000', in *Everyday Welfare in Modern British History: Experience, Expertise and Activism*, Eds Caitríona Beaumont, Eve Colpus, and Ruth Davidson (Cham, 2024), 95-116.
Delamont, Sara, *Feminist Sociology* (London, 2003).
Delap, Lucy, 'Feminist Bookshops, Reading Cultures and the Women's Liberation Movement in Great Britain, c. 1974–2000', *History Workshop Journal*, 81, 2016, 171–96.
Digby, Anne, *The Evolution of British General Practice, 1850–1948* (Oxford, 1999).
Dingwall, Robert, 'Collectivism, Regionalism and Feminism: Health Visiting and British Social Policy 1850–1975', *Journal of Social Policy*, 6, 3, 1977, 291–315.
———, Rafferty, Anne Marie, and Webster, Charles (Eds), *An Introduction to The Social History of Nursing* (London, 1988).
Douglas, G., 'Psychotic Mothers', *The Lancet*, 267, 6908, 1956, 124–25.
Douglas, J.W.B., and Blomfield, J.M. *Children Under Five* (London, 1958).
Draper, J., Field, S., and Thomas, H., *The Early Parenthood Project: An Evaluation of a Community Antenatal Clinic* (Cambridge, 1984).
Drennan, Vari (Ed.), 'Changing Health Visiting Practice', in *Health Visitors and Groups: Politics and Practice* (Oxford, 1988), 1–30.
Dunn, Judy, 'Unhappy Mothers', *London Review of Books*, 2, 14, 17 July 1980. Retrieved from https://www.lrb.co.uk/the-paper/v02/n14/judy-dunn/unhappy-mothers [Accessed 25 September 2024].
Dyhouse, Carol, 'Good Wives and Little Mothers: Social Anxieties and the Schoolgirl's Curriculum, 1890–1920', *Oxford Review of Education*, 3, 1, 1977, 21–35, 27.
———, *Students: A Gendered History* (Abingdon, 2006).
———, 'Working-Class Mothers and Infant Mortality in England, 1895–1914', *Journal of Social History*, 12, 2, 1978, 248–67.
Eddy, John, and Owen, John, *Obstetrics and Gynaecology in General Practice* (London, 1987).
Editorial, 'As Others See Us', *Health Visitor*, 55, 6, 1982, 265.
Editorial, 'A New Look for a New Decade', *Health Visitor*, 62, 1989, 357.
Editorial, 'The Politics of Poverty', *Health Visitor*, 56, 3, 1983, 81.
Editorial, 'Professional Practice in Perspective', *Health Visitor*, 57, 10, 1984, 289.
Editorial, *Shrew*, 4, 2, 1972, 1–2.
Editorial, 'Tackling Racism in the NHS', *Health Visitor*, 1989, 62, 357.
Eichenbaum, Luise, and Orbach, Susie, 'Separation and Intimacy: Crucial Practice Issues in Working with Women in Therapy', in *Living With The*

Sphinx: Papers from the Women's Therapy Centre, Eds Sheila Ernst and Marie Maguire (London, 1987), 49–67.

———, and Orbach, Susie, *Understanding Women* (Middlesex, 1985).

Elston, Mary Ann, 'Medicine: Half Our Future Doctors?', in *Careers of Professional Women,* Eds Rosalie Silverstone and Audrey Ward (London, 2022 [1980]), 99–139.

Emecheta, Buchi, *Second-Class Citizen* (London, 2021 [1974]).

Enright, Anne, 'Diary: Lessons from Angela Carter', *London Review of Books*, 33, 4, 17 February 2011. Retrieved from https://www.lrb.co.uk/the-paper/v33/n04/anne-enright/diary [Accessed 17 September 2024].

Ernst, Sheila, and Maguire, Marie, 'Introduction', in *Living with the Sphinx: Papers From the Women's Therapy Centre* (London, 1987), 1-29.

Eve, Enid (Ed.), 'Introduction', in *Manual for Health Visitors and Infant Welfare Workers* (New York, 1921), 1–16.

Faludi, Susan, *Backlash: The Undeclared War Against American Women* (New York, 1991).

Fell, Alison, 'Everyday Offensives: Notes on Ideology', *Red Rag*, 6, 1973, 18.

——— (Ed.), 'Introduction', in *Hard Feelings: Fiction and Poetry from Spare Rib* (London, 1979), 1–6.

———, 'Rebel with a Cause', in *Truth, Dare or Promise: Girls Growing Up in the 50s,* Ed. Liz Heron (London, 1985), 11–25.

Field, Susan, et al. 'The Health Visitor's View of Consumer Criticisms', *Health Visitor,* 57, 9, September 1984, 272–73.

Finch, Janet, 'It's Great Having Someone to Talk to: The Ethics and Politics of Interviewing Women', in *Social Researching: Politics, Problems, Practice,* Eds Colin Bell and Helen Roberts (London, 1984), 70–87.

Fleury, P.M., *Maternity Care: Mothers' Experiences of Childbirth* (London, 1967).

Flint, Caroline, 'On the Brink: Midwifery in Britain', in *The Midwife Challenge,* Ed. Sheila Kitzinger (London, 1988), 22–41, 35.

Forman, J.A.S., and Fairbairn, E.M., *Social Casework in General Practice: A Report on an Experiment in a General Practice* (London, 1968).

Forster, Laurel, 'Spreading the Word: Feminist Print Cultures and the Women's Liberation Movement', *Women's History Review*, 25, 5, 2016, 812–31.

Foster, Marie-Claude, 'Health Visitors' Perspectives on Working in a Multiethnic Society', *Health Visitor*, 61, 9, September 1988, 275–78.

Francis, G.M., 'The Health Visitor of the Future', *Royal Society of Health Journal*, 80, 4, 1960, 354–56.

Franklin, L.M., 'An Appraisal of Psychiatry in General Practice', *British Medical Journal,* 2: 5196, 1960, 451–53.
Fraser, Robin C., 'Research Methods in General Practice: A Report on a Course at the College', *Journal of The Royal College of General Practitioners,* 17, 83, 1969, 385–87.
Freely, Maureen, 'Keeping Mum', *Everywoman,* November 1995, 10–12.
Friedan, Betty, *The Feminine Mystique* (New York, 1963).
———, *The Second Stage* (Boston, MA, 1998 [1981]).
Fry, John, Dillane, J.B., Connolly, M.M., and Kuenssberg, E.V., 'Health Visiting and General Practice', *The Lancet,* 284, 7358, 1964, 526–27.
Galloway, J.F., 'Integration of Maternity Services', *The Lancet,* 279, 7242, 1962, 1287–89.
Gavron, Hannah, *The Captive Wife* (London, 1976 [1966]).
Gavron, Jeremy, *A Woman on the Edge of Time* (London, 2016).
Gayle, Marilyn, 'Sex Doesn't Fit, Race Doesn't Fit', in *'68, '78, '88: From Women's Liberation to Feminism,* Ed. Amanda Sebestyen (Dorset, 1988), 116–25.
Gebbie, Nicolas, 'The Woman Health Officer', *Health Education Journal,* 4, 1, 1946, 27–32.
Gieve, Katherine (Ed.), 'And Not to Count the Cost', in *Balancing Acts: On Being a Mother* (London, 1989), 41–51.
Giles, Judy, 'Help for Housewives: Domestic Service and the Reconstruction of Domesticity in Britain, 1940–50', *Women's History Review,* 10, 2, 2001, 299–324.
Godber, George, 'The Effect of Specialisation on Maternity Services', *The Lancet,* 281, 7290, 1963, 1061–66.
Goldberg, D.P., *The Detection of Psychiatric Illness by Questionnaire: A Technique for the Identification and Assessment of Non-Psychotic Psychiatric Illness* (Oxford, 1972).
Goodwin, Shirley, 'Practising Prevention: The Health Visitor and prevention', *British Medical Journal (Clinical Research Edition),* 285, 6336, 1982, 181–84.
Gordon, Tuula, *Feminist Mothers* (Hampshire, 1990).
Gough, Ian, 'Thatcherism and the Welfare State', in *The Politics of Thatcherism,* Eds Stuart Hall and Martin Jacques (London, 1983), 148–68.
Gould, Julius, 'The Power of Politics', in *Penguin Social Sciences Survey 1968,* Ed. J. Gould (Middlesex, 1968), 9–10.
Graham, Hilary, and McKee, Lorna, *The First Months of Motherhood: Summary Report of a Survey of Women's Experiences of Pregnancy, Childbirth, and the First Six Months After Birth* (London, 1980).

———, and Oakley, Ann, 'Competing Ideologies of Reproduction: Medical and Maternal Perspectives on Pregnancy', in *Concepts of Health, Illness and Disease: A Comparative Perspective*, Eds Caroline Currer and Meg Stacey (London, 1986), 99–115.

———, 'Coping: Or How Mothers Are Seen and Not Heard', in *On the Problem of Men*, Eds Scarlet Friedman and Elizabeth Sarah (London, 1982), 101–16.

———, *Hardship and Health in Women's Lives* (Hertfordshire, 1993).

———, 'Mothers' Accounts of Anger and Aggression Towards their Babies', in *Psychological Approaches to Child Abuse*, Ed. N. Frude (London, 1980), 39–51.

———, 'Prevention and Health: Every Mother's Business, A Comment on Child Health Policies in the 1970s', in *Sociology of the Family: New Directions for Britain*, Ed. Chris Harris. Sociological Monograph No. 28 (Keele, 1979), 160–85.

———, 'Surveying Through Stories', in *Social Researching: Politics, Problems, Practice,* Eds C. Bell and H. Roberts (London, Boston, MA, Melbourne, and Henley, 1984), 104–24.

Gray, Denis Pereira, 'History of The Royal College of General Practitioners – The First 40 Years', *British Journal of General Practice*, 42, 354, 1992, 29–35.

———, *Forty Years On: The Story of the First 40 Years of The Royal College of General Practitioners* (London, 1992).

Greig, Anne, 'I Am a Mum…', *Health Visitor,* 57, 9, 1984, 268.

Grey, Daniel, 'Women's Policy Networks and The Infanticide Act 1922', *Twentieth Century British History,* 21, 4, 2010, 441–63.

Gupta, Rahila, 'Giving Birth Again', in *Balancing Acts: On Being a Mother,* Ed. Katherine Gieve (London, 1989), 94–106.

Gurr, Myra, and Hansen, Anne, 'NEWPIN: An Opportunity for Positive Change', *Psychiatric Bulletin*, 21, 8, 1997, 480–82.

Hadfield, Stephen, 'A Field Survey of General Practice, 1951–2', *British Medical Journal*, 2, 683, 1953, 684–706.

Haggett, Ali, *Desperate Housewives, Neuroses and the Domestic Environment, 1945–1970* (Abingdon, 2016 [2012]).

———, *A History of Male Psychological Disorders in Britain, 1945-1980* (Basingstoke, 2015).

Halsey, A.H., *A History of Sociology in Britain: Science, Literature and Society* (Oxford, 2004).

Hamilton, James Alexander, *Postpartum Psychiatric Problems* (St. Louis, MO, 1962).

Hardie, Victoria, 'The World Became a More Dangerous Place', in *Balancing Acts: On Being a Mother,* Ed. Katherine Gieve (London, 1989), 52–72.

Hardyment, Christina, *Dream Babies: Child Care from Locke to Spock* (Oxford, 1984).
Harne, Lynne, 'From 1971: Reinventing the Wheel', in *'68, '78, '88: From Women's Liberation to Feminism,* Ed. Amanda Sebestyen (Dorset, 1988), 63–71.
Harris, Cindy, and Scruggs, Marianne, 'Castor Oil, Epidurals and Home Births', in *Women's Health: A Spare Rib Reader,* Ed. Sue O'Sullivan (London, 1987), 316–17. [Originally published in *Spare Rib,* 38, August 1975.]
Hatch, Stephen, and Hinton, Teresa, *Self-Help in Practice* (Sheffield: Joint Unit for Social Services Research, Sheffield University, 1986).
Hayward, Rhodri, 'Desperate Housewives and Model Amoebae: The Invention of Suburban Neurosis in Inter-War Britain', in *Health and the Modern Home,* Ed. Mark Jackson (London, 2007), 42–62.
——, 'Sadness in Camberwell: Imagining Stress and Constructing History in Post-War Britain', in *Stress, Trauma and Adaptation in the Twentieth Century,* Eds David Cantor and Edmund Ramsden (Rochester, NY, 2014), 320–41.
——, *The Transformation of the Psyche in British Primary Care, 1870–1970* (London, 2015).
Hegarty, A.B., 'Post-Puerperal Recurrent Depression', *British Medical Journal,* 1, 4914, 1955, 637–40.
Heggie, Vanessa, 'Health Visiting and District Nursing in Victorian Manchester; Divergent and Convergent Vocations', *Women's History Review,* 20, 3, 2011, 403–22.
Hendrick, Harry, *Child Welfare: England 1872–1989* (London and New York, 1994).
——, *Children, Childhood and English Society, 1880–1990* (Cambridge, 1997).
Henley, Alix, *Asian Patients in Hospital and at Home* (Kent, 1979).
Hennessy, Deborah, 'Parent Support Groups', *Nursing: The Add-on Journal of Clinical Nursing,* 2, 19, 1983, 552–54.
Heron, Liz (Ed.), 'Introduction', in *Truth, Dare or Promise: Girls Growing Up in the 50s* (London, 1985), 1–9.
——, 'The Mystique of Motherhood', in *No Turning Back: Writings from the Women's Liberation Movement 1975–80,* Ed. Feminist Anthology Collective (London, 1981), 138–40.
Hobsbawm, Marlene, in *Once a Feminist: Stories of a Generation* (London, 1990), 121–25.
Hoggart, Richard, *The Uses of Literacy: Aspects of Working-Class Life* (London, 1957).
——, 'The Welfare State Appearance and Reality', *Social Work,* 17, 1, 1960, 13–17.

Holden, Katherine, 'Family, Caring and Unpaid Work', in *Women in Twentieth-Century Britain*, ed. Ina Zweiniger-Bargielowska (Essex, 2001), 134–48.

Holden, Jenifer, Sagovsky, Ruth, and Cox, John, 'Counselling in a General Practice Setting: Controlled Study of Health Visitor Intervention in Treatment of Postnatal Depression', *British Medical Journal*, 298, 6668, 1989, 223–26.

Holden, Jenifer, Sagovsky, Ruth, and Cox, John, 'Health Visitors and Postnatal Depression [with Reply]', *British Medical Journal*, 298, 6676, 1989, 831.

Horder, J., et al., 'The Management of Stress Disorders in General Practice', *Practitioner*, 177, 1956, 729–43.

Howells, J.G., 'Neurosis in the Ordinary Family [Review]', *Health Education Journal*, 27, 2, 1968, 105.

Huang, Marie R., 'Issues in General Practitioner Authority in The National Health Service', in *The Sociology of the NHS*, Ed. Margaret Stacey. Monograph 22 (Keele, 1976), 23–42.

Hubback, Judith, *Wives Who Went to College* (London, 1957).

Hughes, Martin, et al., *Nurseries Now: A Fair Deal for Parents and Children* (Harmondsworth, 1980).

Hunt, John H., 'General Practice in the World Today and its Academic Needs', *The Lancet*, 284, 7349, 1964, 29–32.

———, 'The Renaissance of General Practice', *British Medical Journal*, 1, 5027, 1957, 1075–82.

Illingworth, Cynthia, 'The Emotional State of Mothers in the First Three Months After the Birth of a Baby', *Health Visitor*, 62, 2, November 1989, 340–42.

Jackson, Sue, 'Networking Women: A History of Ideas, Issues and Developments in Women's Studies in Britain', *Women's Studies International Forum*, 23, 2000, 1–11.

Jackson, Mark (Ed.), 'Stress in Post-War Britain: An Introduction', in *Stress in Post-War Britain, 1945–85* (New York, 2015), 1–15.

Jeffreys, Sheila, 'Against Therapy', in *Women's Health: A Spare Rib Reader*, Ed. Sue O'Sullivan (London, 1987), 142–45.

Jephcott, Pearl, *Married Women Working* (London, 1962).

Johnson, D.A.W., 'A Study of the Use of Antidepressant Medication in General Practice', *The British Journal of Psychiatry*, 125, 2, 1974, 186–92.

Jolly, Margaretta, *Sisterhood and After: An Oral History of the UK Women's Liberation Movement, 1968–Present* (Oxford, 2019).

Jones, Roger, and Fitton, Peter, 'General Practice Research: Deaths and Entrances', *British Journal of General Practice*, 48, 426, 1998, 873.

Jones, Lucy, *Matrescence: On the Metamorphosis of Pregnancy, Childbirth and Motherhood* (London, 2023).
Jordanova, L.J., 'Mental Illness, Mental Health: Changing Norms and Expectations', in *Women in Society: Interdisciplinary Essays*, Ed. Cambridge Women's Studies Group (London, 1981), 95–114.
Kagan, G., 'Psychoneuroses in General Practice', *Practitioner*, 182, 1090, 1959, 489–500.
Kedward, H.B., and Cooper, Brian, 'Neurotic Disorders in Urban Practice: A Three Year Follow-ip', *Journal of The College of General Practitioners*, 12, 1966, 148.
Kellner, Robert, 'Neurotic Symptoms in Women: Attendances in a General Practice', *British Journal of Psychiatry*, 112, 1966, 75–77.
Kelsey, Amanda, 'The Making of Health Visitors: An Historical Perspective, Part I', *International History of Nursing Journal*, 5, 3, 2000, 44–50.
———, 'The Making of Health Visitors: An Historical Perspective, Part II', *International History of Nursing Journal*, 6, 2, 2001, 66–70.
Kempe, Margery, *The Book of Margery Kempe*, Ed. B.A. Windeatt (London, 2005).
Kern, Leslie, *Feminist City: Claiming Space in a Man-Made World* (London, 2020).
Kessel, Neil, 'Who Ought to See a Psychiatrist?', *The Lancet*, 281, 7290, 1963, 1092–95.
King, Laura, 'Future Citizens: Cultural and Political Conceptions of Children in Britain, 1930s-1950s', *Twentieth Century British History*, 27, 3, 2016, 389–411.
Kirby, Jill, *Feeling the Strain: A Cultural History of Stress in Twentieth-Century Britain* (Manchester, 2019).
Kitzinger, Sheila, *A Passion for Birth* (London, 2015).
———, *The Experience of Childbirth*. 4th Ed. (London, 1978 [1962]).
———, *The Experience of Childbirth*. 5th Ed. (Middlesex, 1986).
———, 'Women's Experiences of Birth at Home', in *The Place of Birth*, Eds Sheila Kitzinger and John Davis (Oxford, 1978), 135–56.
———, *Women as Mothers* (Glasgow, 1978).
Kitzinger, Jenny, 'Strategies of the Early Childbirth Movement: A Case-Study of the National Childbirth Trust', in *The Politics of Maternity: Services for Childbearing Women in Twentieth-Century Britain*, Eds Jo Garcia, Robert Kilpatrick, and Martin Richards (Oxford, 1990), 92–115.
Klein, Rudolf, *The New Politics of the NHS: From Creation to Reinvention* (London, 2013).
Knott, Sarah, 'Theorizing and Historicizing Mothering's Many Labours', *Past & Present*, 246, Suppl. 15, 2020, 1–24.

———, *Mother Is a Verb: An Unconventional History* (New York, 2019).
Kreitman, Norman, KI. Pearce, and Ryle, Anthony, 'The Relationship of Psychiatric, Psychosomatic and Organic Illness in a General Practice', *The British Journal of Psychiatry*, 112: 487, 1966, 569–79.
Kumar, R., 'Neurotic Disorders in Childbearing Women', in *Motherhood and Mental Illness*, Eds R. Kumar and Ian Brockington (London, 1982), 71–118.
Lambert, Caitlin, "The Objectionable Injectable': Recovering the Lost History of the WLM Through the Campaign Against Depo-Provera', *Women's History Review*, 29, 3, 2019, 520–39.
Langhamer, Claire, 'Love, Selfhood and Authenticity in Post-War Britain', *Cultural and Social History*, 9, 2, 2012, 277–97.
———, *The English in Love: The Intimate Story of an Emotional Revolution* (Oxford, 2013).
———, 'The Meanings of Home in Postwar Britain', *Journal of Contemporary History*, 40, 2, 2005, 341–62.
———, 'Who the Hell Are Ordinary People?' Ordinariness as a Category of Historical Analysis', *Transactions of The Royal Historical Society*, 28, 2018, 175–95.
Laslett, Peter, 'Mothering', *London Review of Books*, 3, 14, 6 August 1981. Retrieved from https://www.lrb.co.uk/the-paper/v03/n14/peter-laslett/mothering [Accessed 20 September 2024].
Lawrence, Jon, *Me Me Me? The Search for Community in Post-War England* (Oxford, 2019).
———, "'Inventing The 'Traditional Working Class': A Re-Analysis of Interview Notes from Young and Willmott's *Family and Kinship in East London*', *The Historical Journal*, 59, 2, 2016, 567–93.
Lawton Tonge, W., et al., 'Prevalence of Neurosis in Women', *British Journal of Preventive and Social Medicine*, 15, 4, 1961, 177–79.
Lee, Ellie, *Abortion, Motherhood, and Mental Health: Medicalising Reproduction in the United States and Great Britain* (New York, 2003).
Leeds Revolutionary Feminist Group, 'Every Single Academic Feminist Owes Her Livelihood to the WLM', WRRC Summer School, Bradford, 1979.
Lethbridge, Nemone, 'News: Postscript to Baby Blues', *Spare Rib*, 21, 1974, 17.
Lewis, Aubrey, 'Foreword', in *Psychiatric Illness in General Practice*. 2nd Ed. Eds Michael Shepherd, Brian Cooper, Alexander C. Brown, and Graham Kalton (Oxford, 1981 [1966]), v–vi.
Lewis, Jane, 'Anxieties About the Family and the Relationships Between Parents, Children and the State in Twentieth-Century England',

in *Children of Social Worlds*, Eds Martin Richards and Paul Light (Cambridge, 1988), 31–54.

———, 'Introduction', in *The Goals of Social Policy: Conference Papers*, Eds Martin Bulmer, Jane Lewis, and David Piachaud (London, 1989), 131–40.

———, 'The Failure to Expand Childcare Provision and to Develop a Comprehensive Childcare Policy in Britain During the 1960s and 1970s', *Twentieth Century British History*, 24, 2, 2013, 249–74.

———, 'The Social History of Social Policy: Infant Welfare in Edwardian England', *Journal of Social Policy*, 9, 4, 1980, 463–86.

———, *The Politics of Motherhood: Child and Maternal Welfare in England, 1900–1939* (London, 1980).

———, *Women in Britain Since 1945* (Oxford, 1993).

Lock, Stephen, 'Self Help Groups: The Fourth Estate in Medicine?', *British Medical Journal*, 293, 6562, 1986, 1596–600.

Loudon, Irvine, 'General Practitioners and Obstetrics: A Brief History', *Journal of the Royal Society of Medicine*, 101, 11, 2008, 531–35.

Macintyre, Sally, 'The Management of Childbirth: A Review of Sociological Research Issues', *Social Science and Medicine*, 11, 8, 1977, 477–84.

———, 'Some Notes on Record Taking and Making in an Antenatal Clinic', *The Sociological Review*, 26, 3, 1978, 595–612.

Mahoney, Kate, *Feminist Mental Health Activism in England, c.1968–95* (Manchester, 2023).

Mahony, Chris, 'Obituary: Sandler, Merton', *British Medical Journal*, 4, 349, 2014, 6609.

Maitland, Sara, *Why Children?* Ed. Stephanie Dowrick and Sibyl Grundberg (London, 1980), 78–91.

Malone, Mary, 'A History of Health Visiting and Parenting in the Last 50 Years', *International History of Nursing Journal*, 5, 3, 2000, 30–43.

Malos, Ellen, *The Politics of Housework* (Cheltenham, 1995 [1980]).

Mandler, Peter, 'Educating the Nation IV: Subject Choice', *Transactions of the Royal Historical Society*, 27, 2017, 1–27.

———, 'Good Reading for the Million: The 'Paperback Revolution' and the Co-production of Academic Knowledge in Mid Twentieth-Century Britain and America', *Past & Present*, 244, 1, 2019, 235–69.

———, 'The Rise of the Social Sciences in British Education, 1960–2016', in *The History of Sociology in Britain: New Research and Revaluation*, Ed. Plamena Panayotova (Switzerland, 2019), 218–99.

Marcus, Piri, 'Motherhood: A Letter', in *Sweeping Statements: Writings from The Women's Liberation Movement 1981–83*, Eds H. Kanter et al. (London, 1984), 296–98.

Marinker, Marshall, "What Is Wrong" and "How We Know It": Changing Concepts of Illness in General Practice', in *General Practice Under the National Health Service: 1948–1997,* Eds I. Loudon, J. Horder, and C. Webster (Oxford, 1998), 5–91.

Marland, Hilary, *Dangerous Motherhood: Insanity and Childbirth in Victorian Britain* (New York, 2004).

———, "Drowned in a Sea of Inhumanity": Natural Childbirth, Postnatal Depression and the National Childbirth Trust, 1956–80s', *Social History of Medicine*, 37, 1, 2004, 69-92.

———, 'A Pioneer in Infant Welfare: The Huddersfield Scheme 1903–1920', *Social History of Medicine*, 6, 1, 1993, 25–50.

Martin, F.M., Brotherston, J.H., and Chave, S.P., 'Incidence of Neurosis in a New Housing Estate', *British Journal of Preventative Social Medicine*, 11, 4, 1957, 196–202.

Maternity in Great Britain: A Survey of Social and Economic Aspects of Pregnancy and Childbirth. Joint Committee of the Royal College of Obstetricians and Gynaecologists and the Population Investigation Committee (London and New York, 1948),

McCarthy, Helen, 'Career, Family and Emotional Work: Graduate Mothers in 1960s Britain', *Past & Present*, 246, Suppl. 15, 2020, 295–317.

———, *Double Lives: A History of Working Motherhood in Modern Britain* (London, 2020).

———, 'Feminism, Selfhood and Social Research: Professional Women's Organizations in 1960s Britain', in *Precarious Professionals: Gender, Identities and Social Change in Modern Britain*, Eds Heidi Egginton and Zoë Thomas (London, 2021), 287–304.

———, 'Social Science and Married Women's Employment in Post-War Britain', *Past & Present*, 233, 1, 2016, 269–305.

McCloskey Deirdre, 'Paid Work', in *Women in Twentieth Century Britain*, Ed. Ina Zweiniger-Bargielowska (Harlow, 2001), 165–79.

McConville, Agnes, 'Setting Up a Parenting Group', *Health Visitor*, November 1989, 62, 2, 338–39.

McEwan, Margaret, *Health Visiting: A Textbook for Health Visitor Students*, 2nd ed. (London, 1957).

McIntosh, James, 'Models of Childbirth and Social Class: A Study of 80 Working Class Primigravidae', in *Midwives, Research and Childbirth*, Vol. 1, Eds Sarah Robinson and Ann M. Thomson (London, 1995 [1989]), 189–214.

McIntosh, Tania, *A Social History of Maternity and Childbirth: Key Themes in Maternity Care* (Abingdon, 2012).

McKears Jane, 'Group Support for Young Mothers', *Health Visitor*, January 1983, 56, 1, 16.

McKibbin, Ross, 'Social Class and Social Observation in Edwardian England', *Transactions of The Royal Historical Society,* 28, 1978, 175–99, 178.
McWhinney, Ian, 'The Primary Physician in a Comprehensive Health Service: Further Reflections After a Visit to the United States', *The Lancet,* 289, 7481, 1967, 91–96.
Michaels, Paula, 'Childbirth and Trauma, 1940s–1980s', *Journal of the History of Medicine and Allied Sciences,* 73, 1, 2018, 52–72.
Millett, Kate, *Sexual Politics* (London, 1985 [1971]).
Mills, Enid, *Living with Mental Illness: A Study in East London* (London, 1962).
Mirza, Heidi Safia, *Black British Feminism: A Reader* (London and New York, 1997).
Mitchell, Juliet, *Psychoanalysis and Feminism* (Harmondsworth, 1974).
Mold, Alex, *Making the Patient-Consumer: Patient Organisations and Health Consumerism in Britain* (Manchester, 2015).
Moorhead, Joanna, *New Generations: 40 Years of Birth in Britain* (Cambridge, 1996).
Morrell, Carol, 'On Not Being the Hostess with the Mostest', *Spare Rib,* 16, 1973, 37–38.
Moulds, Valerie, et al., 'Innovations by a Primary Health Care Team 2. A Postnatal Group for First-Time Mothers', *Health Visitor,* August 1983, 56, 8, 296–97.
Mount, Ferdinand, *The Subversive Family* (London, 1982).
Mowbray, R.M., et al., 'The General Practitioner's Attitude to Psychiatry', *Scottish Medical Journal,* 6, 7, 1961, 314–21.
Muir, Annette, 'On Having Children', *Shrew,* January 1970.
Myrdal, Alva, and Klein, Viola, *Women's Two Roles* (London, 1956).
Nash, Jennifer C., 'The Political Life of Black Motherhood', *Feminist Studies,* 44, 3, 2018, 699–712.
National Childbirth Trust, *The Emotions and Experiences of Some Disabled Mothers* (London, 1984/1985), 19–20.
Nava, Mica, 'Looking Back: '1968', Women's Liberation and the Family', *Free Associations,* 78, 2020, 53–71.
———, 'The Family: A Critique of Certain Features', in *The Body Politic: Women's Liberation in Britain 1969–1972,* Ed. M. Wandor (London, 1972), 36–44.
———, "1968' and The Women's Liberation Movement in Britain', *Moving the Social* 64, 2020, 37.
Newson, John and Elizabeth, *Patterns of Infant Care in an Urban Community* (Harmondsworth, 1976 [1963]).

Nicholson, Paula, 'Motherhood and Women's Lives', *Introducing Women's Studies: feminist theory and practice* ed. Diane Richardson and Victoria Robinson (Basingstoke, 1993), 201–23.

———, 'Understanding Post-Natal Depression: A Mother-Centred Approach', *Journal of Advanced Nursing* 12, 1990, 689–95.

Nicholson, Nigel, 'A Day with a Health Visitor', *British Medical Journal*, 1, 4929, 1955, 299–301.

Noakes, Lucy, *Dying for the Nation: Death, Grief and Bereavement in Second World War Britain* (Manchester, 2020).

O'Brien, P., 'Obstetrics in a General Practice, 1949–1963', *The Journal of the College of General Practitioners*, 8, 3, 1964, 281–303.

O'Connell, P.E., 'The Education and Training of Health Visitors', *Journal of the Royal Sanitary Institute*, 74, 12, 1954, 1131–36.

O'Reilly, Andrea (Ed.), *Feminist Mothering* (Albany, NY, 2008).

———, *Maternal Thinking: Philosophy, Politics, Practice* (Toronto, 2009).

O'Sullivan, Sue, 'Discussing Childbirth', in *Women's Health: A Spare Rib Reader*, Ed. Sue O'Sullivan (London, 1987), 303.

———, '*From 1968*', '68, '78, '88: From Women's Liberation to Feminism, Ed. Amanda Sebestyen (Dorset, 1988), 51–62.

———, *I Used to Be Nice* (London, 1996)

———, in *Once a Feminist: Stories of a Generation* (London, 1990), 214–226.

———, 'Passionate Beginnings: Ideological Politics 1969–72', *Feminist Review*, 11, 1, 1982, 70–86.

Oakley, Ann, *Becoming a Mother* (Oxford, 1979).

———, 'Interviewing Women: A Contradiction in Terms?', in *Doing Feminist Research*, Ed. Helen Roberts (London, 1981), 30–61.

———, *Women Confined: Towards a Sociology of Childbirth* (Oxford, 1980).

———, and Chamberlain, G., 'Doctors, Maternity Patients and Social Scientists', *Birth*, 12, 1985, 161–66.

———, *Father and Daughter: Patriarchy, Gender and Social Science* (Bristol, 2014).

———, *Housewife* (London, 1990 [1974]).

———, *The Sociology of Housework* (Oxford, 1974).

———, 'Interviewing Women Again: Power, Time and the Gift', *Sociology*, 50, 1, 2016, 195–213.

———, *Man & Wife: Richard and Kay Titmuss: My Parents' Early Years* (London, 1996).

———, 'Medical and Social Factors in Postpartum Depression', *Journal of Obstetrics and Gynaecology*, 1, 1981, 182–87.

———, 'A Small Sociology of Maternal Memory', *The Sociological Review*, 64, 3, 2016, 533–49.

———, *Social Support and Motherhood* (Oxford, 1992).

———, 'The Sociology of Childbirth: An Autobiographical Journey Through Four Decades of Research', *Sociology of Health and Illness*, 38, 5, 2016, 689–705.

———, *The Sociology of Housework* (Bristol, 2019 [1974]).

———, *Taking It Like a Woman* (London, 1984).

———, 'Women and Health Policy', in *Women's Welfare Women's Rights*, Ed. Jane Lewis (London and Sydney, 1983), 103–29.

———, 'Women's Studies in British Sociology: To End at Our Beginning?', *The British Journal of Sociology*, 40, 3, 1989, 442–70.

Ong, Bie Nio, 'Child Abuse: Are Abusing Women Abused Women?', in *Feminist Practice in Women's Health Care*, Ed. Christine Webb (Chichester, 1986), 163–82.

———, *Our Motherhood: Women's Accounts of Pregnancy, Childbirth and Health Encounters. A Family Service Units discussion paper* (London, 1983).

OWAAD, 'Black Women and Health', in *No Turning Back: Writings from the Women's Liberation Movement 1975–80* ed. Feminist Anthology Collective (London, 1981), 145–49.

Owen, G.M., 'Health Visiting', in *Nursing, Midwifery and Health Visiting Since 1900*, Eds Peta Allan and Moya Jolley (London, 1982), 92–105.

Palfreeman, Shirley, 'Mother and Toddler Groups Among 'At Risk' Families', *Health Visitor*, 1982, 55, 9, 455–59.

Pascall, Gillian, 'Women and the Family in the British Welfare State: The Thatcher/Major Legacy', *Social Policy & Administration*, 31, 1997, 290–305.

Pasmore, H. Stephen, 'Psychiatry in General Practice', *The Lancet*, 271, 7019, 1958, 524–26.

———, 'The Stabilizing Role of the General Practitioner', *British Journal of Clinical Practice*, 12, 1959, 311–13.

Paterson, Laura, 'I Didn't Feel Like My Own Person': Paid Work in Women's Narratives of Self and Working Motherhood, 1950–1980', *Contemporary British History*, 33, 3, 2019, 405–26.

Peffer, Linda, *Dutiful Daughters: Women Talk About Their Lives*, Eds Jean Mcrindle and Sheila Rowbotham (Middlesex, 1979), 378–89.

Perkins Gilman, Charlotte, *The Yellow Wallpaper* (London, 2008 [1892]).

Phoenix, Ann, 'Practicing Feminist Research: The Intersections of Gender and 'Race' in the Research Process', in *Researching Women's Lives from a Feminist Perspective*, Eds Mary Maynard and June Purvis (London, 1994), 49–71.

Pitt, Brice, "Atypical' Depression Following Childbirth', *British Journal of Psychiatry*, 114, 1968, 1325–35.

———, *Enjoying Motherhood: How to Have a Happy Pregnancy* (London, 1978).

Pixner, Stef, 'For Therapy', *Spare Rib*, 69, 1978, 20–21.

Platt, Jennifer, 'The History of the British Sociological Association', *International Sociology* 17, 2, 2002, 179–98.

———, 'The Women's Movement and British Journal Articles, 1950–2004', *Sociology* 41, 5, 2007, 961–75.

Political and Economic Planning, *Family Needs and the Social Services* (London, 1961).

Pollitt, Katha, 'Dream On', *London Review of Books*, 25, 17, 11 September 2003. Retrieved from https://www.lrb.co.uk/the-paper/v25/n17/katha-pollitt/dream-on [Accessed 25 September 2024].

Posner, Tina, 'The Development of Self Help Organizations: Dilemma and Ambiguities', in *Self Help and Social Welfare: England and West Germany*, Eds S. Humble and J. Unell (London and New York, 1989), 51–61.

Price, Jane, *Motherhood: What It Does to Your Mind* (London, Sydney, and Wellington, 1990 [1988]).

Purves, Libby, *How Not to Be a Perfect Mother* (London, 1988).

Rantzen, Esther, 'Foreword', in *Depression After Childbirth: How to Recognise and Treat Postnatal Illness*, Ed. Katharina Dalton (Oxford, 1989 [1980]), v–vi.

Rapoport, R., and Rapoport, R.N., *Dual-Career Families* (Harmondsworth, 1971).

Rathbone, B., *Focus on New Mothers: A Study of Antenatal Classes* (London, 1973).

Rawnsley, K., and Loudon, J.B., 'The Attitudes of General Practitioners to Psychiatry', *The Sociological Review*, 5, 1 suppl, 1957, 49–60.

Ree, Janet, *Once a Feminist: Stories of a Generation*, Ed. Michelene Wandor (London, 1990), 93–106.

Rich, Adrienne, *Of Woman Born: Motherhood as Experience and Institution* (New York, 1986 [1976]).

Riley, Denise, *War in the Nursery: Theories of the Child and Mother* (London, 1983).

Rivett, Geoffrey, *From Cradle to Grave: Fifty Years of the NHS* (London, 1998).

Roberts, Helen (Ed.), 'Ten Years on', in *Doing Feminist Research* (London, 1990 [1981]), xiii–xxi.

———, 'Women and their Doctors: Power and Powerlessness in the Research Process', in *Doing Feminist Research* (London and New York, 1988 [1981]), 7–29.

———, and Woodward, Diana, 'Changing Patterns of Women's Employment in Sociology: 1950–80', *The British Journal of Sociology*, 32, 4, 1981, 531–46.

———, 'Some of the Boys Won't Play Any More: The Impact of Feminism on Sociology', in *Men's Studies Modified: The Impact of Feminism on the Academic Disciplines*, Ed. Dale Spender (Oxford, 1981), 73–81.

Roberts, Llywelyn, Davies, I.G., and Corner, Beryl D., *Textbook for Health Visitors* (London, 1951).

Roberts, Michèle, *Paper Houses: A Memoir of the '70s and Beyond* (London, 2008).

Robinson, Jane, *An Evaluation of Health Visiting* (London: Council for The Education and Training of Health Visitors, 1982).

———, 'The Role Dilemma of Health Visiting', *Health Visitor*, 1983, 56, 1, 22–24.

Rocheron, Yvette, 'The Asian Mother and Baby Campaign: The Construction of Ethnic Minorities' Health Needs', *Critical Social Policy*, 8, 22, 1988, 4–23.

Rodger, Ferguson, 'The Management of the Neuroses in General Practice', *Glasgow Medical Journal*, 32, 2, 1951, 48–49.

Römer, Felix, 'Poverty, Inequality Statistics and Knowledge Politics Under Thatcher', *English Historical Review*, 137, 585, 2022, 513–51.

Rose, Jacqueline, *Mothers: An Essay on Love and Cruelty* (London, 2018).

Rowbotham, Sheila, *The Past Is Before Us* (Boston, MA, 1989).

———, 'To Be or Not to Be: The Dilemmas of Mothering', *Feminist Review*, 31, 1989, 82–93.

———, and McCrindle, Jean (Eds), *Dutiful Daughters: Women Talk About Their Lives* (Middlesex, 1989).

Rowe, Marsha (Ed.), 'Introduction', in *Spare Rib Reader: 100 Issues of Women's Liberation* (Middlesex, 1982), 13–22.

Rowntree, Seebohm, *Poverty: A Study in Town Life* (London, 1902 [1901]).

Royal College of Midwives, *Preparation for Parenthood* (Taunton, 1966).

Ryle, Anthony, *Neurosis in the Ordinary Family: A Psychiatric Survey* (London, 1967).

———, 'Personal View', *British Medical Journal*, 1, 5647, 1969, 840.

———, 'Psychoanalysis and Cognitive Analytic Therapy', *British Journal of Psychotherapy*, 10, 3, 1994, 402–4.

———, 'The Psychological Disturbances Associated With 345 Pregnancies in 137 Women', *The British Journal of Psychiatry*, 107, 447, 1961, 279–86.

———, Grant, D.M., Rea, J.N., and Faulkner, Hugh C., 'Nurses in General Practice', *British Medical Journal*, 1, 5238, 1961, 1541.

———, *Diary from the Edge, 1940–1944: A Wartime Adolescence* (London, 2014).

———, 'The Neuroses in a General Practice Population', *The Journal of the College of General Practitioners*, 3, 3, 1960, 313–28.

———, 'Therapeutic Abortion', *British Medical Journal*, 1, 5176, 1960, 878–79.

———, 'Whither Natural Childbirth?', *British Medical Journal*, 1, 4915, 1955, 725.

———, and Hamilton, Madge, 'Neurosis in Fifty Married Couples: Assessed from General Practice Records, Interviews by a Psychiatric Social Worker and the Use of the Cornell Medical Index', *Journal of Mental Science*, 108, 1962, 265–73.

Saeger, Ann, 'The Ten Commandments for Health Visitors', *Health Visitor*, January 1988, 61, 1, 15.

Sanders, Deirdre, and Reed, Jane, *Kitchen Sink, or Swim? Women in the Eighties: The Choices* (Harmondsworth, 1982).

Sandler, Merton (Ed.), *Mental Illness in Pregnancy and the Puerperium* (Oxford, 1978).

Sarachild, Kathie, 'Consciousness-Raising: A Radical Weapon', in *Feminist Revolution*, ed. Kathie Sarachild (New York, 1978), 144–50.

———, 'A Program for Feminist "Consciousness Raising"', *Notes from the Second Year: Women's Liberation, 1970*, ed. Shulamith Firestone, 78–80, available at http://library.duke.edu/digitalcollections/wlmpc_wlmms01039/.

Sargant, William, Review of *Depressive Disorders in the Community* by C.A.H. Watts, *World Medicine*, August 1966, n/p.

Saunders, Mary, *Health Visiting Practice* (Oxford, 1968).

Savage, Mike, 'Changing Social Class Identities in Post-War Britain: Perspectives from Mass Observation', *Sociological Research Online*, 12, 3, 6, 2007, doi:10.5153/sro.1459.

———, 'Elizabeth Bott and the Formulation of Modern British Sociology', *The Sociological Review*, 56, 4, 2008, 579-605.

———, *Identities and Social Change in Britain Since 1940: The Politics of Method* (Oxford, 2010).

———, 'History and Sociology: A Twenty-First Century Rapprochement?', *Twentieth Century British History*, 33, 3, 2022, 416–31.

Saville, P.R., 'Psychotherapy and The General Practitioner-II', *British Medical Journal*, 1, 5011, 1957, 158–60.

Schaffer, H.R., 'Social Development in Early Childhood', in *Psychology for Nurses and Health Visitors*, Ed. John Hall (London and Basingstoke, 1988 [1982]), 165–81.

Scott, Ann, 'Why Is Your Magazine So Depressing?', *Spare Rib*, 34, 1974, 8.

Scott-Samuel, A., et al., 'The Impact of Thatcherism on Health and Well-Being in Britain', *International Journal of Health Services*, 44, 1, 2014, 53–71.

Seaton, Andrew, 'Against the 'Sacred Cow': NHS Opposition and the Fellowship for Freedom in Medicine, 1948–72', *Twentieth Century British History*, 26, 3, 2015, 424–49.

——, *Our NHS: A History of Britain's Best Loved Institution* (New Haven, CT, 2023).

Segal, Lynne, *Is the Future Female? Troubled Thoughts on Contemporary Feminism* (London, 1987).

——, *Making Trouble: Life and Politics* (London, 2007).

——, 'The Politics of the Family: Laing and Esterson in Context', *Journal of Psychosocial Studies,* 11, 1, 2018, 104–25.

——, *Straight Sex: The Politics of Pleasure* (London, 1994).

Seton, Frances, 'Opening Myself to Change', *Spare Rib*, 44, 1976, 30–32.

Shapira, Michal, *The War Inside: Psychoanalysis, Total War, and the Making of the Democratic Self in Postwar Britain* (Cambridge, 2013).

Sharpe, Sue, *Double Identity: The Lives of Working Mothers* (Middlesex, 1984).

——, 'The Role of the Nuclear Family in the Oppression of Women', in *Body Politic: Women's Liberation in Britain 1969–1972,* Ed. M. Wandor (London, 1972), 138–45.

Shaw, L.A., 'Impressions of Family Life in a London Suburb (Studies of a general practice IV)', *The Sociological Review*, 2, 2, 1954, 179–94.

Shepherd, Michael, et al., 'Minor Mental Illness in London: Some Aspects of a General Practice Survey', *British Medical Journal*, 2, 5421, 1964, 1359–63.

——, 'Preface to the Second Edition', in *Psychiatric Illness in General Practice*, Eds. M. Shepherd, B. Cooper, A. C. Brown and G. W. Kalton. New material by M. Shepherd and A. W. Clare. 2nd edn. (Oxford, 1981 [1966]), vii.

——, *Psychiatric Illness in General Practice* (London, 1966).

——, Fisher, Michael, Stein, Lilli, and Kessel, WIN, 'Psychiatric Morbidity in an Urban Group Practice [Abridged]', *Proceedings of the Royal Society of Medicine*, 52, 4, 1959, 269–74.

Simms, Madeleine, and Smith, Christopher, 'Teenage Mothers: Some Views on Health Visitors', *Health Visitor,* 57, 9, 1984, 269–70.

Simpson, Julian M., *Migrant Architects of the NHS: South Asian Doctors and the Reinvention of General Practice, 1940s-1980s* (Manchester, 2018).

Skegg, D.C., Doll, R., and Perry, J., 'Use of Medicines in General Practice', *British Medical Journal,* 18, 1, 6076, 1977, 1561–63.

Skeggs, Beverley, 'The Dirty History of Feminism and Sociology: Or the War of Conceptual Attrition', *Sociological Review*, 56, 4, 2008, 670–90.

Smith Wilson, Dolly, 'A New Look at the Affluent Worker: The Good Working Mother in Post-War Britain', *Twentieth Century British History*, 17, 2, 2006, 206–29.

Smith, Andrew, 'Future of British Medicine: The Possibilities', *British Medical Journal*, 2, 5548, 1967, 369–70.

Smith, Jennifer, 'Illustrations from The Wellcome Institute Library: The Archive of the Health Visitors' Association in the Contemporary Medical Archives Centre', *Medical History*, 39, 3, 1995, 358–67.

Smith, Rebecca, 'Postnatal Depression', *Spare Rib*, 98, 1980, 46.

Smith, Margaret, 'The Best of Both Worlds?', in *Balancing Acts: On Being a Mother*, Ed. Katherine Gieve (London, 1989), 160–76.

Snaith, R.P., 'The Health Visitor and Prevention', *British Medical Journal (Clinical Research Edition)*, 285, 6340, 1982, 512.

Speed, Bebe, 'Family Therapy's Origins in the UK and Ireland – Date Chart', *Context*, 115, June 2011, 4–12.

Spender, Dale (Ed.), 'Introduction', in *Men's Studies Modified: The Impact of Feminism on the Academic Disciplines* (Oxford, 1981), 1–10.

Spinks, Jenny, 'A Personal View of the ARM', in *Radical Midwifery: Celebrating 21 Years of A.R.M.*, Ed. Margaret Jowitt and Ishbel Kargar (Lancashire: Association of Radical Midwives, 1997), 15–16.

Spray, Jean, 'Brent Feels the Brunt', *Socialist Organiser*, 119, 10 February 1983, 8.

———, 'The Radical Health Visitors Group', in *Health Visitors and Groups: Policy and Practice*, Ed. Vari Drennan (Oxford, 1988), 108–13.

Spring Rice, Margery, *Working-Class Wives* (London, 1981 [1939]).

Stacey, Margaret, 'Social Sciences and the State: Fighting Like a Woman', *Sociology*, 16, 3, 1982, 406–21.

———, 'The Division of Labour Revisited or Overcoming the Two Adams', in *Practice and Progress: British Sociology 1950–1980*, Ed. Philip Abrams, Rosemary Deem, Janet Finch, and Paul Rock (London and New York, 1981), 172–90.

Stanley, Liz (Ed.), *Feminist Praxis: Research, Theory and Epistemology in Feminist Sociology* (London and New York: Routledge, 1990).

———, and Wise, Sue, *Breaking Out: Feminist Consciousness and Feminist Research* (London, 1983).

Starkey, Pat, 'The Feckless Mother: Women, Poverty and Social Workers in Wartime and Post-War England', *Women's History Review*, 9, 3, 539–57.

Stott, Mary, *Women Talking: An Anthology from the Guardian Women's Page, 1922-35, 1957-71* (London, 1987).

Stevenson, J.S.K., 'Maternity Work in a General-Practitioner Unit', *British Medical Journal,* 1, 5240, 1961, 1673–76.
Stewart, John, *Child Guidance in Britain, 1918–1955: The Dangerous Age of Childhood* (London, 2013).
——, 'The 'New Era in Medicine': John Ryle and the Promotion of Social Medicine', *Medical History,* 67, 3, 2023, 247–65.
Stimson, G.V., 'General Practitioners, 'Trouble' and Types of Patients', *The Sociological Review,* 22, 1_suppl, 1974, 43–60.
Stoller, Sarah E., 'Forging a Politics of Care: Theorising Household Work in the British Women's Liberation Movement', *History Workshop Journal,* 2018, 85, 95–119.
——, *Inventing the Working Parent: Work, Gender, and Feminism in Neoliberal Britain* (Cambridge, MA, 2023).
Summerfield, Penny, 'Women and War in the Twentieth Century', in *Women's History: Britain, 1850–1945, an Introduction,* Ed. June Purvis (London, 2000), 307–32.
Sutcliffe-Braithwaite, Florence, and Thomlinson, Natalie, 'Vernacular Discourses of Gender Equality in the Post-War British Working Class', *Past & Present,* 254, 1, 2022, 277–313.
Tanner, Barb, and Rob, Jo, 'What Do ARM Midwives Want?', in *Radical Midwifery: Celebrating 21 Years of A.R.M.,* Ed. Margaret Jowitt and Ishbel Kargar (Lancashire: Association of Radical Midwives, 1997), 18–19.
Taylor Allen, Ann, *Feminism and Motherhood in Western Europe, 1890–1970: The Maternal Dilemma* (Basingstoke, 2005),
Taylor, Barbara, *The Last Asylum* (London, 2015).
Taylor, Stephen, *Good General Practice: A Report of a Survey* (London, 1954).
——, 'Psychiatric Research: A New 'Mental Million', *British Medical Journal,* 1, 5338, 1963, 1107–11.
——, 'The Suburban Neurosis', *The Lancet* 23, 5978, 1938, 759–62.
Taylor, Stephen, and Chave, Sidney, *Mental Health and Environment* (London, 1964).
Tew, Marjorie, *Safer Childbirth? A Critical History of Maternity Care* (London, 1998 [1990]).
Thane, Pat, 'Unmarried Motherhood in Twentieth-Century England', *Women's History Review,* 20, 2, 2011, 11–29.
Thomas, Clayton, and Gordon, John, 'Psychosis After Childbirth: Ecological Aspects of a Single Impact Stress', *American Journal of the Medical Sciences,* 238, 1959, 238–63.
Thomas, Phoebe, and Sullivan, Ann, 'A Mothers' and Babies' Group in a Family Health Clinic', *Health Visitor,* 1983, 56, 8, 299–300.

Thomlinson, Natalie, *Race and Ethnicity in the Women's Movement in England, 1968–1993* (Basingstoke, 2016).
Thompson, June, Briscoe, Monica E., and Clare, Anthony W., 'The Health Visitor and Prevention', *British Medical Journal (Clinical Research Edition)*, 285, 6343, 1982, 739–40.
Thomson, Mathew, *Psychological Subjects: Identity, Culture, and Health in Twentieth-Century Britain* (Oxford, 2006).
———, 'Psychology and the 'Consciousness of Modernity' in Early Twentieth-century Britain', in *Meanings of Modernity: Britain from the Late-Victorian Era to World War II*, Eds Martin Daunton and Bernhard Rieger (London, 2001), 97–115.
Timbury, Morag C., and Ratzer, Maria A., 'Glasgow Medical Women 1951–4: Their Contribution and Attitude to Medical Work', *British Medical Journal*, 2, 5653, 1969, 372–74.
Timms, Noel, 'Knowledge, Opinion and the Social Services', *The Sociological Review*, 9, 3, 1961, 361–65.
———, *Psychiatric Social Work in Great Britain (1939–1962)* (London, 1964).
———, 'The Public and the Social Worker: Results of a Pilot Research Project', *Social Work*, 19, 1, 1962, 3–7.
Titmuss, Richard, 'The Limits of the Welfare State', *New Left Review*, 1, 27, September–October 1964, 28–37.
Todd, Selina, 'Family Welfare and Social Work in Post-War England, C.1948—C.1970', *The English Historical Review*, 129, 537, 2014, 362–87.
Tomes, Nancy, 'Feminist Histories of Psychiatry', in *Discovering the History of Psychiatry*, Eds Mark Micale and Roy Porter (Oxford, 1994), 348–83.
Torkington, Protasia, 'Black Women and the NHS', in *Sweeping Statements: Writings from the Women's Liberation Movement 1981–83*, Eds Hannah Kanter, Sarah Lefanu, Shaila Shah, and Carole Spedding (London, 1984), 92–96.
Vaux, Anna, 'Motherblame', *London Review of Books,* 20, 10, 21 May 1998. Retrieved from https://www.lrb.co.uk/the-paper/v20/n10/anna-vaux/motherblame. [Accessed 25 September 2024].
Vellacott, Julia, 'Motherhood in the Imagination', in *Balancing Acts: On Being a Mother*, Ed. Katherine Gieve (London, 1989), 177–203.
Vickers, Geoffrey, 'Medicine, Psychiatry, and General Practice', *The Lancet*, 285, 7394, 1965, 1021–27.
Vinten, Gerald, '1. Who Holds the Purse Strings?', *Health Visitor*, 1983, 56, 3, 94–96.
Wagorn, Judith, 'Health Visiting', *Nursing: The Add-on Journal of Clinical Nursing*, June 1982, 2, 2, 54.

Wallsgrove, Ruth, 'Choosing to Fit In... or Not Fit In', *Spare Rib*, 65, 1977, 13.
Walters, Diane, 'Who's Birthing the Baby – Postnatal Depression and Maternity Hospitals', *Spare Rib*, 118, 1982, 22–23.
Wandor, Michelene, 'A Diary in Keeping', in *'68, '78, '88: From Women's Liberation to Feminism*, Ed. Amanda Sebestyen (Dorset, 1988), 1–4.
———, 'Family Everafter', *Spare Rib*, 5, 1972, 10–13.
Ward, A.W., 'Careers of Medical Women', *British Medical Journal*, 284, 6308, 1982, 31–33.
Ward, Tony, 'The Sad Subject of Infanticide: Law, Medicine and Child Murder, 1860–1938', *Social & Legal Studies*, 8, 2, 1999, 163–80.
Waters, Rob, *Thinking Black: Britain, 1964–1985* (Oakland, CA, 2018).
Watson, G.I., ''What?' and 'How Often?' in Medical Research', *The Journal of The College of General Practitioners* 7, 1, 1964, 24.
Watts, B.M., 'The Influence of Home Conditions During the First Five Years of Life on the Physical and Mental Health of Children', *Research Newsletter*, 1956 Os-4, (11), 63–75.
Watts, C.A.H, 'The Incidence and Prognosis of Endogenous Depression', *British Medical Journal*, 1, 4980, 1956, 1392–97.
———, *Depressive Disorders in the Community* (Bristol, 1966).
———, 'The Blue Plague', *The Journal of the Royal College of General Practitioners*, 22, 117, 1972, 233–39.
———, *Depression: The Blue Plague* (London, 1973).
———, 'Looking Back at *Psychiatry in General Practice*', *Bulletin of the Royal College of Psychiatrists*, 10, 7, 1986, 162–65
———, and Watts, B.M., *Psychiatry in General Practice* (Devon, 1994 [1952]).
Webster, Charles, 'Psychiatry and The Early National Health Service: The Role of The Mental Health Standing Advisory Committee', in *150 Years of British Psychiatry, 1841–1991*, Eds G.E. Berrios and Hugh Freeman (London, 1991), 103–6.
———, *The Health Services Since the War, Volume I: Problems of health care: The National Health Service Before 1957* (London, 1988).
———, *The Health Services Since the War, Volume II. Government and Healthcare: The National Health Service 1958–79* (London, 1996).
———, *The National Health Service: A Political History* (Oxford, 1998).
Webster, Wendy, *Imagining Home: Gender, Race and National Identity, 1945–1964* (Abingdon, 2023 [1998]).
Weiss, Robert, 'Neurosis in The Ordinary Family [Review]', *Social Science & Medicine* 5, 4, 1971, 411–14.
Welburn, Vivienne, *Postnatal Depression* (Glasgow, 1983 [1980]).
Welshman, John, 'Family Visitors or Social Workers? Health Visiting and Public Health in England and Wales 1890–1974', *International History of Nursing Journal*, 2,4, 1997, 5–22.

———, 'The Social History of Social Work: The Issue of the 'Problem Family'', 1940–70', *The British Journal of Social Work*, 29, 3, 1999, 457–76.

West, Michael A., Jones, Avril, and Savage, Yvonne, 'Stress in Health Visiting: A Quantitative Assessment', *Health Visitor*, September 1988, 61, 9, 269–71.

Whelehan, Imelda, *Modern Feminist Thought: From Second Wave to 'Post Feminism'* (Edinburgh, 1995).

White, Jessica, 'Child-Centred Matriarch or Mother Among Other Things? Race and the Construction of Working-Class Motherhood in Late Twentieth-Century Britain', *Twentieth Century British History*, 33, 4, 2022, 498–521.

Wilkinson, Greg, 'The General Practice Research Unit at the Institute of Psychiatry', *Psychological Medicine*, 1989, 19, 787–90.

Williams, Jan, Twort, Hazel, and Bachelli, Ann, 'Women and The Family', in *The Body Politic: Women's Liberation in Britain 1969–1972*, Ed. M. Wandor (London, 1972), 31–36.

Williams, Paul, and Clare, Anthony, 'Social Workers in Primary Health Care: The General Practitioner's Viewpoint', *The Journal of The Royal College of General Practitioners* 29, 206, 1979, 554–58.

Wilton, Tamsin, 'Madness and Feminism: Bristol Crisis Service for Women', in *Feminist Activism in the 1990s*, Ed. Gabriele Griffin (London, 1995), 28–40.

Wing, J.K., and Hailey, Anthea, *Evaluating a Community Psychiatric Service: The Camberwell Register, 1964–71* (London, 1972).

Winnicott, D.W., *The Child and The Family*, Ed. Janet Hardenberg (London, 1957).

Wise, Sue, 'Becoming A Feminist Social Worker', in *Feminist Praxis: Research, Theory and Epistemology in Feminist Sociology*, Ed. Liz Stanley (London and New York, 1990), 236–49.

Witz, Anne, *Professions and Patriarchy* (London, 1992).

Women's Studies Group (Ed.), , 'Women's Studies Group: Trying to do Feminist Intellectual Work', in *Women Take Issue: Aspects of Women's Subordination*, Centre for Contemporary Cultural Studies(London, 1978), 7–17.

World Health Organization, The Role of Public Health Officers and General Practitioners in Mental Health Care: Eleventh Report of the Expert Committee on Mental Health, No. 235 (1962).

Worth, Eve, 'Women, Education and Social Mobility in Britain during the Long 1970s', *Cultural and Social History*, 16, 1, 2019, 67–83.

Wortis, Rochelle P., 'Child-Rearing and Women's Liberation', in *The Body Politic: Women's Liberation in Britain 1969–1972*, Ed. M. Wandor (London, 1972), 124–30.

Young, Michael, and Willmott, Peter, *Family and Kinship in East London* (London, 2007 [1957]).
———, *The Symmetrical Family* (London, 1980 [1973]).
Yuill, Mary E., 'Medical Research and General Practice', *British Medical Journal*, 2, 4356, 1944, 26.
Zweiniger-Bargielowska, Ina (Ed.), 'Housewifery', in *Women in Twentieth Century Britain* (Essex, 2001), 149–64.

Websites

APNI. 'History'. Retrieved from https://apni.org/history/ [Accessed 1 November 2023].
Bowes, Claire. 'Janet Balaskas: Campaigner for Active Birth Movement', *BBC News*, 4 April 2012. Retrieved from www.bbc.co.uk/news/health-17589544. [Accessed 29 August 2024].
Carter, Angela. 'Notes from a Maternity Ward', *New Statesman*, 24 September 2015 [December 1983], https://www.newstatesman.com/long-reads/2005/09/notes-from-a-maternity-ward [Accessed 1 June 2023].
Conservative Manifesto 1979. Retrieved from http://www.margaretthatcher.org/document/110858 [Accessed 5 May 2023].
Cox, J. 'Brice Pitt: in Memoriam', Marcé Society, March 2021. Retrieved from https://marcesociety.com/wp-content/uploads/2021/05/Brice-Pitt-In-Memoriam.pdf [Accessed 21 July 2023].
Crockford, S. 'In the Beginning, We Demanded'. Retrieved from https://www.bl.uk/collection-items/in-the-beginning-we-demanded#:~:text=Sue%20Crockford%20was%20a%20member,The%20film%20A%20Woman's%20Place [Accessed 1 July 2023].
Eliot, J. *In Personal Histories of The Second Wave of Feminism Summarised From Interviews*. By Viv Honeybourne and Ilona Singer, Volumes One and Two, Feminist Archive South, 91. Retrieved from http://feministarchivesouth.org.uk/wp-content/uploads/2013/02/Personal-Histories-of-The-Second-Wave-of-Feminism.pdf [Accessed 10 August 2023].
National Health Service. 'Postnatal Depression'. Retrieved from https://www.nhs.uk/conditions/post-natal-depression/ [Accessed 1 April 2018].
National Health Service. 'Postpartum Psychosis'. Retrieved from https://www.nhs.uk/mental-health/conditions/post-partum-psychosis/ [Accessed 7 June 2022].
Oakley, A. 'Interview with Social Science Space', 4 February 2013. Retrieved from https://www.socialsciencespace.com/2013/04/podcast-ann-oakley-on-womens-experience-of-childbirth/ [Accessed 14 January 2023].

Page, Lesley. 'Kitzinger (née Webster), Sheila Helena Elizabeth (1929–2015), Anthropologist and Childbirth Activist', *Oxford Dictionary of National Biography*, 10 January 2019. Retrieved from www.oxforddnb.com/view/10.1093/odnb/9780198614128.001.0001/odnb-9780198614128-e-110338. [Accessed 28 August 2024].

Parliamentary Debates and HMSO Publications

Day Nurseries, HC Deb 12 June 1947 Vol 438 cc1457–66.

Department of Health, an Inquiry into Health Visiting: Report of A Working Party on The Field of Work, Training, and Recruitment of Health Visitors (London: HMSO, 1956).

General Practice, Report of a W.H.O. Expert Committee, World Health Organization: Technical Report Series, No. 267. Geneva (London: HMSO, 1964).

Infanticide Act, HMSO, 1938.

Perinatal Mortality and Morbidity, HL Deb 2 May 1978 Vol 391 cc122–67.

Play Groups, HC Deb 25 May 1971 Vol 818 cc229–30.

Report of The Committee on Local Authority and Allied Personal Social Services, CMND. 3703 (London: HMSO, 1968).

Social Science Research Council, HC Deb 22 November 1965 Vol 721 cc165–201.

The Family Doctor, HC Deb 22 January 1964 Vol 687 cc1230–42.

The Field of Work of the Family Doctor: Report of The Sub-Committee (London: HMSO, 1963).

Index

abortion 26, 138, 139, 166
Abrams, Lynn 24, 32, 96, 99, 129, 130, 133, 139, 169, 171, 184, 208
active birth movement 165, 175
AIMS *see* Association for Improvements in the Maternity Services
Alibhai, Yasmin 22–23, 32
Allaun, Frank (MP) 21
ambivalence 10, 22, 139, 142, 158, 189, 200, 205, 218, 219
anger 5, 11, 80, 144, 151, 156, 164–165, 187, 201, 205, 213, 219
antenatal clinic 211
antidepressants 1, 13, 34, 46, 47, 61, 75, 105, 124, 155 *see also* drugs
Ardill, Sue 146
Asian Mother and Baby Campaign 31–32
Association for Improvements in the Maternity Services (AIMS), 2, 104, 125, 165
Association for Post-Natal Illness (APNI) 97, 99, 123–125, 126, 127, 135, 136,
Association of Radical Midwives (ARM) 104, 164–165, 175, 196

baby blues 5, 94, 156, 161, 162
backlash 17, 30
Balint Movement 45, 60

Balint, Michael *see* Balint Movement
Bardon, Desmond 104, 131
Battersby, Audrey 141–142, 14
BBC 10, 26, 79, 94, 95, 113, 161, 162, 174, 196, 212, 235
Beaumont, Caitríona, 26, 30, 97, 118, 129, 130, 135
Becoming a Mother 14, 29, 2, 57, 74, 86, 90, 91, 198, 206, 211, 212, 213
 formatting in 194
 Looking Back at Becoming a Mother 72, 86, 90, 91
Bedford College 13–14, 181, 182, 183
Berry, Liz, 8
Black Parents Movement 23
Black Power 138
boredom 2, 9, 94, 116, 128, 165, 182
Borkman, Thomasina 7
Bourke, Joanna 57, 194–195, 206, 212
Bowlby, John 10, 34, 37, 52, 109, 137, 150, 157
breakdown 6, 20, 94, 157, 167
breastfeeding 5, 17, 37, 137, 201
Briance, Prunella 99, 101 *see also* National Childbirth Trust (NCT)
Brighton 114, 116–123
British Sociological Association (BSA) 185–186, 189, 192, 193, 208

British Way of Birth 57, 58, 88, 91, 95, 102, 129, 131
Bruley, Sue 169, 173
Bryce, José 67–68

cabbage 121, 122
Cain, Ruth, 9
Captive Wife, The 52, 111, 181–185 *see also* Hannah Gavron
Carby, Hazel V., 166, 176
Carstairs, G.M. 44, 60
Carstairs, G.M. 44, 60
Carter, Angela 215, 220
Caversham Centre 51–52
Centre for Contemporary Cultural Studies 176, 190, 210
Charlotte Perkins Gilman 2
Charlton, Val 142, 170, 175
child guidance 9, 10, 27
childbirth 4, 5, 9, 13, 14, 19, 37–40, 50, 51, 54, 76, 85, 99, 101–102, 161, 162–165, 177, 178, 194–200, 204–206, 215–216
  caesareans 5, 39, 161, 163
  induction 163, 196, 212
  medicalisation 13, 85, 195
  'natural' childbirth 99, 100, 101, 162, 163
  use of forceps in 39, 65, 163, 197
childminders 17, 18, 30, 109
Christmas 21, 72, 126
cities 5, 83
Comer, Lee 145, 157, 158, 171, 173
Comport, Maggie 106, 131, 132, 197–198, 213
consciousness raising 150, 154, 173
Conservative Party 81, 84, 98, 112, 130,
contraception 3, 51, 138, 139, 166
coping 49, 65, 203, 204–205, 214
council estate 21, 200

Council for the Education and Training of Health Visitors 83
Cox, John 53, 64, 67, 87
Cranbrook Report (1959) 38, 101, 163
Currer, Caroline 201, 213
Cusk, Rachel 219

Dally, Ann 140, 141, 144, 169
Dalton, Katharina 128, 129
daycare *see* nurseries
debt 21, 110
Delpech, Clare 123, 124, 135
Delphy, Christine 189, 210
demonstration 118–119, 165
Depo-Provera 21, 99
depression 1, 2, 5, 18, 19, 36, 40, 45, 46, 49, 50, 51, 73, 74, 95, 146, 155, 157, 158, 159, 160, 162, 164, 165, 177, 187, 189, 197, 199, 200, 201 *see also* postnatal depression
Depressives Associated 2, 126, 162, 174
Dick-Read, Grantly 99, 101, 130, 163
divorce 3, 107, 108, 210
domestic labour *see* housework
drugs 42, 46, 47, 49, 155, 156, 162, 195

Edinburgh Postnatal Depression Scale 53, 67, 87, 124
Edinburgh Women's Liberation Group 139–140
Eichenbaum, Luise, 172, 173
emotions 5, 24, 43, 57, 131, 138, 147, 154, 155, 157, 206
  politicisation of 8, 108, 128
  sharing of 79
  visibility and expression of 99, 165, 168,
employment *see* paid work
England 3, 38, 39, 58, 61, 70, 88, 91, 107, 111, 129, 130, 130, 135, 157, 171, 122, 179
Enright, Ann 220

Index

expertise 2, 3, 4, 6, 7, 8, 9, 14, 17, 24, 25, 36, 52, 55, 74, 75, 78, 86, 94–97, 99, 101–102, 105, 107, 123, 125–128, 139, 150, 164, 179, 187, 203, 206, 216, 220

family
  changing size of 15, 16, 19, 156–157
  nuclear 3, 108, 156, 157, 159, 168, 173
  proximity to 48, 180
fathers 108, 158, 163, 164, 217
Fell, Alison 142, 147, 170, 171
female doctors 35–36
feminist
  magazines and journals 6, 139, 148, 149, 154, 160, 220
  see also Shrew, Spare Rib, Red Rag, Feminist Review
  bookshops 188, 209
  sociology 87, 177–214
Feminist Review 173, 187
fiction 23, 171, 218, 220
Finch, Janet 193, 210, 211
Fletcher, Ronald 183
Fleury, Phyllis Mary 39, 57
Freely, Maureen 168, 176
Friedan, Betty 24, 32, 140, 168, 176, 178, 190, 206
Frost, Shirley 109–110, 133
Fry, John 43, 90

Gavron, Hannah 14, 52, 111, 115, 181–185, 202 *see also Captive Wife, The*
Gavron, Jeremy 182, 183
General Practice Research Unit (GPRU) 46, 47, 60
Gieve, Katherine 26, 28, 30, 105, 171
Gillie Report (1963) 43
Goodwin, Shirley, 84
Graham, Hilary 193, 199, 201–204, 213
Gupta, Rahila 146–147

Hall, Stuart 92, 141, 143, 170, 239
Hamilton, Madge 51, 62
Hardie, Victoria 6, 7, 25
Harne, Lynne 146, 171
hate
  for child 198
  for health visitors 76
  for the home 184
  for way of life 142
health education 80, 163, 20
Health Visitors' Association (HVA), 54, 136, 66, 69, 84, 87, 93, 128, 136
  financial struggles of 85
  origins of 68–71
Heron, Liz 143, 146, 170, 171, 173
heterosexuality 22, 81, 107, 217, 159
higher education 12, 19, 118, 185, 68
  adult 189
  discrimination in and limitations of 23, 186
  expansion 12, 118, 185,
  impact of 12, 19, 109, 112, 122, 138, 145, 178, 179, 190, 207
Hobsbawm, Marlene 143, 170
Hoggart, Richard 52–53, 63, 66, 87
hormones 5, 161, 197, 199
hospitals
  and feelings 23, 50, 100,
  and general practice 33, 38, 39, 41,
  children in 186–187
  closures of 84, 215
  giving birth in 13, 38–40, 53, 65, 100, 101, 102, 163, 195–197, 199, 215, 99–101
  treatment of mental health struggles in 150, 167, 167, 44, 49, 78
housewife 13, 15, 18, 24, 48, 96, 115, 121, 141, 142, 143, 145, 146, 159, 185, 187, 190
housewifery *see* housewife; housework

housework 14, 15, 16, 111, 159, 160, 204
Hubback, Judith 44, 207

infanticide 9, 27
Inventing Motherhood 140, 169
see also Ann Dally

Jameson Committee 70–71
Jephcott, Pearl 207

Kentish Town 50–51, 62, 182
King, Truby F, 9
Kitzinger, Jenny 100
Kitzinger, Polly 164
Kitzinger, Sheila 4, 18, 19, 162–163, 186, 206, 217
Klein, Viola 16

Laura Ashley 107
Leach, Penelope 128
Lee, Ellie, 5
Leeds Revolutionary Feminist Group, 188, 210
Leman, Grahame 111, 112, 113, 133, 134, 135
Lethbridge, Nemone 26, 161–162, 174
Lewis, Jane 29, 62, 82, 88, 133, 194, 212
Llewlyn Davies, Margaret 20, 31
Lock, Stephen 98, 130
London School of Economics (LSE) 12, 169, 134, 183, 185, 186, 204
London Women's Liberation Workshop 150, 155
loneliness 2, 5, 13, 40, 48, 55, 61, 65, 73, 75, 79, 80, 86, 94, 105, 106, 110, 114, 115, 116, 120, 122, 127, 134, 136, 155, 158, 164, 167, 182, 184, 195, 208
love 3, 10, 27, 63, 104, 114, 147, 155–156, 158, 217, 220
    worries about 161, 215, 145

Macintyre, Sally 189, 194, 210, 211, 212
Maitland, Sara 155–156, 171, 173
Marcus, Piri 150, 172
Marcé Society for Perinatal Mental Health 55, 64
Marland, Hilary 26, 56, 88, 104, 129, 131
Marriage 3, 9, 10, 12, 27, 55, 19, 122, 141, 145, 157, 183, 186, 189, 194, 66
Marriage Guidance Council 1, 9, 37
McCarthy, Helen 25, 29, 30, 114–115, 134, 181, 207, 211
Meet-A-Mum-Association (MAMA) 79, 94, 95, 98, 107, 123, 124, 126, 132, 162
midwives 6, 38, 40, 54, 69, 100, 101, 160, 163, 164, 165, 196, 203, 204. *See also* Association of Radical Midwives
Mother and Baby 2
mother and baby unit 95
Mothers
    Asian 166–167, 176, 201
    Black and ethnic minority 18, 21–24, 104, 165–167, 176
    disabled 104, 49, 193, 211
    experiencing disappointment 19, 145, 161
    lone 3, 18, 68, 74, 75, 83, 91, 92, 107–110, 130, 132, 133, 139, 166
    middle-class 2, 8, 11, 14, 15, 16, 18–21, 68, 76, 82, 106, 107, 115, 117, 155, 161, 166, 182, 200, 208, 217, 218
    romanticisation of 76, 180, 182, 137
    single or unsupported *see* lone
    working-class 14, 18–21, 26, 31, 48, 52, 68, 69, 76, 77, 80, 82, 88, 116, 117, 159–160, 180–182, 197, 202, 207
Mothers in Action 99, 107–110, 123, 132

Mothers Talking about Postnatal Depression 103–106, 131, 132
Mount, Ferdinand 81
Myrdal, Alva 16

National Baby 39
National Baby Week 69, 89
National Childbirth Trust (NCT) 2, 96, 99, 101–107, 123, 126, 128, 162, 163, 165, 193 *see also* Briance, Prunella
National Health Service (NHS) 3, 20, 21–22, 23, 37–39, 41–44, 50, 82–83, 84–86
  Love for 86
National Housewives Register 98, 184,
Nava, Mica 137–138, 139, 143, 155, 169, 170, 173, 176, 187, 209
NCT *see* National Childbirth Trust
Neurosis in the Ordinary Family 49, 51–52, 59, 63 *see also* Anthony Ryle
New Baby 54, 136
new town 49, 106
Newpin 79, 85, 91
Newson, John and Elizabeth 11, 28, 39, 57, 75–76, 91, 207
newspapers, national 6
  local 7, 49, 78, 94, 96, 97, 106, 113, 124–127, 216, 219
Nicholson, Paula 176, 204, 214
nightmares 197
nuclear annihilation 124
nurseries 17, 18, 30, 90, 108, 109, 120, 135, 138, 139, 144, 173

Oakley, Ann 11, 12–16, 24, 28, 29, 30, 32, 49, 57, 62, 72, 74, 76, 86, 87, 91, 115, 134, 177, 178, 180–181, 183, 186, 189–214
Obstetric
  care 144
  list 38
  patients 194
  practice 38,
  procedures 198
  service 38, 57
One O'Clock Club 141
Ong, Bie Nio 200, 202–203, 213
Orbach, Susie 172, 173
ordinariness 7, 24, 53, 96–97, 108, 125–128, 129, 132, 136, 179, 184, 186, 219
Organisation of Women of Asian and African Descent (OWAAD) 167, 176
O'Sullivan, Sue 142, 154, 157, 158, 159, 170, 172, 173, 174, 175

Peel Report (1970) 101, 163
Pitt, Brice 67, 77, 87, 91
playgroups 24, 111, 139, 141
Postnatal Committee (NCT), 103, 128, 131, 132
postnatal depression 1, 2, 5, 6, 13, 17, 20, 23, 53, 67, 71, 73, 78, 85, 94–96, 97, 99, 102–106, 123–126, 128, 149, 155–162, 165, 167, 178, 196–199, 200, 204, 217, 220
Postnatal Depression: Focus on a Neglected Issue (1996) 128
poverty 19, 20, 31, 81, 82, 87, 91, 92, 202
pregnancy 4, 5, 14, 37, 40, 51, 70, 72, 155, 200, 203
prescription 1, 13, 46, 47, 49, 61, 75, 105, 162
prescription *see* drugs
Price, Jane 99
Priestley, Diana 110–119, 133, 134, 135
protest *see* demonstration
Purves, Libby 168, 176

racism 18, 21, 22, 23, 31, 77, 84, 92, 166, 167, 176, 201
Radical Health Visitors Group (RHVG) 83–84, 101 *see also* Spray, Jean
Rantzen, Esther 94–96, 129

Readers' Digest 41
Red Rag 142, 157, 170, 173
Ree, Janet 147, 138
Rich, Adrienne 11, 12, 28, 137, 169, 206
Roberts, Helen 186, 187, 192, 209, 211
Roberts, Michèle 141, 170
Rolling Stones, The 18
Rose, Jaqueline 8
Rowbotham, Sheila 146, 155, 157, 159, 171, 173, 174
Royal College of General Practitioners, 34, 42–43, 46, 58, 59
Ryle, Anthony 44, 49, 50–52, 53, 59, 62, 63
Ryle, John 50, 116
Ryle, Miriam 50

Safer Childbirth: A Critical History of Maternity Care see Marjorie Tew
Sandler, Merton 124, 135
Savage, Mike 179, 206, 207
Scotland 3, 7, 38, 70, 71, 94, 98, 100, 125, 126, 127, 169, 197
Second World War 4, 9, 10, 15, 17, 35, 36, 39, 48, 59, 77, 96
sedatives *see* drugs and Valium
Segal, Lynne 143, 144, 145, 146, 170, 171, 172, 185, 208
self-help 4, 6, 12, 26, 41, 78, 79, 86, 94–136, 150, 153, 162
sex 9, 138, 146, 159, 171
sexism 183, 192
Sharpe, Sue 173, 177, 179, 207
Shepherd, Michael 46, 60, 61, 63, 64
Short, Renée (MP) 118
Shrew 148, 151, 153, 171–173
Skeggs, Beverley 189, 205–206, 209, 210, 214
sleep deprivation 5, 155, 199
  exhaustion 155, 199
  tiredness 202
social services 57, 72, 86, 90, 110, 112, 196

social work 43, 63, 66, 69, 71, 77, 87, 89, 91, 96, 186, 220
social worker 12, 51, 62, 66, 71, 75, 80, 87, 91, 188
Spare Rib 64, 148, 149, 151, 152, 154, 159, 160, 161, 163, 170–175
Spender, Dale 191, 205, 209, 211, 214
Spinks, Jenny 164, 174
Spock, Benjamin 10
Spray, Jean 84, 92, 93
Spring Rice, Margery 20, 91, 207
Stacey, Margaret 186–187, 192, 209, 210, 211
Stanley, Liz 87, 179, 188, 191, 207, 210, 211
stigma
  around distress 24, 26, 96, 105–106, 162
  around employment 16
stress 40, 43, 47, 56, 61, 204, 205
suburban
  housewives (discontent of) 24, 112
  neurosis 9, 27, 47–49, 55, 61, 62, 64
survey 6, 11, 14, 39, 40, 48, 49, 51, 68, 72, 77, 78, 95, 97, 102, 114–117, 120–123, 183, 186, 192, 200

Tavistock Institute of Human Relations 37, 114, 115, 134, 135
Taylor, Barbara 5–6
Taylor, Dr Stephen 48, 49, 55, 58, 61, 62, 64
teenage mothers 74, 87, 90
television 7, 26, 48, 95, 135, 162, 100
Tew, Marjorie 195–196, 212
Thatcher, Margaret 92, 118, 119, 130, 166, 173, 176
  Thatcherism 81, 92
That's Life 95
The Doctor, His Patient and the Illness see Balint Movement

The Feminine Mystique see Betty Friedan
therapy 149
  family 37, 56
  feminist 151, 154, 152–154, 172
  psychotherapy 47, 58, 60, 87
Thomson, Mathew 27, 132, 148, 171, 172
Titmuss, Richard 12, 28, 86, 93, 180, 183
Torkington, Protasia, 23
tranquilisers 24, 46, 49, 155 *see also* drugs
trauma 20, 31

Valium 18, 75, 162, 185 *see also* drugs; antidepressants
violence
  feelings of 155, 158
  of motherhood 22, 202,
  within families 168, 201–202

Wages for Housework 123
Wales 3, 38, 70, 78, 88, 91, 94, 107, 186, 208
Wandor, Michèlene 143, 149, 169, 170, 171, 172, 173, 174, 176
Watts, Beatrice (B.M) 33–36, 48, 53
Watts, C.A.H (Arthur) 33–34, 36, 42, 44–47, 50, 53, 54
Waumsley, Liz 103, 106, 131, 132
Welburn, Vivienne 1–2, 40–41, 54, 74, 101, 219
welfare state 3, 8, 10, 12, 37, 66, 81, 82, 179, 220
Wiggins, Meg 14, 72, 76, 87, 90, 91
Williams, Jan 141, 174

Wilson, Amrit 166–167
Winnicott, Donald 10, 12
Wise, Sue 66, 87, 188, 191, 210
Women and Mental Health Conference (1977) 151
Women's liberation movement 6, 23, 112, 137–140, 169–176
  and childbirth 162–165
  and postnatal depression 155–162
  and sociology 177, 181, 187, 188, 205, 209–210
  Black women and 166–167
  mothers and the origins of the movement 140–148, 168
  mothers' organisations distancing from 118, 121
  politicisation of feeling 148–155, 168–169
  Ruskin conference (1970) 143
Women's Studies 172, 176, 189, 190, 210, 211
Woodward, Diana 186, 48
work (paid) 3, 13, 15–18, 19, 24, 35, 48, 52, 73, 86, 107, 111, 112, 114, 116, 120, 121, 122–123, 178, 179, 186, 202, 207, 209, 217
Working Association of Mothers (WAM) 99, 110–123, 133–135
World Health Organisation (WHO) 98
Wortis, Rochelle (Sheli) 137, 150, 172

Young, Michael 30, 48, 61, 62, 180, 207
Younghusband Report (1959) 71

EU authorised representative for GPSR:
Easy Access System Europe, Mustamäe tee 50,
10621 Tallinn, Estonia
gpsr.requests@easproject.com

www.ingramcontent.com/pod-product-compliance
Ingram Content Group UK Ltd.
Pitfield, Milton Keynes, MK11 3LW, UK
UKHW021823140426